D0151826

THE ENCYCLOPEDIA OF

MEMORY AND MEMORY DISORDERS

Second Edition

Carol Turkington and
Joseph R. Harris, Ph.D.

Facts On File, Inc.

The Encyclopedia of Memory and Memory Disorders, Second Edition

Copyright © 2001 by Carol Turkington

Facts On File, Inc.
132 West 31st Street
New York NY 10001

Library of Congress Cataloging-in-Publication Data

Turkington, Carol.
The encyclopedia of memory and memory disorders / Carol Turkington and Joseph Harris—2nd ed.
p.cm.
Includes bibliographical references and index.
ISBN 0-8160-4141-5 (hardcover : alk. paper)
1. Memory—Encyclopedias. 2. Memory disorders—Encyclopedias.
I. Harris, Joseph, 1951 Dec. 20– II. Title.
BF371. N55 2001
153.1'2'03—dc21   00-052806

Text and cover design by Cathy Rincon

Printed in the United States of America

VB FOF 10 9 8 7 6 5 4 3 2

This book is printed on acid-free paper.

CONTENTS

FOREWORD

For psychologists in general, and for psychologists working with memory function in particular, we live in fascinating but frustrating times. Easily half of the articles in my "To Be Read" file have something to do with memory or memory disorders. Five of the six psychological evaluations I recently completed for individuals seeking Social Security disability benefits were for applicants claiming a disorder related to memory.

As we complete the revision of this volume, researchers have just announced completion of a major part of the Human Genome Project. They promise that we will shortly be able to unlock many of the mysteries of how thinking processes develop, as well as develop vaccines and cures for many of the diseases and genetic abnormalities that cause the cognitive disorders that plague us. At the same time, we continue to puzzle over the nature and mechanisms of memory as well as the causes of and cures for disorders such as Alzheimer's and Parkinson's disease.

Researchers still search frantically for a "smart pill" or "memory pill" that will help students perform better in school and elderly patients regain some of their lost memory. We are seeing rapid advances in our ability to scan and map the brains of living patients without having to wait until autopsy, but we still argue over the nature of attention-deficit hyperactivity disorder, learning disabilities and normal versus abnormal changes in cognition that come with aging.

In this revision of the 1994 volume, Carol Turkington and I have attempted to update previous entries with new findings, provide updates of diagnostic and treatment tools, as well as add new topics that reflect the current state of knowledge of memory and memory disorders. We have attempted to strike a balance between comprehensive coverage appropriate for professionals seeking information pertinent to their fields and a broad coverage appropriate for students and general readers who do not want to get lost in technical jargon or drown in an esoteric "alphabet soup." We have strived to make the entries readable and informative.

As I look back on the additions to the body of knowledge about memory and memory disorders that we have experienced between the previous edition and this, I cannot help but marvel at the additions in our knowledge that will likely come about between this revision and the next.

I can't wait.

—Joseph R. Harris, Ph.D.

INTRODUCTION

Throughout history, memory has worn many guises. To the ancient Greeks and Romans, memory was the source of political success. To later memory experts, it was the path to spiritual fulfillment. To countless preliterate tribes, memory carried the key to the history of their people.

With the advent of the alphabet, of the written word, of typewriters and computers and satellites, memory no longer holds the mystical, spiritual magic it offered our ancestors. For many in today's world, a good memory is nothing more than a sort of intellectual shorthand, an easier way to study, to succeed in business, to live an organized life.

But in a deeper sense, there is far more to memory than recalling dates, finding car keys or cramming for a history final. It is our memory that transforms a series of unconnected moments into a continuous unified whole, linking us to our past and pointing the way into the future.

We are compassionate because we remember what it is to feel pain. We buttress our lives against disaster because we remember what disaster has cost in the past. Our memory gives us a future more secure than creatures who are doomed to repeat their past simply because they cannot remember it. It can rescue us from a fate that awaits those destined to obliteration because they cannot adapt to changed circumstances.

Our memory has made possible the development of philosophy and science and song. More personally, it is the repository of our deepest emotions and our most compelling experiences. After all, it is our memory that holds the scent of the sea wind, the sound of a child's laughter, the image of the beloved. In the final analysis, it is our memory that makes us fully human, because it distills the rich diversity of experience into the essence of the soul.

This book has been designed as a guide and reference to a wide range of terms related to memory and to additional information and addresses of organizations that deal with memory and memory disorders. It is not a substitute for prompt assessment and treatment by experts trained in the diagnosis of memory problems.

In this new, revised edition, we have tried to present the latest information in the field of memory disorders. All-new topics include

mad cow disease
Creutzfeldt-Jakob disease (both classical and variant)
prions
Lewy body dementia
ADHD and memory
cell phones and memory
football and memory loss
smart drugs
the proteins of Alzheimer's (tau, amyloid beta, apolipoprotein)
Alzheimer's drugs
organic mental disorders
plasticity

In addition, almost every entry has been revised, many with extensive updates, including a total revision of entries on memory itself, plus the newest information on Alzheimer's disease, such as the most recent findings in the etiology of Alzheimer's and the newest four-drug treatments for the disease recently approved by the Food and Drug Administration. Other updated information includes details on the latest findings about mild cognitive impairment and its possible link to Alzheimer's disease, the newest information on aging and memory loss, and how to tell what's normal and what may be pathological when it comes to memory problems.

Readers will also find the latest information on a wide range of other memory-related disorders and revised details on vitamins and memory loss, memory and brain development, memory of child abuse, stress, transient ischemic attacks, nootropic drugs, and much more. In addition, the revised edition discusses the newest information on the link between medications and memory loss, diet and dementia, attention deficit hyperactivity dis-

order and memory and includes a complete discussion of the wide variety of memory tests now available.

The appendixes have been completely updated, including all addresses and phone numbers of organizations. In addition, Internet addresses for the websites of relevant organizations have been provided.

Information in this book comes from the most up-to-date sources available and includes some of the most recent research in the field of memory disorders. Readers should keep in mind, however, that changes occur very rapidly in this field. A bibliography has been provided for readers who seek additional sources of information. All entries are cross-referenced, and appendices provide additional information.

—Carol Turkington
Cumru, Pennsylvania

abaissement du niveau mental A term meaning "lowering of the level of consciousness" invented by French psychiatrist Pierre Janet to describe the weakening control of consciousness prior to DISSOCIATION. Today this term usually refers to ALTERED STATES OF CONSCIOUSNESS.

Janet believed this altered state of consciousness was found not just in dissociation but also in multiple personality, trances and automatic writing. He used the term to describe the weakening of willful control of consciousness and the subsequent dissociation into autonomous parts that might not be aware of each other.

Swiss psychoanalyst Carl Jung picked up Janet's term to describe schizophrenia; Jung believed this lowering of consciousness was the root of the mental disorder. In 1902 in Paris Jung became a student of Janet and was influenced by Janet throughout his life.

While Janet wrote widely in French, very few of his works have been translated into English. (See also JANET, PIERRE.)

abreaction Emotional release or discharge after recalling a painful experience that has been repressed because it was consciously intolerable. A therapeutic effect sometimes occurs through partial discharge or desensitization of the painful emotions and increased insight. (See also REPRESSED MEMORIES; REPRESSION.)

absentmindedness Failure to register information because of preoccupation with other thoughts. This kind of forgetting is not the same thing as the inability to recall information, which means that the information has been registered and stored. In absentmindedness, the information was never registered in the first place, so it can't be recalled.

While everyone may be absentminded occasionally, as people age they tend to become more absentminded. The phenomenon occurs most often in familiar surroundings, during habitual automatic activities that don't require much attention and when the mind is distracted or preoccupied with outside stress.

If absentmindedness is due primarily to not paying attention, it can be averted by putting more energy into registering information. People who always forget where they put their keys might try saying out loud, "I'm putting my keys down HERE," as they set them down. Then the keys should be looked at, while noticing what is being done. The only cure for absentmindedness is finding better ways to pay attention to daily activities.

abstract memory This term refers to a person's general store of knowledge. This type of memory has a huge capacity for storing meanings of events and objects. Its center is believed to be located in the CORTEX, the brain's outer gray layer. Damage to the temporal, parietal and occipital cortex affects abstract memory in different ways.

acalculia A specific impairment in dealing with arithmetical concepts.

accident neurosis See AMNESIA, SIMULATED.

acetylcholine A type of neurotransmitter (a chemical that transmits messages between nerve cells) that may play a role in learning and memory by helping brain cells in the CORTEX retain the imprint of incoming information. (See NEUROTRANSMITTERS AND MEMORY.) Acetylcholine is vital for the transmission of messages from one nerve cell to another, and the neurotransmitter is found at all nerve-muscle junctions as well as at many other sites in the nervous system. Its action is called cholinergic. Low levels of this chemical may cause forgetfulness.

Scientists discovered its role in memory when studying ALZHEIMER'S DISEASE patients, whose memory problems underlie their disease. Scientists speculate that Alzheimer's patients forget because their brains contain low levels of acetylcholine.

acetyl-L-carnitine (ALC) A molecule found naturally in the body responsible for carrying fats into the mitochondria (the energy-producing part of the cells) and regarded by some scientists as one of the most promising chemicals for the treatment of ALZHEIMER'S DISEASE.

Long-term administration of ALC, which is found in many common foods (including milk), has preserved spatial memory in aged rats. Some studies suggest that ALC also may play an important part in protecting the brain from the effects of aging. One study has found that ALC helps nourish certain receptors in the brain that are important for learning. In addition, other animal research suggests that ALC interferes with the formation of lipofuscin, a substance that is associated with a reduction of cognitive ability in the aged.

In human studies, ALC has been found to increase short-term memory, attention span and alertness of those with Alzheimer's disease and other forms of senility. It also is said to increase the brain levels of choline acetyltransferase and to increase dopamine activity. (Dopamine deficiencies in the brains of Alzheimer's patients are believed to be the primary reason behind low levels of ACETYL-CHOLINE, which can lead to muddy thinking, confused memory, slow reflexes and depression. [See DEPRESSION AND MEMORY.])

After studying 30 Alzheimer's patients and ALC, researchers at Columbia University concluded that ALC may retard the deterioration in some cognitive areas in patients with Alzheimer's disease.

ALC has been available in Italy since 1986, where it is classified as a NOOTROPIC DRUG and is used to treat Alzheimer's disease and age-associated

memory impairment. Recent studies at the University of Modena in Italy found that ALC improved cognitive performance in 279 elderly patients and that the cognitive gains persisted long after the treatment ended. In tests of cognitive function, emotional state and relational behavior, patients showed gains on all measures when compared to a placebo group. (See also CHEMICALS AND MEMORY LOSS.)

acquisition The process of encoding or recording information in the first stage of the memory process (followed by storage and retrieval/recall). If a person can't remember something, it may be because the information was never recorded in the first place (a failure of acquisition), although it is most likely a problem of retrieval.

acrostic A mnemonic technique (also called first-letter mnemonics) in which the first letters from a word or phrase are used to create a new phrase that is easier to remember. To remember the names of the Great Lakes, an acrostic would be: Happy Old Mares Exercise Some (Huron, Ontario, Michigan, Erie, Superior). (See also FIRST-LETTER CUEING; MNEMONICS; MNEMONIC STRATEGIES.)

ACTH (adrenocorticotropic hormone) A hormone that aids in memory retention and concentration. Produced by the anterior part of the pituitary gland, ACTH stimulates the adrenal cortex to release various corticosteroid hormones. ACTH also is necessary for the maintenance and growth of adrenal cortex cells.

A combination of ACTH and melanocyte-stimulating hormone (MSH) have been studied as a possible "memory pill" helpful in treating some types of mental retardation, hyperactive children and adults with SENILE DEMENTIA; however, its use also has serious side effects.

ACTH stimulates the adrenal cortex to increase production of the hormones hydrocortisone, aldosterone and androgen. ACTH production is controlled partly by the hypothalamus and partly by the level of hydrocortisone in the blood; when ACTH levels are too high, hydrocortisone production is increased, which suppresses the release of

ACTH from the pituitary gland. If levels are too low, the hypothalamus releases its hormones, stimulating the pituitary gland to increase ACTH production. ACTH levels increase in response to stress, emotion, injury, infection, burns, surgery and a decrease in blood pressure.

ADH   See VASOPRESSIN.

ADHD and memory   Some children with attention deficit hyperactivity disorder (ADHD) also may have problems with memory that are unrelated to that disorder and which require separate assessment. These children frequently show short-term memory deficits, including problems remembering math facts, spelling words and other reading-related tasks. Professionals treating them may incorrectly attribute such difficulties to the ADHD and not evaluate for other undiagnosed learning disorders.

What this means, according to researchers, is that experts should assess children for learning disorders—including disorders of memory—when they evaluate for ADHD. Proper psychological tests can reveal whether a child has problems learning because of ADHD-related poor listening skills, or because of problems in short-term memory caused by another learning disorder. In fact, the two problems may coexist. This is why many children continue to have problems with learning and memory even after they begin treatment targeted specifically at their ADHD.

Because there is no known drug to correct short-term memory problems, children diagnosed with these types of problems will need special help and instruction in more-efficient learning strategies, along with any treatment they are receiving specifically for their ADHD. One particular pitfall that parents and teachers may encounter is advice to punish the very forgetfulness that is beyond the child's control.

Researchers also discovered that during memory tasks, adults with ADHD were not using the brain regions that they should have been. Subjects without ADHD showed increased activity in certain brain regions including the right frontal cortex and the anterior cingulate, when engaged in short-term memory tasks. The right frontal cortex is probably involved in retrieving information, and the anterior cingulate may help by suppressing unnecessary information in normal subjects. Healthy subjects also showed increased activity in the hippocampus when the short-term memory task required more thought and when they were having problems answering the questions.

In contrast, subjects with ADHD showed more activity in the basal ganglia, an area typically associated with response readiness and motor control. This finding suggests that individuals with ADHD rely on less-efficient regions of the brain to perform short-term memory tasks.

Ad Herennium   The standard Roman text on memory written by an unknown author in 80 B.C., this is the earliest existing how-to book on rhetoric. The text, which includes a section on MNEMOTECHNICS, was written for rhetoric students and had a profound influence on some of the greatest thinkers of the ancient world.

Rhetoric students learned effective communication, especially effective public speaking. Since paper and books were expensive and scarce, rhetoric students had to learn ways to remember their speeches without referring to notes. In the *Ad Herennium*, the author describes an astonishing system of recalling facts, known as the Method of Loci, in which people can recall facts by arranging scenes in a space they have committed to memory and placing the things to be remembered in those rooms.

Students would first imagine a space in a quiet building they knew well. (Often rhetoric students searched for very large buildings with interesting architecture and committed these buildings to memory.) Then students would mentally lodge associative images in this space. When they wanted to recall information, they would take an imaginary walk through the space, looking at the images and remembering the associations. For example, if a lawyer wished to memorize details of a case, he might begin with an intruder hitting his victim. In order to remember this, he would imagine himself walking into his memory palace, stopping at the first architectural detail—a staircase—and imagining a picture of the intruder standing on the steps, hitting the victim. He would proceed through the memory palace, lodging other facts throughout the building. When it came time to call up the facts of the case, he would simply enter the memory palace in his mind; when he encountered the staircase, he would immediately remember the *association* of the intruder standing on the steps, hitting the victim.

The book discusses one of the classic rules of artificial memory: The aids must be unusual—even bizarre—in order to be memorable. The book's author notes that things in life that are boring, banal and ordinary are soon forgotten because the mind has not been stirred; but we are likely to remember the marvelous or novel, the base, dishonorable, unusual, great or ridiculous.

The *Ad Herennium* is the only complete source for the Roman and Greek art of memory, and was the primary transmitter of this classical art to the Middle Ages and the Renaissance, where the book enjoyed great popularity because it was thought to have been written by CICERO.

While the *Ad Herennium* gives general rules for memory systems, however, it does not give many concrete examples of images that a person could use to aid memory. The book's author apparently believed that a person should generate his or her own images and not use the pictures or associations of others.

adrenaline   See EPINEPHRINE.

adrenocorticotropic hormone (ACTH)   See ACTH.

advance knowledge and witness perception
Having some sort of knowledge about an event before it happens can influence how people view that event—what they see and what they pay attention to. (See also AGE AND EYEWITNESS ABILITY; EYEWITNESS TESTIMONY; MEMORY FOR EVENTS.)

age and eyewitness ability   A slight decline in recall and recognition ability may begin to occur at about age 60. Eyewitnesses over age 60 perform more poorly than do somewhat younger people, and some decrease in performance has been found on many tasks between ages 40 and 60.

But although some tasks, such as memory for details, may weaken slightly with age, other cognitive skills are maintained. In addition, there are great individual differences among people. Therefore, while performance on some tasks may decline somewhat as people age, performance on others—memory for logical relationships or the ability to make complex inferences, for example—does not deteriorate.

In addition, age may affect whether a witness is susceptible to potential biases and misleading information. Researchers always have believed children are both highly suggestible and particularly inaccurate, and studies suggest that younger children are very much more suggestible than older children or adults. (See also CROSS-RACIAL WITNESS IDENTIFICATION; EYEWITNESS TESTIMONY; GENDER AND EYEWITNESS ABILITY; MEMORY FOR EVENTS.)

age-associated memory impairment (AAMI)
See MILD COGNITIVE IMPAIRMENT.

age regression, hypnotic   A hypnotic technique that directs the subject mentally to return to childhood; it is not uncommon for the subject to take on childlike qualities, with changes in voice, handwriting and gestures. Often the subject of age regression spontaneously may relive a painful or traumatic experience of childhood.

The first published report of age regression appeared in 1883 in the *Revue Philosophique* by Charles Richet, who suggested to a subject that he was six years old again. This report set off a plethora of age-regression suggestions, which became popular during the 1890s as one type of "personality alteration" (similar to the "double personality" also being explored at that time).

Estimates are that about 43 percent of individuals respond positively to age-regression suggestions, much higher than the 15 percent of people who are considered to be highly hypnotizable.

Many researchers now believe that any time age-regression techniques are used to elicit memories, the subsequent memories may be either fact or fantasy—or a mixture of both. Clinically, therapists don't really care whether the memory is fact or fiction, since it is believed that treating a person's fantasies of the past can be just as effective as treating the documented reality of that past.

Hypnotized subjects are not consciously lying, according to memory expert Martin Orne, M.D. When subjects are regressed to age five, they really believe they are children and they will respond as they believe five-year-olds would. While subjects feel they are children, they are not really children; instead, the subjects are role playing with all of their heart, Orne says—but not all of their mind.

One of the hallmarks of HYPNOSIS is translogic, or a decrease in critical judgment. It is translogic that causes a hypnotized subject to copy down a complicated dictation in a childish scrawl—but with perfect spelling beyond the capability of any child. An adult who is consciously trying to mimic a child would not make the mistake of copying a complicated paragraph without inserting some spelling errors.

Scientists can test hypnotic memories by testing the reactions of regressed subjects and comparing them to actual behavior exhibited by children of the same "age." Most regressed subjects demonstrate that they react as they expect children of that age would react, not as true children act.

aging and memory As a person ages, the functioning of the memory process begins to slow down, affecting different types of memory in different ways. There could be a whole host of reasons why this memory deterioration occurs: malnutrition, depression, medications—or a range of organic problems in the aging brain itself.

Causes

Researchers have come up with several possible reasons for this age-related memory deterioration, although none has been proven conclusively. First of all, there are a range of reversible reasons for an age-related loss: depression, medications (especially the BENZODIAZEPINES used to treat anxiety), dietary irregularities, thyroid deficiency, alcohol and marijuana.

But there are also a wide range of organic reasons that underlie this type of memory loss. While scientists once thought that age brought an irreversible loss of cells in the cerebral cortex, they have now completely changed their minds. Today

researchers believe that major cell loss appears to be in a tiny region toward the front of the brain called the basal forebrain and in the HIPPOCAMPUS and AMYGDALA, which control memory and learning. Loss of these cells causes a drop in the production of the neurotransmitter ACETYLCHOLINE, vital to memory and learning. Alzheimer's disease patients, for example, have marked decreases in this vital neurotransmitter.

Unfortunately, the hippocampus—probably one of the most important brain structures involved in memory—is highly vulnerable to aging. Studies have found that up to 5 percent of the nerve cells in the hippocampus evaporate with each decade past middle age. This could mean a loss of up to 20 percent of total hippocampal nerve cells by the time people enter their 80s.

Damage to this area of the brain may be a result of stress hormones such as cortisol, made in the adrenal glands. Research with rats at Stanford University and the University of Kentucky have found that stress-induced increases in cortisol prematurely age the hippocampus. Excessive amounts of free radicals (toxic forms of oxygen) also can build up as a person ages, damaging the hippocampus.

It may be that as the brain ages, the speed with which information is processed decreases so that retrieving stored material takes longer. Or memory problems may occur because of dying neurons or decreased production of neurotransmitters (chemicals like acetylcholine that allow brain cells to communicate with each other).

Memory problems also may be linked to the fact that as a person ages, the brain shrinks and the cells become less efficient, according to neuroscientist Mark Shapiro, M.D., of the Neuroscience Laboratory of the National Institute on Aging in Bethesda, Maryland. In addition, things can happen to the brain to accelerate its decline—a person can be genetically unlucky, be exposed to toxins such as lead or make bad choices in life, as by smoking and drinking to excess. All those things will accelerate memory decline.

Or it could be that an aging person's ability to retrieve memories may be impaired directly. Studies have shown that older people may have problems recalling a list of words but have no problem picking out those previously seen words from a longer list. Because they can recognize these previously seen words, it is obvious that the memory of the words has been stored somewhere in the brain—it is just harder to retrieve them (remember) than recognize them (picking from a list). In this case, a list may serve as a visual cue to help a person retrieve the memory.

Age-related memory problems also may be due to differences in ENCODING (storing information). Those people with the best ability to remember at any age tend to cloak new information with details, images and "cues." When they are introduced to a new acquaintance, for example, they notice the physical appearance of the person and link it in some way to the person's name, fitting the introduction into a context they already understand. Researchers have discovered that with age, a person is less able to organize this information effectively, perceiving less and noticing fewer details. In fact, researchers have documented a drop in effective encoding strategies during the 20s and traced a further, more gradual decrease over the life span. For these reasons, older people have the most difficulty when attempting unfamiliar tasks that require rapid processing—such as learning how to program a videocassette recorder or operating a computer.

About half of elderly men and women with severe intellectual impairment have ALZHEIMER'S DISEASE; another fourth suffer from vascular disorders (especially multiple strokes) and the rest have a variety of problems, including BRAIN TUMOR, abnormal thyroid function, infections, pernicious anemia, adverse drug reactions and abnormalities in the spinal fluid. (See STROKE.) A good diagnosis is important because all of these other disorders can be treated.

Symptoms

The chief decline in mental ability among healthy older people is in "executive function"—the ability to perform several tasks at once or to switch back and forth rapidly between tasks.

And while semantic memory (general vocabulary and knowledge about the world) often stays sharp through the 70s, memory for names (especially those not used frequently) begins to decline after age 35. While short-term memory does not decline as a person ages, long-term and episodic memory (remembering the time and place something occurred) does deteriorate.

The elderly also suffer from SOURCE AMNESIA (forgetting where something was learned). Spatial visualization skills (the ability to recognize faces and find one's car) already has begun to wane by the time a person enters the 20s.

An older person's ability to recall memories from long ago does not necessarily have anything to do with memory; the memories are not being remembered from long ago, but merely from the last time the story was told. This is why memories that have been retrieved many times may be distorted.

The Good News

While some specific abilities do decline with age, overall memory remains strong through the 70s; research studies have shown that the average 70-year-old performs as well on such a test as do 25 to 30 percent of 20-year-olds. In fact, many older people in their 60s and 70s score significantly better in verbal intelligence than young people.

There is significant proof that memory loss is not an inevitable part of aging, according to experts at Harvard University. Studies of nursing home populations controlled for age bias and excess anxiety showed that patients were able to make significant improvements in memory through rewards and cognitive challenges.

While some memory loss is common, it is usually benign and memory function diminishes only slightly with the years. Physical exercise and mental stimulation improve mental function in some people. Animal studies in California reveal that rats living stimulating lives, with plenty of toys in their cages, have larger brain cells and longer dendrites.

"One may not learn or remember quite as rapidly during healthy late life, but one may learn and remember nearly as well," says Dennis Selkoe, M.D., co-director of the Center for Neurologic Diseases at Brigham and Women's Hospital in Boston.

So while it is true that the brain does become less effective as a person ages, it is generally because of disuse rather than disease. And just as it's possible to strengthen a muscle by lifting weights, it's also possible to challenge the brain to become more efficient.

"The use-it-or-lose-it principle applies not only to maintaining muscular flexibility, but to high levels of intellectual performance as well," says psychologist K. Warner Schaie, Ph.D., director of the Gerontology Center at Pennsylvania State University. Dr. Schaie, who's been tracing the mental meanderings of 4,000 people for more than 30 years, is an international authority on mental stimulation and the aging brain. He believes that by running through some daily mental drills—sort of like practicing scales on a piano—a person can prevent intellectual breakdown. In fact, he's discovered that you can reverse a downward mental slide through a combination of mental gymnastics and problem-solving skills.

Only recently have scientists figured out that a person's brain doesn't gradually self-destruct during aging—that there is some choice over when, and how much, mental ability is lost, says gerontologist Robert Butler, M.D., director of the National Institute on Aging and winner of the Pulitzer Prize for his book *Why Survive? Being Old in America* (1985). "There is no overall decline with age," Butler says. "In fact, judgment, accuracy and general knowledge may increase."

Researchers once thought that by age 13 a person's brainpower began a slow downward spiral until—by about age 70 or 80—there would be barely enough brain cell wattage to power a penlight. More recent studies have exploded that myth.

Schaie's long-term study has looked at how older people handle skills ranging from identification of a rotated object to finding the square root of 243. He found that after about age 30, most people reach a plateau that is usually maintained until about age 60; after that, there are small declines depending on ability and sex. It's not until the 80s that any sort of serious mental slowdown occurs.

The capacity to focus on a task or follow an argument remains strong throughout life. The bad news, according to some neuropsychologists, is that memory may decline by 50 percent between ages 25 and 75. But the good news is that wisdom does not decline.

Preventing Memory Problems

It is possible to slow down a memory decline, some experts say. Evidence from animal research suggests that stimulating the brain can not only stop cells from shrinking, it can actually increase brain size. Studies show that rats living in an enriched environment had larger outer brain layers, with larger, healthier neurons. The rats also had brains with more cells responsible for providing food for the neurons. Those rats kept in a barren cage with nothing to play with were listless and had smaller brains.

Some scientists now believe that humans can also improve their brain function and even reverse a decline by challenging themselves with active learning or by living in an "enriched" environment. In fact, stimulating environments can even counteract the brain shrinkage due to old age.

In addition, research has found that exercised brain cells have more dendrites (the branchlike projections that allow the cells to communicate with each other). With age, a stimulating environment encourages the growth of these dendrites, and a dull environment lowers their number. That's why scientists believe that a person's socioeconomic status often predicts mental decline, since people who don't have a lot of disposable income often can't afford very stimulating environments. Researchers conclude that fewer, smaller brain cells is the price a person pays for failing to stimulate the brain.

In the Future

Someday, researchers suggest, it will be possible to go to a doctor and get a personally designed "exercise plan" for the brain to prevent mental skills from deteriorating, much the way a physical therapist might devise a treatment plan to help a trick knee or bad back.

Interestingly, researchers have discovered that older people best remember things and events that occurred from the ages of 25 to 40 rather than after age 50. This is probably because most of a person's life goals were begun during those years: jobs, relationship, children, marriage. It's not that life gets dull in middle age, but it has become routine—and the brain is far better at remembering details of a wedding day than thoughts during a bridge game last Tuesday. This is related to the FLASHBULB MEMORY phenomenon, in which an extremely emotional event is remembered clearly years later. Everyone remembers what he or she was doing when President Kennedy was shot, although not much will be remembered about the day before or after.

Part of the reason why momentous events are imprinted so strongly in the brain is that it's more than likely that a person was paying attention when they occurred. As generations of students have found out, no matter how well material is presented, if they are not paying attention they probably won't remember it. This is also why most people immediately forget a person's name when introduced—they are so busy looking at the new person, making initial judgments and trying to make pleasant conversation, that they forget the name quickly.

There are probably as many memory aids as there are things to be remembered. As far back as the late 19th century, psychologist William James was busy coming up with ways to put some pizzazz into his brain cells. He came to the conclusion that it's possible to improve memory by improving the way facts are memorized . . . which is why every music teacher since has translated the notes of the scale (E, G, B, D, F) into "Every Good Boy Does Fine."

But no matter what method is used to remember the name of the new neighbor, a zip code or the third law of quantum mechanics, the amount of time spent trying to remember is crucial. Researchers have found it's always better to sit down once or twice a day to try to remember things than to try to cram ten hours of study in at one time. People pay attention to what interests them. If older people must read and remember something, they should try to find a room where they can read without too many distractions. Also, it helps to be an active reader, reading a sentence as a critic would, ready to locate an inconsistency, checking against what is already known.

If a memory problem is caused by any sort of brain disease, memory strategies aren't going to help. But if the brain is structurally healthy, odds are these strategies will provide some improvement in memory and problem-solving skills.

NORMAL MEMORY CHANGES WITH AGE

- *Reduced attention span:* Problems paying attention and ignoring distractions in the environment
- *Slowed thinking process:* Particularly apparent when dealing with new problems or a problem that needs an immediate reaction
- *Fewer memory strategies:* Older people don't use as many cues and associations as younger people
- *Longer learning time*

MEMORY THAT DOESN'T NORMALLY CHANGE

- *Short-term memory*
- *Semantic memory*
- *Retention of well-known information*
- *Searching technique:* Searching may take longer, but the technique doesn't change
- *Interference:* New information in one area competes with original information, which makes it hard to break old habits

---

agnosia A neurological condition in which patients fail to recognize objects even though they show no signs of sensory impairment. The problem in recognizing objects is often restricted to particular types of stimuli, such as colors or objects, and may take quite subtle forms. For example, in facial agnosia (PROSOPAGNOSIA) patients cannot recognize a familiar face, but they can recognize the person's voice. Even odder, some facial agnosics can't recognize their own faces in a mirror, although their concept of self is intact; it is just that the face in the mirror and the connection to the self has vanished. There are indications that patients with facial agnosia also may have problems recognizing other classes of stimuli (such as makes of cars or species of birds).

Because an object can be recognized only if the sensory information about it can be interpreted, a person must be able to recall memorized information about similar objects. Agnosia is caused by damage to those parts of the brain responsible for this necessary interpretative and memory recall. The most common causes of this type of brain damage are stroke and head injury. In addition, tumors of the parietal lobe of the cerebral hemispheres also frequently cause agnosia.

Sigmund Freud invented the term *agnosia*, meaning "state of not knowing." It can be contrasted with APHASIA (inability to recall words and construct speech).

In addition to facial agnosia, there are other types: In *visual agnosia*, the patient is unable to verbally identify visual material, even though he or she may be able to indicate recognition of it by other means (such as gestures). In *color agnosia*, a patient can't recognize colors; if asked to pick out a blue sweater, he or she cannot do so. There is nothing wrong with a color agnosic's eyesight and he or she is not color blind; it is just that colors are devoid of meaning.

There are a wide variety of agnosias for sound (sensory agnosia): These can include *pure word deafness*, the inability to recognize spoken words although the patient can read, write and speak, and react to other sounds. In *cortical deafness*, the patient has problems discriminating all kinds of sounds.

Somatosensory agnosia is the inability to recognize objects by shape or size. ANOSOGNOSIA is the inability to recognize the fact that you are ill; a patient may feel sick but cannot make the connection between the symptoms and the perception "I'm sick."

Reduplicative paramnesia, or CAPGRAS SYNDROME, is a rare disorder in which patients fail to recognize other people and places they know well. The effect can be induced by showing a patient a picture and then, a few minutes later, producing the same picture again. A patient with reduplicative paramnesia may say she has seen a similar picture but insist that it is definitely not the one she is now looking at. This disorder is believed to have a psychological origin, although more recent research suggests there may be an organic cause. It is typically associated with CONFABULATION, speech problems and a denial of illness.

agraphia   The loss or reduction of the ability to write, despite normal hand and arm muscle function, as a result of brain damage to the part of the brain concerned with writing.

Writing requires a complex sequence of mental processes, including the selection of words, recall from memory of how these words are spelled, formulation and execution of necessary hand movements and visual checking that written words match their representation in the brain.

Researchers believe these processes take place in a number of connected brain areas; damage to any of these areas (usually within the left cerebral hemisphere) can cause an agraphia of different types and severity. The most common reasons for such damage are head injury, stroke and brain tumors.

Agraphia rarely occurs on its own, but often is accompanied by alexia (loss of the ability to read) or expressive APHASIA (general disturbance in speaking).

While there is no specific treatment for agraphia, some of the lost writing skills may return sometime after the stroke or head injury. (See also ALEXIA; APRAXIA; DYSPHASIA.)

AIDS dementia complex (ADC)   A complicated DEMENTIA syndrome made up of different nervous system and mental symptoms found somewhat commonly in people infected with HIV (the virus that causes AIDS). It becomes more common with advancing disease. ADC is not a true opportunistic infection, but one of the few conditions caused directly by the HIV virus. It is believed to be fairly uncommon in early stages of HIV infection, but is found more commonly in AIDS patients with system-wide symptoms.

In AIDS, the central nervous system can be damaged by a number of things, including opportunistic infections, direct effects of HIV in the brain and the toxic effects of drug treatments. A patient with ADC has HIV viruses that actively infect brain cells. ADC consists of many progressive conditions that can be mistaken for other problems, such as depression, drug-induced side effects or specific opportunistic infections that affect the brain, such as toxoplasmosis or lymphoma.

At present, there is no reliable data estimating the percentage of AIDS patients who may eventually develop ADC. Although several studies in the mid-1980s suggested that between 10 percent and 70 percent of people with AIDS may develop the condition, more recent anecdotal reports indicate there are fewer patients with ADC since drug therapy has become standard. Patients who do have the syndrome tend to be sicker; ADC has become a disease of late-stage AIDS.

Symptoms

Early symptoms include apathy, loss of interest, poor concentration, forgetfulness and depression. Later symptoms involve short- and long-term memory loss, social withdrawal, slowed thinking, short attention span, irritability, apathy, weakness, poor coordination, impaired judgment and personality change. Because there are many different manifestations of ADC, the syndrome is poorly understood and has been reported and described in a variety of conflicting ways. The U.S. Centers for Disease Control considers HIV encephalopathy (dementia) an AIDS-defining condition.

Diagnosis

To diagnose ADC accurately, a patient must have mental status exams, a spinal tap and one of the standard scans (CT, MRI or SPECT). These tests may also help doctors tell the difference between ADC and other brain disorders such as meningitis or toxoplasmosis.

A mental status examination is designed to reveal problems such as short- or long-term memory loss and problems with orientation, concentration and abstract thinking, as well as mood swings. A spinal tap of cerebrospinal fluid (CSF) may reveal the typical mild elevations of certain proteins and of white blood cells common among ADC patients. In addition, the amount of HIV virus in the spinal fluid seems to be linked with progressive dementia in children.

Brain scans that may help diagnose the condition include CT, MRI and SPECT (single-photon emission computerized tomograms). In ADC-affected patients, CT scans usually show signs of atrophied brain tissue, whereas MRIs can detect white matter disease in the brain. SPECT scans are the newest way to diagnose ADC by using a radioactive material to measure blood flow in the brain; the scan also can show if anti-HIV therapy has improved the blood flow of the brain.

Treatment

The drug AZT is the most effective treatment and prevention of HIV activity in the brain because it crosses the blood-brain barrier. Several groups have reported an improvement in cognitive functions with AZT. Larger doses (1,000 mg) of AZT appear to be necessary to treat ADC, although many of the sickest patients can't tolerate such high doses. Another approach is direct injections of AZT into the spinal canal. One study found that of eight patients receiving AZT injections, five showed neurological improvements.

Psychiatric drugs are often used to treat other symptoms, including antipsychotics, antidepressants, anti-anxiety drugs, psychostimulants, anti-manic drugs and anticonvulsants. While these drugs don't affect the underlying condition, they may ease some symptoms. Haloperidol (Haldol) is often indicated for alleviating ADC symptoms, although it has many side effects. Ritalin (methylphenidate) has been used successfully to treat apathy and to boost energy, concentration and appetite.

In the Future

Nimodipine is one of the few drugs under development specifically for treating ADC. Nimodipine (Nimotop) is commercially available as a pill, and prescribed to treat cerebral hemorrhages. In test tube studies, nimodipine counteracts the toxic effects of the HIV protein. Because nimodipine can cause low blood pressure, careful monitoring is required.

akashic records   This concept is a description of "divine memory" described in ancient texts from Tibet, Egypt and India. It refers to a cosmic data bank of all universal happenings recorded on a sort of "ether"—an invisible unmanifested medium through which visible light passes as a manifestation of vibration. The name comes from the Sanskrit word *Akasha,* meaning "unshining light" or black light of radiation, referring to primordial substance.

alcohol amnestic disorder   See KORSAKOFF'S SYNDROME.

alcohol and memory   Alcoholism is one of the most serious and prevalent medical problems in the United States, and brings with it serious memory problems. Statistics suggest that at least 12 to 15 percent of the population may be alcoholics, and even a few drinks four times a week will lower the ability to remember.

Short-term memory loss is a classic problem among patients who abuse alcohol, which impairs the ability to retain new information. This potential deficit is based not on the number of ounces drunk per day but on each individual's tolerance for alcohol. In studies at the University of California at Los Angeles, scientists discovered that people over age 40 experienced the most memory problems after drinking—but even people age 21 to 30 experienced some memory loss.

In addition, women appear to be more susceptible to the toxic effects of alcohol, especially in relation to their short-term memory performance. Among alcoholics, women also seem to suffer from both verbal and spatial cognitive problems, whereas men seem to be affected only by spatial cognitive difficulties.

Chronic alcohol abuse may result in Wernicke's Encephalopathy, a condition characterized by the sudden onset of confusion, coordination problems, loss of sensation and impaired reflexes. (See WERNICKE-KORSAKOFF SYNDROME.)The level of consciousness progressively decreases, and without treatment, this syndrome may lead to coma and death.

If treatment is not begun early enough, Korsakoff's psychosis (or syndrome) may result. With this disorder, sufferers experience severe amnesia, apathy and disorientation. Recent memories are affected more than distant memory; often patients cannot remember what they did even a few moments ago, and they may make up stories to cover for their loss of memory.

Some researchers believe that people who are frequently drunk and sober may experience state dependency (also called compatibility); that is, things learned in one state or context are impossible to remember in another. For example, on the following day an alcoholic will not remember activities at a party while drunk—but can recall them when drunk again. This type of state dependency is why witnesses are sometimes brought to the scene of a crime to help them remember details.

Most alcohol-induced memory problems seem to disappear when the person stops drinking,

although a lifetime of abuse may cause irreversible damage. When investigators tested alcoholics after four or five weeks of treatment, their memory performance was much better. (See also BLACKOUTS, ALCOHOLIC; KORSAKOFF'S SYNDROME; STATE-DEPENDENT LEARNING.)

alcohol idiosyncratic intoxication   A marked behavioral change (usually to aggressiveness) caused by drinking an amount of alcohol insufficient to induce intoxication in most people. This behavior change, which is usually atypical for the person, is usually followed by AMNESIA for the period of intoxication.

Some experts believe the phenomenon is really a dissociative disorder in which aggressive and destructive behaviors are likely to be prominent. (See also ALCOHOL AND MEMORY; BLACKOUTS, ALCOHOLIC; KORSAKOFF'S SYNDROME.)

alexia   The inability to recognize and name written words by a person who had been literate, severely disrupting the ability to read. The disability is caused by brain damage from stroke or head injury to a part of the cerebrum. It is considered to be a much more serious reading disability than dyslexia. (See also AGRAPHIA; APHASIA; APRAXIA; DYSLEXIA AND MEMORY; DYSPHASIA.)

alphabetical searching   A type of verbal method for improving memory in which the subject works through the alphabet in the hope that a particular letter will act as a retrieval cue for a forgotten word or name. Alphabetical searching is believed to be effective only when the person already has a great deal of information about the word (its length, whether it is common, the number of syllables, etc.).

altered states of consciousness   Qualitative alterations in the overall pattern of mental functioning, so that the person feels consciousness is radically different from the way it normally functions.

Alzheimer, Alois (1864–1915)   German neuropathologist who first diagnosed Alzheimer's disease in 1906 during the autopsy of a 55-year-old patient who had died with severe dementia. Alzheimer's, a disease characterized by progressive loss of memory, had never before been isolated as a brain disorder.

During the autopsy, Alzheimer noted two abnormalities in the woman's brain—neuritic plaques and NEUROFIBRILLARY TANGLES.

Alzheimer worked with colleagues Emil Kraepelin and Franz Nissl in the research lab at the Psychological Clinic of the University of Munich, where they conducted research on the underlying disease processes in the nervous system that caused DEMENTIA PRAECOX. While Nissl invented new staining techniques to better study nerve cells, Alzheimer discovered the disease process for Alzheimer's disease. Alzheimer also served as a professor at Breslau University in Poland from 1912 until he died in 1915.

Alzheimer's Association   The largest national, nonprofit organization dedicated to research for the causes, prevention, cure and treatment of ALZHEIMER'S DISEASE and related disorders and to providing support and education to 4 million patients and their families.

In 1980 seven independent caregiver groups joined to form the Alzheimer's Disease and Related Disorders Association to help families who endure the financial, physical and emotional tolls of Alzheimer's disease. The association has become the nation's leading nonprofit health organization. In 1988 the organization changed its name from ADRDA to the Alzheimer's Association.

The group also helps set up chapters at the local level, advocates for improved public policy and legislation and provides patient and family service to help present and future victims and caregivers.

Through its national chapter and volunteer network, the association sponsors 1,600 support groups and other services for America's 4 million patients, families and caregivers.

The association publishes a quarterly *Alzheimer's Association Newsletter* and produces educational brochures, books and publications for patients, family members and professionals.

Through its medical and scientific advisory board, the association promotes and funds re-

search; its Autopsy Assistance Network helps families make the difficult decision about autopsy to confirm the diagnosis of Alzheimer's disease.

In addition to its Chicago headquarters, the association maintains an office in Washington, D.C. to ensure that the needs of patients and families are taken into consideration as legislation and public policy are developed. Each year the association presents Congress and the president with a National Program to Conquer Alzheimer's Disease.

For more information, contact the Alzheimer's Association, 919 North Michigan Avenue, Suite 1100, Chicago, IL 60611-1676; phone (312) 335-8700; TTD (312) 335-8882; website http://www.alz.org. A nationwide 24-hour hotline—(800) 272-3900—provides information and referrals to local chapters.

Alzheimer's Association Autopsy Assistance Network, The   A network designed to assist families with the difficult decision of autopsy, which is the only way to confirm the diagnosis of ALZHEIMER'S DISEASE (AD). The network provides families with information regarding autopsy and helps in obtaining a confirmed diagnosis. It also provides tissue for AD research and establishes diagnosis for the purpose of clinical and epidemiological studies. The network was established because families needed support and guidance in making the decision and planning for an autopsy.

There are two major reasons for autopsy. One is the ongoing research need for tissue. Also, to aid in more reliable studies and statistics on the prevalence of dementia, it is important that the cause of death be listed accurately on the death certificate.

The Alzheimer's Association Medical and Scientific Advisory Board recommends that the body organs of the patient with Alzheimer's disease *not* be donated for transplant purposes.

All states require a signed autopsy permit; in some states, it is possible to presign a permit, but the decision for brain autopsy must be confirmed verbally at the time of death. Permit forms are available from the pathologist or hospital. The pathologist will arrange the details of the autopsy.

Family members can expect a written autopsy report from the pathologist, neuropathologist or research center within a reasonable time after the patient's death.

Legally, the next of kin or guardian is the person to make the autopsy decision. If the spouse is deceased, the oldest child is considered next of kin. In instances where Alzheimer's disease is suspected, only the brain tissue is examined for diagnosis.

The autopsy is performed in the hospital, if that is where death occurs; if the patient dies in a nursing home, the pathologist will make other arrangements.

Alzheimer's disease   A progressive, neurodegenerative disease characterized by loss of function and death of nerve cells in several areas of the brain, leading to loss of mental functions such as memory and learning. Alzheimer's disease is not a normal part of aging, nor is it inevitable. It is the most common cause of DEMENTIA, a condition that leads to the loss of mental and physical functions.

Alzheimer's affects 4 million Americans, but experts believe that number could increase to more than 22 million by 2025 as the population grows and as people live longer and longer. The numbers will explode by more than threefold by the year 2050, according to some estimates. However, about 60,000 Alzheimer's patients are younger than 60; this condition is known as "early onset Alzheimer's disease." (See ALZHEIMER'S DISEASE IN YOUTH).

The disease, which kills 120,000 Americans each year, is the fourth leading cause of death among the elderly, following heart disease, cancer and stroke. It is the most common of the more than 70 forms of dementia.

It is characterized by an accumulation of twisted protein fragments inside nerve cells in the cortex (gray matter) of the brain, which appear under the microscope as a tangle of filaments called NEUROFIBRILLARY TANGLES. These tangles are one of the characteristic structural abnormalities found in the brains of Alzheimer patients; they were first described in 1906 by German neurologist Alois Alzheimer, M.D., who discovered them after performing an autopsy on the brain of a 55-year-old woman with dementia. In addition, other brain changes common in Alzheimer's disease include groups of degenerated nerve endings in the cortex called plaques that disrupt the passage of electro-chemical signals in the brain. The larger the number of plaques and tangles, the greater the disturbance in intellectual function and memory. Upon autopsy, the presence of plaques and tangles is the only definite way to diagnose Alzheimer's.

Risk Factors

So far, only two risk factors have been identified with Alzheimer's disease: age and family history. The risk of getting Alzheimer's disease rises with age, doubling in each decade after age 65. Average age at diagnosis is about 80; only one or two people in 100 have Alzheimer's at age 65, but that risk increases to about one in five by age 80. By age 90, half of all Americans have some symptoms. It's also true that people with relatives who develop Alzheimer's disease are more likely to develop the disease themselves.

The incidence of Alzheimer's is about the same for all races, but women are more likely than men to develop the disease, in part because they live longer. Head injury also has been linked with the disease, since some studies have found the condition occurs more often among those who have had traumatic head injuries earlier in life. Finally, lack of education seems to be linked to Alzheimer's. Research suggests that the more years of formal education a person has, the less likely he or she is to develop Alzheimer's later in life.

Symptoms

Alzheimer's disease begins slowly with mild forgetfulness that leads to problems finding the right word. Ever so gradually, it progresses to an inability to recognize objects, and ultimately, to an inability to use even the simplest of things, such as a hairbrush. This gradual degeneration often lasts more than 10 years. A person with mild dementia can usually live independently with only minor problems in work or social activities. As the dementia continues, however, the patient may seem capable, but independent living becomes increasingly dangerous. The person may begin to dress carelessly and neglect work and family responsibilities. He may leave the stove or iron turned on and become lost while away from home.

As the dementia becomes severe, eventually the person must be constantly supervised. As short-term memory falters, the person can no longer perform everyday tasks such as zipping a zipper. In later stages of the condition, the person may string together unrelated words into meaningless sentences.

Eventually, the failing nervous system affects the entire body, and the patient becomes completely incapacitated and even unable to eat. Death usually occurs as the result of pneumonia or an infection.

Memory problems aren't the only symptom, however. Behavioral symptoms are also quite common in Alzheimer's disease, since the damage to the brain from this condition can cause a person to act in different or unpredictable ways. Some people become anxious or aggressive, while others engage in repetitive behavior. Other behavioral symptoms may include agitation, combativeness, delusions, depression, hallucinations, insomnia and wandering.

Alzheimer's vs. Normal Memory Problems

One of the problems with the beginning symptoms of Alzheimer's is that so many of the symptoms appear, in much milder forms, as part of normal human habits. The following are some of the differences between normal behavior and Alzheimer's symptoms:

- Memory loss: The memory loss of Alzheimer's often affects daily life and job skills. It's normal to occasionally forget a task or a person's name, but frequent forgetfulness or unexplainable confusion at home or in the workplace may signal something's wrong.

- Problems with familiar tasks: It's normal to forget a pan on the stove, but people with Alzheimer's might not only forget to serve a meal, but also forget they made it.

- Language problems: A person with Alzheimer's disease may forget simple words or substitute inappropriate words, so that sentences become hard to understand.

- Disorientation: It's normal to momentarily forget the day of the week, but people with Alzheimer's disease get lost on their own street.

- Poor judgment: A person with Alzheimer's may dress inappropriately, such as wearing pajamas to the workplace.

- Abstract thinking problems: Recognizing numbers or simple adding or subtracting becomes impossible.

- Misplacing things: A person with Alzheimer's disease may put flour in the cat's bowl, and then not know how it got there.

- Rapid mood or behavior swings.

- Personality changes: A person with Alzheimer's can change dramatically, either suddenly or over a period of time and become suspicious or fearful.

Diagnosis

Alzheimer's disease is a complex illness characterized by a range of gradual, subtle changes that make it difficult to diagnose. Because of the many other disorders that can be confused with Alzheimer's disease, a comprehensive clinical evaluation is essential to arrive at a correct diagnosis of symptoms that look like those of Alzheimer's disease.

While the only definite way to diagnose Alzheimer's disease is an autopsy and there is no single diagnostic test that can detect Alzheimer's disease, doctors at specialized centers can correctly diagnose the disease 80 percent to 90 percent of the time. They do this by combining physical and neuropsychological testing with caregiver input and the doctor's judgment. Often, the diagnosis will involve a primary care physician together with a psychiatrist or neurologist.

Typically, a doctor will try to assess for the presence of Alzheimer's by asking 10 simple questions that seek to identify if the person knows who he is or where he is. In addition, however, tests of visual memory may help diagnose the condition, since people with Alzheimer's begin to lose immediate visual memory sooner than is expected in normal aging, and long before other markers of dementia are noticeable. Visual memory is the ability to remember and reproduce geometric patterns, for example. One way to test visual memory would be to ask a patient to draw the face of a clock with the hands pointing to a certain hour.

Evaluations commonly performed include:

- A medical history describing current mental or physical conditions, prescription drugs and family health history.

- A mental status evaluation to assess the patient's sense of time place, person and situation, and the ability to remember, understand, communicate and calculate. In early-stage Alzheimer's, screening of mental status may not detect symptoms.
- A physical exam that evaluates nutritional status, blood pressure and pulse.
- A neurological examination that tests the brain and spinal cord for evidence of other neurological disorders.
- A brain scan to search for other possible causes of dementia, such as a stroke. In early stages of Alzheimer's, these results are often "normal."
- Blood and urine tests to provide more information about problems other than Alzheimer's that may be causing dementia.
- Neuropsychological evaluations test memory, reasoning, vision-motor coordination and language function, and may provide the only evidence of dementia, especially in the early stages.
- Psychiatric evaluation, which provides an assessment of mood and other emotional factors that could mimic dementia or may accompany Alzheimer's disease.

Brain scan changes become more evident as the disease progresses, which is why a scan in the first stages of the disease can't by itself be used to make a definite diagnosis. It can, however, help rule out some other disorders that mimic Alzheimer's. In later stages, CAT scans often reveal changes characteristic of Alzheimer's disease, including shrunken brain tissue with widened tissue indentations and enlarged cerebral fluid-filled chambers.

A new method to test for Alzheimer's disease in people with signs of dementia is now available, which checks cerebrospinal fluid for proteins associated with the disease, and determines what version a person has of the ApoE gene. The National Institute on Aging notes that while the gene test may be useful in diagnosing someone with symptoms, it shouldn't be used for anyone else because the limits of the test are not known.

Of course, not all memory changes or complaints in later life signal Alzheimer's disease or mental disorder. Many memory changes are only temporary, such as those that occur with bereavement or any stressful situation that makes it difficult to concentrate. In fact, older people are often accused or accuse themselves of memory changes that are not really taking place.

Causes

No one yet knows exactly what causes Alzheimer's disease; indeed, it may well be that there is not one single cause but several factors that affect different people differently. Understanding its underlying mechanisms will provide the basis for advances in all other areas of research, including diagnosis, treatment, prevention and care.

Many types of dementia involve the degeneration of neurons, which lose their ability to communicate and die, which affects brain function. But scientists aren't sure what triggers the neuron degeneration in Alzheimer's. At least five major theories about the cause of Alzheimer's are currently under investigation:

- chemical
- genetic
- viral
- autoimmune
- blood-brain problems.

CHEMICAL THEORIES

Deficiencies

One of the ways in which brain cells communicate with one another is through chemicals called neurotransmitters. In 1976, researchers discovered that levels of the neurotransmitter acetylcholine dropped up to 90 percent in people with Alzheimer's, and the number of synaptic connections between neurons was reduced by about 40 percent. It could be, however, that the drop in acetylcholine and other neurotransmitters may happen late in Alzheimer's as a result of the disease process rather than a cause.

In any case, drugs whose side effects lower acetylcholine levels in the brain can cause reversible memory problems. These treatments have included lecithin, choline, PHYSOSTIGMINE, deprenyl, TACRINE (Cognex) and others, used alone or in different combinations with one another.

Toxicity

One of the most well-known and controversial theories concerns aluminum, which became a suspect when scientists found aluminum in the brain tissue of people who had Alzheimer's. There was concern that environmental levels of these metals may in some way trigger the disease.

But scientists who've studied environmental aluminum sources from antacids and antiperspirants to cooking pots and drinking water haven't found a link between aluminum and Alzheimer's. Most researchers believe that aluminum is an effect of the disorder rather than its cause. It's also possible that some of the aluminum supposedly found in brain tissue actually came from the special substances used in the lab to study the brain tissue.

Other experts are concerned that too much zinc might be related to Alzheimer's disease. Recent studies found that zinc triggered clumping of the protein beta-amyloid, very similar to the plaques found in the brains of people with Alzheimer's. More research is being done in this area.

Some scientists are studying the possibility of food toxins as another cause, since two amino acids found in the seeds of certain legumes in Africa, India and Guam may cause brain damage, enhancing the action of a neurotransmitter implicated in Alzheimer's. Another possibility is demoic acid found in some shellfish, which also stimulates the neurotransmitter linked to the disease.

Mutant Proteins

For nearly a century, scientists have wondered whether the brain lesions associated with Alzheimer's cause the disease—either the plaques that litter the empty spaces between nerve cells or the stringy tangles that erupt from within those cells.

In the mid-1980s, researchers discovered beta-amyloid, a generic name for a class of sticky proteins, in the plaques of Alzheimer's patients. A short time later, four research teams found the gene that makes the protein; it turns out that beta-amyloid is a fragment of a much larger protein called amyloid-precursor protein (APP), which is involved in cell membrane function.

Beta-amyloid protein is produced by cells throughout the body, but it's found in large amounts in the brain. The normal function of beta-amyloid remains mysterious, however; scientists don't know what it does, but they do know it occurs in two lengths, and that in the brain the slightly longer version is more likely to clump into plaques.

What happens in Alzheimer's disease is that for some reason, the brain suddenly identifies tiny bits of beta-amyloids as foreign, and immune cells try to clear them away. The result is a state of chronic inflammation that progressively injures nearby nerve cells. Among the powerful weapons the brain's immune system brings to bear against the beta-amyloid bits are oxygen-free radicals, which is one reason many think that antioxidants like vitamin E may be helpful against Alzheimer's.

Researchers are intrigued by beta-amyloid plaques because they occur early in the disease, before there is any damage to surrounding brain cells—and the plaques appear 10 to 20 years before symptoms develop. Although scientists don't know the ultimate cause of brain cell death, mounting evidence suggests that a form of beta-amyloid protein may be the culprit.

While scientists know that plaques are made of beta-amyloid, the tangles are made of another kind of protein called tau. (See TAU PROTEIN.) The key question scientists need to resolve is the relationship between beta-amyloid and tau. It's also important to discover if beta-amyloid and tau are the triggers of the disease, or merely the byproduct of some neurological process gone terribly awry.

While scientists don't know for sure what beta-amyloid does, they do know that tau protein plays a critical role in the brain. The internal support structure for nerve cells depends on the normal functioning of tau, which functions like the rungs of a ladder, holding the two parallel branches of axons apart. When something happens to the brain and tau suddenly starts to twist and collapse, the axons shrivel and die. In 1998, researchers discovered a form of dementia associated with mutations of the tau gene. People with these mutations didn't develop any of the plaques traditionally associated with Alzheimer's disease—but when they died, their brains were riddled with tangles.

Growth Factors

Some experts suspect that naturally occurring substances that affect the nervous system may contribute to the dysfunction or death of brain cells in Alzheimer's. It could be that the reason brain cells die in Alzheimer's patients is a decline in growth-promoting factors that maintain the functioning of brain cells—or a spontaneous increase in factors that are toxic to brain cells.

Experiments in aged rats indicate that specific nerve growth factors can stimulate the growth of new synaptic connections in the hippocampus and, as a result, restore some memory loss. Although there could be neurotoxic as well as growth-enhancing effects in the use of NGF, scientists are looking ways to safely use NGF in humans, perhaps through the transplant of genetically engineered cells.

Metabolism

Other research is exploring whether changes or an imbalance in the metabolism of certain elements like calcium in brain cells may be part of the process by which the cells degenerate and die in Alzheimer's disease.

Neurons use calcium to help transmit signals in the brain, but too much calcium can kill a cell. Some scientists think that excessive levels of calcium may be the cause of cell death in Alzheimer's patients. This may be caused by a number of problems, such as a defect in the structure that stores calcium in the cell, or those that pump it out of the cell.

In another metabolic theory, experts suspect the hormone called glucocorticoid, which normally enhances the manufacture of glucose (sugar) and reduces inflammation in the body. Animal studies have suggested that long exposure to glucocorticoids contribute to cell death and dysfunction in the hippocampus.

GENETIC THEORIES

It's quite clear that genes are involved in at least a few types of Alzheimer's disease in some way; some experts suspect that genes may be involved in more than half of all cases of Alzheimer's. Several

genetic markers have been identified on chromosomes 21 and 14 in a small number of families in which Alzheimer's disease has occurred with unusual frequency at relatively early ages. The mutant APP gene is found on chromosome 21; the single change in its DNA sequence occurred in the vicinity of the beta-amyloid fragment. Two more early-onset Alzheimer's genes (presenilin-1 and presenilin-2) were later found on chromosome 14. Like APP, these genes were dominant (a child who received just one gene from either parent would inevitably get the disease).

In 1992, scientists found a particular form of the APOLIPOPROTEIN E (ApoE) gene on chromosome 19 in families in which the disease has tended to develop at later ages. The ApoE lipoprotein is one of the many workhorses of the body's cholesterol-transport system.

Although there are three forms of ApoE (e2, e3 and e4), only ApoE-4 is associated with late-onset Alzheimer's cases and is considered to be a major risk factor for the disease. But unlike APP and the presenilins, it is a susceptibility gene—this means that people who carry it don't invariably develop Alzheimer's.

Experts think that other factors, such as diabetes or atherosclerosis, boost the chance that gene carriers will develop Alzheimer's. If they do, however, their brains appear to be more riddled with plaques and tangles than those of Alzheimer's patients who carry slightly different versions of the ApoE gene. In addition, ApoE-4 seems to have a broad impact on the health of nerve cells. For example, people who carry two copies of ApoE-4 have more trouble recovering from strokes and head injuries, and are more likely to sustain brain damage during heart surgery.

Scientists are trying to identify environmental factors that may help protect people who carry genes like ApoE-4. It's clear that these genes alone aren't enough to cause Alzheimer's. They are simply risk factors, which means that lifestyle choices, such as high-cholesterol diets, could be just as important.

While ApoE-4 may contribute to the development of more than 60 percent of all late-onset Alzheimer's cases, that leaves 40 percent caused by something else. For this reason, scientists assume there must be other Alzheimer's-susceptibility genes.

Indeed, they may be well on the way to discovering more. In late spring 2000, another mutant gene—this one causing inflammation—was discovered to be associated with Alzheimer's disease. Scientists know that genes produce a protein called interleukin-1 (Il-1) that promotes inflammation. This protein is produced in the brains of Alzheimer's patients. Now researchers have found that several variations of the gene can significantly increase the risk of developing Alzheimer's disease. One variation of the gene, called A-2, increases the risk threefold if a person receives a copy from each parent. Furthermore, if a person has two copies of this A2 gene and in addition has another variation of that gene called B2, their risk increases 10-fold for developing that disease.

Scientists think this may help explain why anti-inflammatory drugs have helped to ease symptoms in some Alzheimer's patients.

However, the full extent of the hereditary nature of Alzheimer's disease remains unclear. Many people are affected with this disease who don't have a strong family history. Moreover, the genetic factors associated with the disease vary from family to family. It may be that there are a number of subtypes of Alzheimer's disease, with differing risk factors and causes for each.

Down Syndrome and Alzheimer's

Autopsies of all individuals with Down syndrome over the age of 35 show brains filled with amyloid plaques and neurofibrillary tangles. In fact, nearly every person with Down syndrome who lives to the age of 60 or more will develop dementia. Moreover, compared to the general population, people with Down syndrome will begin to develop symptoms of Alzheimer's at a much younger age—usually by the late 40s or early 50s.

Scientists don't know why people with Down syndrome are vulnerable to Alzheimer's, but they suspect it could be related to the fact that these patients produce too much beta-amyloid protein—the major component of plaques.

The gene for the protein that produces beta-amyloid is found on chromosome 21—and Down syndrome patients have an extra copy of this chromosome. This means that instead of having two copies, individuals with Down syndrome have three copies of the gene that produces beta-amyloid. It's likely that the overproduction of beta-amyloid ultimately leads to its buildup in the brain in the form of plaques.

AUTOIMMUNE THEORY

The body's immune system protects against potentially harmful foreign invaders—but it can sometimes begin to attack its own tissues by mistake, producing antibodies to its own cells. This is called an autoimmune response, and it is responsible for many diseases, such as lupus and probably multiple sclerosis.

Some experts speculate that certain changes in aging brain cells might trigger an autoimmune response that produces symptoms of Alzheimer's in vulnerable individuals. In fact, some antibrain antibodies have been identified in the brains of those with Alzheimer's disease, but scientists aren't sure what this means since these antibodies also have been found in the brains of people without Alzheimer's disease. Even if changes are occurring in brain cells to trigger an autoimmune response, what originally set off these brain cell changes is not known.

VIRUS THEORY

Because a slow-acting virus has been identified as a cause of some brain disorders that closely resemble Alzheimer's disease (such as CREUTZFELDT-JAKOB DISEASE), some scientists think a slow virus may be causing Alzheimer's disease. Various researchers have suggested that suspicious brain tissue changes in Alzheimer's disease may be caused by a virus. But no virus has been isolated from the brains of those with Alzheimer's disease, and no immune reaction has been found in the brains of Alzheimer's patients like that found in patients with other viral dementias.

BLOOD VESSEL THEORY

Some experts think that Alzheimer's may be caused by defects in blood vessels supplying blood to the brain or potential defects in the blood-brain barrier (a protective membrane-like mechanism that keeps foreign bodies or toxins in the blood outside the brain).

There have been several reports of a possible association between serious head injuries involving a loss of consciousness and later onset of Alzheimer's disease. It could be, some experts theorize, that these traumas might injure the blood-brain barrier in some way.

Treatment

Three drugs have been approved by the FDA to treat loss of memory and decline in abilities such as thinking and reasoning: tacrine (Cognex), available by prescription since 1993; DONEPEZIL (Aricept), available since 1996; and RIVASTIGMINE (Exelon), approved in 2000. A fourth drug, galantamine (Reminyl), is under FDA review. All these drugs work by increasing the brain's supply of acetylcholine, a neurotransmitter chemical that is deficient in people with Alzheimer's. (Galantamine also affects some of the brain's receptors that respond to acetylcholine).

However, none of these drugs will cure Alzheimer's, nor do they stop progression of the disease. They are approved for treatment of mild to moderate Alzheimer's and may not be as useful for people in more advanced stages. Currently, there is no known way to predict whether or not a patient will benefit from any of these drugs. Because of this uncertainty, doctors and patients' families must weigh the potential benefits, risks and costs associated with use of these drugs.

Problem behaviors are also a part of Alzheimer's disease, and there are several kinds of treatments to help control this problem as well. Non-drug treatment of behavioral symptoms is recommended as a first option, since these symptoms are best modified without the use of medication. Indeed, some medications can induce further dementia symptoms. Changes in lighting, color and noise can greatly affect behavior—dim lighting may make some people with Alzheimer's uneasy, while loud or erratic noise often causes confusion and frustration. Patients should stay active for as long as possible, establishing a routine for bathing, dressing, cooking, cleaning and laundry. Creative leisure activities may include singing, playing music, painting, walking, playing with a pet or reading.

Unfortunately, non-drug treatments don't always work. Severe behavioral symptoms may be treated with medication. In some cases, drugs for the treatment of cognitive symptoms (donepezil or tacrine) may also improve behavioral problems.

Several other drugs can treat problem behaviors, including antipsychotics such as haloperidol (Haldol); anti-anxiety drugs such alprazolam (Xanax), buspirone (BuSpar) or diazepam (Valium); or many of the newest antidepressants such as fluvoxamine (Prozac), nefazodone (Serzone) or paroxetine (Paxil). As with any other drugs, these treatments can cause undesirable side effects.

In addition to drugs, some experts think that maintaining mental fitness may delay onset of dementia. In one study of a large order of nuns, the sisters had significantly lower rates of Alzheimer's, even though their average age is 85 and many are in their 90s.The study is interesting because most other environmental factors affecting the nuns, such as diet and environment, are no different from those among the lay population. What is different is that many of the nuns have advanced academic degrees and lead an intellectually challenging life into old age.

Some researchers believe that lifelong mental exercise and learning may promote the growth of additional synapses, the connections between neurons, and delay the onset of dementia. Other researchers argue that advanced education gives a person more experience with the types of memory and thinking tests used to measure dementia. This advanced level of education simply may help some people "cover" their condition until later.

Although Alzheimer's disease isn't curable or reversible, there are ways to ease symptoms. Not every person with this illness must move to a nursing home. Many patients (especially those in the early stages of the disease) are cared for at home. When to transfer a patient to a nursing home is a decision to be carefully considered by the family.

Prevention

A vaccine that prevents and reduces the buildup of plaque in the brains of mice has been proven safe in humans, according to researchers from Elan Pharmaceuticals. But scientists stressed it's far too soon to tell if the vaccine will actually work. Experts theorize that the vaccine, which is made from beta-amyloid protein, would stimulate a person's immune system to recognize and attack the protein. However, even if the vaccine works on humans, it would not be a cure but a preventive therapy. People who have established Alzheimer's disease have lost significant amounts of brain cells and probably would not regain function of those cells with this kind of treatment.

Despite the vaccine's promise, there are a number of reasons the method that worked in mice may not prevent or halt Alzheimer's in humans. First, the plaques may be a symptom of the disease, rather than the cause. In addition, Alzheimer's patients have other changes in the brain that the mice don't fully exhibit, such as tangles of protein inside nerve cells.

Another vaccine developed by researchers at Brigham and Women's Hospital in Boston prevents the plaque buildup in the brain.

While both vaccines show promise, it could be years before an Alzheimer's vaccine is approved.

Vitamin E Some researchers believe this antioxidant vitamin may protect memory from the effects of disease and prevent its onset. In one study of Alzheimer's patients at the University of California/San Diego, very high doses of the vitamin did slow down the progression of symptoms. However, at this time vitamin E is not recommended specifically for the treatment of Alzheimer's because there is no direct evidence that it prevents the disease.

Vitamin E is an antioxidant and may prevent nerve cell damage by destroying toxic free radicals (byproducts of normal cell metabolism). Some scientists think free radicals are discharged by immune cells that are in the brain responding to chronic brain inflammation from Alzheimer's. The free radicals may attach to molecules in the nerve cell membrane and disrupt function.

However, because vitamin E has other health benefits, researchers say there is no reason not to take it. However, vitamin E has been associated with increased bleeding in vulnerable patients, so patients taking vitamin E should discuss it with a doctor.

Estrogen Estrogens have strong effects on the brain; indeed, women often complain of memory problems during pregnancy and perimenopause, when estrogen levels fluctuate. Some experts suspect that Alzheimer's disease in older women may be related to estrogen deficiency, because estrogen may interact with nerve growth factors and delay the degeneration of neurotransmitters that facilitate memory and learning.

It is true that studies have shown that hormone replacement therapy (which includes estrogen) can boost a woman's performance on memory tests, and may reduce the chance of getting Alzheimer's. On the other hand, estrogen may increase the risk of breast cancer, gallbladder disease, high blood pressure and stroke, so it is often not recommended for women with a history of any of these conditions.

Recent studies show that estrogen replacement after menopause can reduce a woman's risk of developing Alzheimer's by 30 percent to 50 percent. In June 1997, the report of a long-term study from the National Institute on Aging (NIA) documented that estrogen replacement therapy in postmenopausal women was associated with a 50 percent reduction in the risk of developing Alzheimer's disease. In all, 472 women were studied for 16 years. Another NIA study documented the effects of estrogen in slowing the decline of visual memory in 288 women. The study showed that women who received ERT during the memory testing period performed better than women who had never taken estrogen.

Scientists still don't understand how estrogen lowers the risk of Alzheimer's disease or delays the onset of symptoms. It may help brain cells survive, slowing the onset of the disease, or it may help prevent the formation of beta-amyloid fibers (a protein associated with neuron damage) in the brain. Another theory claims that estrogen works as an antioxidant to protect nerve cells.

Unfortunately, research also suggests that taking estrogen may help women prevent the onset of the condition, but it doesn't work for women who already have been diagnosed with the condition.

Anti-Inflammatory Drugs The fact that people with arthritis seem to suffer less from Alzheimer's suggested to some researchers that this may be due to the arthritis patients' use of anti-inflammatory drugs, which could limit brain scarring and also reduce the inflammation caused by a type of gene (Interleukin-1) that boosts inflammation. Of all the common nonsteroidal anti-inflammatory drugs (NSAIDs), ibuprofen may be the most effective. In one study of 1,686 people it appeared to lower the incidence of Alzheimer's by 50 to 75 percent.

A study released in June 1996 showed that the NSAIDs ibuprofen (Advil, Motrin, Nuprin), naproxen sodium (Aleve) and indomethacin (Indocin) reduced risk of Alzheimer's by 30 percent to 60 percent. Doctors think brain inflammation occurs as one stage in the development of Alzheimer's. Investigators were uncertain why aspirin, which is also an anti-inflammatory drug, and acetaminophen (Tylenol), which is not, had no effect.

The study reinforced an earlier one that compared NSAID use in twins, which found that a twin who used NSAIDs regularly was 10 times less likely to develop Alzheimer's than the twin who wasn't taking an NSAID.

However, because of the risk of gastrointestinal bleeding, doctors don't recommend taking NSAIDs solely to prevent Alzheimer's until more research confirms these results.

Ginkgo Biloba The extract from the leaves of the ginkgo biloba tree have been used in Chinese medicine for centuries as a memory tonic. Extracts of the ginkgo leaves are one of the most popular herbal supplements in the United States, and are among the most widely prescribed treatments in Germany and France. Some studies have documented the safety and efficacy of ginkgo in treating patients with mild to moderate Alzheimer's, although experts agree more research is needed.

Ginkgo biloba is the oldest living tree species in the world. Extracts are made up of flavone glycosides, several terpene molecules unique to the tree and organic acids. Scientists believe the special terpenes improve circulation in the brain, and extracts are thought to have both anti-inflammatory and antioxidant properties. A study now under way at the National Center for Complementary and Alternative Medicine is currently investigating whether the plant can prevent common types of age-related memory problems.

In the Future . . .

Discovery of a previously unknown lesion characteristic of Alzheimer's disease may lead research-
ers to further understand the disease process and how intervention therapies may be designed. This lesion, called AMY plaque, may play a role in the onset and progression of Alzheimer's.

Diagnosis

New tests that look for biological markers for the disease have recently become available to measure spinal fluid levels of proteins associated with Alzheimer's. While these tests may ultimately prove useful, they can't yet be relied on for accurate diagnosis.

New imaging techniques that are still primarily research tools offer other new possibilities of earlier, more accurate diagnoses. Positron emission tomography (PET), single-photon emission computerized tomography (SPECT), and magnetic resonance spectroscopy imaging (MRSI) allow doctors to see interactions of brain chemicals, such as neurotransmitters and their receptors, at the molecular level.

New Treatments

Researchers are studying dozens of compounds in the search for medications to treat symptoms of Alzheimer's disease. Several experimental drugs have begun to show promise in enhancing nerve cell communications, regulating defective cell processes, protecting nerve cells from damage brought on by Alzheimer's and repairing nerve cells in the brain.

While today's treatments only ease symptoms, the next generation of treatments may delay onset or slow progression by protecting nerve cells for longer periods of time. In recent experiments, vitamin E, nonsteroidal anti-inflammatory drugs (NSAIDs), and estrogen have shown promise in delaying the onset of disease.

Although use of these treatments in individuals with Alzheimer's is still experimental, some have shown improved cognition or behavior with few side effects when taken in moderation.

Prevention

Researchers hope eventually to be able to inoculate individuals with Alzheimer's disease markers with engineered genes to prevent the condition.

Alzheimer's Disease and Related Disorders Association   Former name of the ALZHEIMER'S ASSOCIATION.

Alzheimer's disease in youth   While the disease is generally thought of as an older person's problem, Alzheimer's disease (AD) can strike those in their 30s, 40s or 50s. The behavioral symptoms are the same no matter when the disease strikes, but the younger patient with AD *is* different.

Younger patients may have more problems expressing thoughts and feel even more frustration at the situation. In addition, while the symptoms may be noticed, they will often be confused with psychiatric disorders or thought of as some sort of "midlife crisis." This preconceived idea that AD is an "old person's disease" may lead even the physician to disregard AD as a possible diagnosis. In this event, a second opinion should be obtained from a physician who is familiar with the diagnosis of dementia-type illnesses.

Families are encouraged to seek legal advice as soon as possible after receiving a diagnosis; this is even more important for the family of younger patients, because of the possibility of children still living at home.

While a person with AD finds that friendships often fade away as the disease progresses, younger patients may find friends breaking away even sooner because they are faced with the reality that AD can strike someone their own age.

The Alzheimer's Association provides a brochure, "Dealing with the Younger Alzheimer's Patient," that describes expected changes in the younger patient's physical and emotional behavior. For a free copy or for referral to a family support group, the association can be called: (800) 272-3900.

Alzheimer's Disease Research Center Program   The National Institute on Aging currently funds 12 Alzheimer's Disease Research Centers in a program designed to understand the disorder's etiology and treatment.

Each center serves as the site for new, expanded studies of the basic clinical and behavioral aspects of Alzheimer's disease. The centers also train scientists and health care professionals new to the field and serve as the link between research and the public. Centers include Duke University, Mt. Sinai School of Medicine, Harvard Medical School/Mass. General Hospital, University of California at San Diego, The Johns Hopkins Medical Institutions, University of Kentucky, University of Pittsburgh, University of Southern California, Case Western Reserve University, University of Washington, Washington University and University of Texas, Southwestern Medical Center.

amnesia   A memory disorder featuring the loss of the ability to memorize and/or to recall information. In most cases of amnesia, the storage of information in long-term memory and/or the recall of this information is impaired.

In many types of amnesia, the patient experiences a gap in memory extending back for some time from the moment of onset of the cause (usually a head injury). Called RETROGRADE AMNESIA, this is principally a deficit of recall, which usually shrinks over time. In addition, a patient may not be able to store information right after damaging the brain; this resulting gap in memory is called ANTEROGRADE AMNESIA. It extends from the onset of amnesia to the time when long-term memory resumes. This gap in memory is usually permanent.

Many theories explain the underlying mechanism of amnesia. It can be caused by damage from a head injury (including concussion) in areas that are concerned with memory function (TRAUMATIC AMNESIA). Other possible causes include degenerative disorders such as ALZHEIMER'S DISEASE or other DEMENTIA, infections (such as encephalitis [see ENCEPHALITIS AND MEMORY]) or a thiamine deficiency in alcoholics leading to KORSAKOFF'S SYNDROME. Amnesia with an organic basis also could be caused by a BRAIN TUMOR, STROKE or a SUBARACHNOID HEMORRHAGE, or certain types of mental illness for which there is no apparent physical damage.

Transient Global Amnesia

This type of uncommon amnesia refers to an abrupt loss of memory from a few seconds to a few hours without loss of consciousness or other impairment. During the amnesia period, the victim cannot store new experiences and suffers a permanent memory gap for the time of the amnesic episode.

There also may be a loss of memory encompassing many years prior to the amnesia attack; this retrograde memory loss gradually disappears, although it leaves a permanent gap in memory that does not usually extend backward more than an hour before onset of the attack. Attacks of transient global amnesia, which may occur more than once, are believed to be caused by a temporary reduction in blood supply in certain brain areas. Sometimes they act as a warning sign for an impending stroke.

The attacks, which usually strike healthy, middle-aged victims, may be set off by many things, including sudden temperature changes, stress, eating a large meal or even sexual intercourse. While several toxic substances have been associated with transient global amnesia, it is believed that the attacks are usually caused by a brief loss of blood flow to regions of the brain involved in memory.

Posthypnotic Amnesia

Amnesia also may occur after HYPNOSIS either spontaneously or by instruction, leaving the memory of a hypnotic trance vague and unclear, much the way a person remembers a dream upon awakening. If a hypnotized subject is told that she will remember nothing upon awakening, she will experience a much more profound posthypnotic amnesia. However, if the patient is rehypnotized and given a countersuggestion, she will awaken and remember everything; therefore, experts believe the phenomenon of posthypnotic amnesia is clearly psychogenic.

The amnesia may include all the events of the trance state or only selected items—or it may occur in matters unrelated to the trance. Memory for experiences during the hypnotic state also may return (even after a suggestion to forget) if the subject is persistently questioned after awakening. This observation led Sigmund Freud to search for repressed memories in his patients without the use of hypnosis.

Psychogenic Amnesia

Several types of amnesia belong in a different class from those caused by injury or disease; called PSY-CHOGENIC AMNESIAS, they are induced by hypnotic suggestion or occur spontaneously in reaction to acute conflict or stress (usually called hysterical). They also may extend to basic knowledge learned in school (such as mathematics), which never occurs in organic amnesia unless there is an accompanying aphasia or dementia. These types of amnesia are completely reversible, although they have never been fully explained.

In one type of MIXED AMNESIA, organic factors may also be involved in the development of psychogenic amnesia, and an accurate diagnosis may be difficult. This complex intermingling of a true organic memory defect with psychogenic factors can prolong or reinforce the memory loss. It is quite common for a brain-damaged patient to experience a hysterical reaction in addition to brain problems. For example, one patient who developed a severe amnesia that impaired the formation of new memories after CARBON MONOXIDE POISONING went on to develop a HYSTERICAL AMNESIA that continued to sustain the memory loss.

In psychogenic amnesia, there is no fundamental impairment in the memory process, registration or retention—the problem lies in accessing stored or repressed (usually painful) memories. This inability to recall painful memories is a protection against bringing into consciousness ideas associated with profound loss or fear, rage or shame.

Usually psychogenic amnesia can be treated successfully by procedures such as hypnosis. Under traumatic conditions, memories can become detached from personal identity, making recall impossible. Modern accounts of hysterical amnesia have been heavily influenced by Sigmund Freud, who attributed it to a need to repress information injurious to the ego.

Freud believed that the memory produces a defense reaction for the individual's own good. This explains why psychogenic amnesia occurs only in the wake of trauma and is consistent with the high incidence of depression and other psychiatric disorders in those who go on to develop psychogenic memory problems.

There are four types of recall problems following trauma: *localized amnesia, selective amnesia, generalized amnesia* and *continuous amnesia*.

Localized amnesia: The failure to recall all the events during a certain period of time (usually the first few hours after a disturbing event).

Selective amnesia: The failure to recall some, but not all, of the events during a certain period of time.

Generalized amnesia: The inability to recall any events from a person's entire life.

Continuous amnesia: Failure to recall events subsequent to a specific time, up to and including the present. (See also ALCOHOL AND MEMORY; AMNESIA, CHILDHOOD; AMNESIA AND CRIME; AMNESIC SYNDROME; ANESTHESIA AND MEMORY; ANTERIOR COMMUNICATING ARTERY ANEURYSM; BLACKOUTS, ALCOHOLIC; BRAIN SURGERY AND MEMORY; CAPGRAS SYNDROME; CHOLINERGIC BASAL FOREBRAIN; CONFABULATION; DIENCEPHALON; DISSOCIATIVE DISORDERS; DRUGS AND MEMORY; ELECTROCONVULSIVE THERAPY AND MEMORY; EMOTIONS AND MEMORY; EPILEPSY; FUGUE; KLÜVER-BUCY SYNDROME; MEDIAL TEMPORAL AMNESIA; MEMORY, DISORDERS OF; SCOPOLAMINE; SOURCE AMNESIA.)

amnesia, childhood   The lack of memories of early childhood (usually before age four in most people). Sigmund Freud believed that repression of infantile sexuality caused this early amnesia. Many modern memory researchers believe it occurs because of a child's lack of sophisticated mental abilities, such as language, which are used to cue memory.

While scientists have now documented that preschoolers and even infants do have memories, they have found that both verbal recall of childhood events and visual memories of familiar faces from childhood are sketchy at best. However, children can remember some things far more accurately than would be expected by simple chance.

While memory for events in particular contexts (episodic memory) may be vague, experts point out that semantic memory (that is, memory for facts and words) is quite strong in early childhood. Very young children easily learn thousands of words and their underlying concepts that make up language. Apparently, the ability to remember both words and events in context seems to require a well-developed prefrontal cortex.

amnesia, normal   See AMNESIA, CHILDHOOD.

amnesia, simulated   A condition related to PSEUDODEMENTIA in which head-injured victims awaiting settlement of compensation claims exaggerate the extent of their memory defect in a bid for higher compensation. It is very difficult to detect malingering, and clinicians must rely on common sense and intuition for a proper diagnosis. (See also PSYCHOGENIC AMNESIA.)

amnesia and crime   According to research, between 23 and 65 percent of murderers claim to have amnesia related to their crime. A great deal of amnesia for crime has a psychogenic origin; that is, the crimes are so horrific that the criminal must not remember in order to remain sane.

But not all criminal amnesia is of a self-protective nature; some criminals do not remember their crimes because they have schizophrenia or depression. In these cases, their amnesia may be an intrinsic part of their illness. In addition, many violent crimes are committed by alcoholics during "blackouts." During such a blackout, the person is not unconscious or stuporous—just drunk. (See also BLACKOUTS, ALCOHOLIC.)

If a defendant claims amnesia for the crime with which he is charged, it could be argued that he is unfit for trial or that he can plead "automatism." This means that the behavior was carried out involuntarily and without conscious intent. Crimes committed during an alcoholic blackout are not included in this plea, since it is assumed that people are aware of the effects of alcohol and are therefore responsible for their actions while drunk.

Amnesia for a crime may be a form of emotional defense that arises after the crime has been committed; this does not therefore imply a lack of conscious involvement during the amnesic period itself.

No cases have been found in which a defendant was acquitted due to an organic amnesic state.

amnesic syndrome   A permanent, global disorder of memory following brain damage from accident or illness that does not result in a general deterioration of memory function, but selectively impairs some aspects of memory while leaving others normal.

For example, patients with this syndrome score very badly on clinical memory tests but perform normally on intelligence tests, such as the Wechsler Adult Intelligence Scale. Therefore, a person with amnesic syndrome will have a memory quotient (MQ) between 20 to 40 points below the IQ. In particular, these patients score very poorly on tests of the retention of novel information (such as paired-associate learning or free recall), but they have no problem understanding a normal-length sentence—they just can't remember it for any length of time. Skills learned before the onset of the syndrome, such as riding a bike or driving, are unaffected.

The amnesic syndrome can be caused by lesions in two distinct parts of the brain: the DIENCEPHALON and the MEDIAL TEMPORAL LOBE of the CORTEX. Damage can be caused by a wide range of problems, including disease, neurosurgery, BRAIN TUMOR or HEAD INJURY, STROKE and deprivation of oxygen (anoxia). It also may be caused by a TRANSIENT ISCHEMIC ATTACK (TIA) that briefly blocks blood flow to the HIPPOCAMPUS.

amusia   The loss of the ability to comprehend or reproduce musical tones.

amygdala   A part of the brain lying within each temporal lobe that is important for memory; its primary function may well be its responsibility for bringing emotional content to memory.

Sensory stimulation from the cortical area enters the limbic system directly through the amygdala and indirectly through the hippocampus via the entorhinal cortex. Lesions to the hippocampus and entorhinal cortex lead to mild memory impairment; lesions to the amygdala and entorhinal cortex produce devastating impairment.

Researchers suggest that associative recall is established through a mechanism that requires information to be carried from the limbic system back to the sensory system—a process mediated by the amygdaloid complex. In some studies animals were required to associate an object with the location in which it first appeared; only those with an intact hippocampus were able to complete the task. This suggests, scientists say, that the hippocampus

serves an associative function with regard to spatial memory.

Some researchers believe that when a perception reaches the cerebral cortex, it will be stored within the amygdala if it arouses emotions (such as fear of a dog)—but other experts disagree.

While most now believe the amygdala does not process memory, it is believed to be a source of emotions that imbue memory with meaning. For example, often the remembrance of a memory or a whole stream of recollection brings with it a burst of emotion—evidence that the amygdala has become involved. (See also HIPPOCAMPUS; MEMORY.)

amyloid precursor protein (APP)   A protein molecule found in the brain, heart, kidneys, lungs, spleen and intestines. The normal function of APP in the body is unknown. In ALZHEIMER'S DISEASE, plaques are made when an enzyme snips APP apart at a specific place and then leaves the fragments—BETA-AMYLOID—in brain tissue where they come together in abnormal deposits.

amytal   See SODIUM AMYTAL.

anemia   A condition in which the concentration of the oxygen-carrying pigment hemoglobin in the blood is below normal. Hemoglobin molecules travel inside red blood cells and carry oxygen from the lungs to the tissues. In severe cases, anemia cuts down on the amount of oxygen carried by the blood, which cuts the amount available to the brain. Memory problems can result.

By far the most common form of anemia is caused by a deficiency of iron, an essential component of hemoglobin. But there also are many other causes of anemia, which is not a disease in itself but a symptom of many other disorders.

Normal blood hemoglobin concentrations are between 14 to 16 grams (g) per 100 milliliters (ml) for men and 12 to 14 g/100 ml for women. Concentrations below 10 can cause headaches, tiredness and lethargy. Concentrations below 8 can cause breathing problems on exercise, dizziness, heart palpitations and angina, and memory problems. Symptoms also depend on how quickly the anemia develops—its sudden development causes immediate symptoms, depending on the degree of blood loss.

Treatment, which will restore the memory to normal function, is aimed to correcting the underlying disorder.

anesthesia and memory Some anesthetized patients may comprehend enough of what is said during surgery to affect their recovery. Language understanding may continue while a person is anesthetized even though explicit recall does not. Nearly all adequate anesthetics produce an AMNESIA that prohibits any recall of memory during surgery; at the same time, auditory function is the last sense to fade under anesthesia. When unexpected recall occurs after surgery with an apparently adequate anesthesia, it usually involves memories for meaningful events that are recalled.

Recent research has found that anesthetized patients recover faster when given positive suggestions. One group was told that they would "want to get out of bed to help your body recover earlier." According to British researchers, this group actually did recover earlier, with fewer complications than a comparison group. However, not all studies have reached the same conclusions, and some physicians are skeptical. While the effects may be subtle, researchers also warn that thoughtless remarks may have very profound consequences.

If patients do not receive sufficient oxygen during anesthesia, they can experience memory disturbances. Even under perfect conditions, memory disturbances may linger for several days after surgery until the medications are eliminated from the system. (See also "FAT LADY" SYNDROME.)

animal memory Not all animals possess a memory in the sense that humans do. Animals farther down on the evolutionary ladder possess a rudimentary perceptive memory, genetically programmed to help them survive, but a productive memory that depends on recall developed later in animal evolution.

Ants, for example, live a deceptively complex life of rigid job descriptions and interrelated socialization patterns, but they are unable to recognize each other based on a memory of past experience.

Instead, they make sure of chemical signals to identify each other; they live their busy little lives based entirely on the way they interpret smells. By extracting a chemical that would normally identify larvae and attaching the chemical to fake larvae, scientists were able to prove that ants could not distinguish fakes from real larvae. To an ant, if it smells like larvae, it is larvae, and ants have no ability to adapt to any other circumstance or possibility.

Birds are farther along, evolutionarily speaking. While they are still largely guided by inborn instincts, they also are able to adapt to their circumstances using recognition based on memory. If a scientist moves eggs from one nest to another, birds can recognize their own eggs and reclaim them: The bird's past experience molds its present behavior. This is the difference between recognition based on memory and identification based on genetically programmed instinct.

Higher animals, however, rely on the adaptive value of the memory to an even greater degree. An elephant stuck in quicksand will, once freed, always remember the danger of quicksand and avoid it. This type of memory based on recognition is memory of the highest order; many animals are not capable of it, and scientists have yet to be able to program any computer to recognize other objects. Animals without such memory cannot adapt their behavior to changing circumstances; their adaptation relies only on natural selection.

aniracetam One of a class of NOOTROPIC DRUGS that some studies suggest may be capable of improving cognitive performance on a number of intelligence and memory tests. Its chemical structure is similar to PIRACETAM, a drug being investigated in the treatment of Alzheimer's disease.

Aniracetam's mechanism of action is unknown, although it does not seem to act directly on the catecholamine, serotonin or acetylcholine neurotransmitter systems.

Aniracetam is not approved for distribution in any country. Other names for aniracetam include Draganon, RO 13-5057 and Sarpul.

Anna O A young Viennese woman and hysteric patient in the late 19th century whose real name was Bertha Pappenheim. She was called Anna O by Josef Breuer and Sigmund Freud, who described her treatment in their book *Studies on Hysteria.*

Anna O was treated by Breuer from 1880 to 1882 for a range of psychosomatic problems and dissociative absences. Freud learned about her case after her treatment by Breuer, but her case led him to the technique of letting patients talk about their problems.

Breuer and Freud did not agree on the fundamental cause of dissociative absences. Breuer insisted they were a form of autohypnosis, while Freud believed they served as a defense mechanism, a protection against harmful thoughts.

Anna O was quite hypnotizable and excellent at self-hypnosis, and Breuer hypnotized her almost daily for hours at a time. Before the onset of her hysteria, she had often hallucinated an alternate world she called her private theater, a fairy-tale world in which she lived her life. If her father had not contracted a fatal case of tuberculosis, she might have spent the rest of her life in her dream world, but she was called upon to stay alert and nurse her father.

Although a bright, energetic woman, her culture expected her to live a life of quiet self-denial. She spent her time tending her dying father, never revealing any emotion and never earning a respite from her duties. Yet despite her resentment, she did not rebel openly. Her father's illness brought about a crisis in her life; she could no longer retreat into her private world, but she couldn't bear her new life, either. First, she experienced a hysterical cough while hearing an orchestra playing as she tended her father. She wished she could be at the party, and then immediately felt guilty for wanting to dance while her father lay dying. She coughed instead and continued to cough whenever she heard music. She had altered her emotional memory; she associated music with happiness, but then remembered her father and despised her wish for fun, changing the association with music.

After six months, she retreated to her bed, where she alternated between consciousness and dissociation. During conscious periods, she seemed normal except that she stayed in bed and exhibited a variety of odd behaviors—speaking only English,

coughing when hearing music, and hating water. When she retreated into her dream world, she lost the abilities of recognition and perception. She did not see or hear people, although Breuer could break through to her and maintain contact by steady speech. Anna did not, however, perceive strangers.

When Breuer brought a colleague to see her, she did not perceive him, and recognized that there was another person in the room only when he blew cigar smoke at her. She looked for the source of smoke, saw the stranger and ran.

Eventually Anna O recovered apparently on her own, although her changed circumstances helped. (Her father died and she entered a sanitarium where she had no responsibilities.) While Breuer's intensive therapy relieved some of her symptoms, she developed others, and when he stopped her treatment she was no better than when she had begun two years before. Many more years passed before she was healthy, but eventually she became an important figure in Austria's feminist movement.

Anna O's case shows that emotional memory failures don't need to have an objective cause—they can be related to a patient's own perceptions. While Breuer could attempt to treat her symptoms, he couldn't address the inequities of Viennese society. (See also BREUER, JOSEF; FREUD, SIGMUND.)

anosognosia   A type of AGNOSIA in which people can't recognize that they are ill because they can't make the connection between the fact of symptoms and the perception "I'm ill."

anterior communicating artery aneurysm   An aneurysm on the anterior communicating artery. When this type of aneurysm bursts, it leads to AMNESIA. While experts are not sure of the location of the critical aneurysm, both the frontal association neocortex and the cholinergic basal forebrain may be affected. The symptoms also may vary, both in the extent of the frontal symptoms and the degree of amnesia.

anterograde amnesia   A loss of the ability to learn, featuring very poor recall and recognition of recently presented information. This is contrasted with RETROGRADE AMNESIA, which is the very poor recall and recognition of information that was acquired before brain damage occurred. (See also AMNESIA.)

anticholinergics and memory   Anticholinergics are a group of ACETYLCHOLINE-blocking drugs that are used to treat irritable bowel syndrome and certain types of urinary incontinence, Parkinson's disease, asthma and other diseases. They also have a reputation as amnesic drugs.

These drugs act as antagonists to the actions of cholinergic nerve fibers (or cells), usually of the parasympathetic nervous system. These cholinergic nerve cells are those that use acetylcholine as their neurotransmitter. Drugs that have anticholinergic effects block the transmission of this neurotransmitter, preventing the communication between nerve cells and altering behavior. Most psychoactive drugs have anticholinergic effects in both the central and the peripheral nervous systems.

Depending on the dose, the anticholinergics SCOPOLAMINE, atropine and glycopyrrolate all can produce sedation and lack of vigilance. The most famous of the memory-clouding anticholinergics is scopolamine, a belladonna alkaloid that is a particularly potent amnesic agent. Other anticholinergics include heterocyclic antidepressants, antipsychotics, antihistamines, antiparkinsonian drugs and some hypnotics.

Research studies suggest that after a patient has received an anticholinergic drug, memory retention remains intact but effortful retrieval is impaired. It is believed that the neurochemical processes disrupted by these drugs are not involved in maintaining information in memory; rather they control the encoding process, which leads to a deficiency of retrieval.

If a patient takes several of these drugs together—or takes too many of any one kind—the combination can cause a crisis called the anticholinergic syndrome. Symptoms of this include dry mouth, constipation, urinary retention, decreased sweating, fever, flushing, discoordination, tachycardia, confusion, delirium, disorientation, agitation, visual and auditory hallucinations,

anxiety, restlessness, pseudoseizures and delusions. Treatment for anticholinergic syndrome is anticholinesterase therapy.

antidiuretic hormone (ADH)   See VASOPRESSIN.

anxiety and memory   Anxiety—the feeling of uneasiness, apprehension or dread—is one of the major causes of memory problems at any age. When anxiety becomes pronounced, it monopolizes a person's attention so that it is impossible to concentrate on anything else. Because the formation of memory is dependent on paying attention, anything that interferes with attention will impair memory.

Anxiety attacks can affect memory. These attacks are a pervasive feeling of anxiety not associated with anything in particular. In fact, this is how most definitions distinguish anxiety from fear, which usually has an object. In the midst of an anxiety attack, the sufferer withdraws from the exterior world and turns inward, focusing on internal turmoil. This is why the person fails to record information the way he or she normally would. When the thought processes are occupied exclusively with negative thoughts, there is no room for other thoughts that could cue memory.

Experts suggest that anxious patients tell themselves "I'm going to calm down and pay strict attention if I want to remember this." Together with relaxation techniques such as deep breathing, this should help calm anxiety enough to facilitate encoding and recall.

aphasia   A neurological condition in which the previously acquired capacity for language comprehension or expression is disturbed due to brain dysfunction that affects the ability to speak and write and/or the ability to comprehend and read. *Aphasia* is a complete absence of these communication and comprehension skills, while *dysphasia* is merely a disturbance in these abilities. A stroke or head injury is the most common cause of brain damage leading to aphasia.

The speech expression problems found in aphasia are different from those problems caused by disease or damage to the parts of the body involved in the mechanics of speech; comprehension problems are not due to hearing or vision difficulties.

Language skills within the brain lie in the dominant cerebral hemisphere; two areas in this hemisphere (Broca's and Wernicke's areas) and the pathways connecting the two are important in language skills. Damage to these areas is the most common cause of aphasia. Other disabilities that may occur with aphasia include AGRAPHIA (writing difficulty) or ALEXIA (word blindness).

While there may be some recovery from aphasia after a stroke or head injury, the more severe the aphasia, the less chance for improvement. Speech therapy is the main remedy.

Broca's Aphasia   While aphasia is a general term covering loss of language ability, there are different ways of classifying its various forms. In BROCA'S APHASIA, the patient has very disturbed speech and will often experience some comprehension problems. Speech is nonfluent, slow, labored, with a loss of normal rhythm.

Wernicke's Aphasia   In WERNICKE'S (RECEPTIVE) APHASIA, the patient has fluent speech but the contents are often meaningless because of poor comprehension. There are often many errors in word selection and grammar, indicating that internal speech also is impaired. Writing may be disturbed too, and spoken or written commands usually are not understood.

Global Aphasia   A patient with GLOBAL APHASIA exhibits total or near-total inability to speak, write or understand spoken or written words. The aphasia usually is caused by widespread damage to the dominant cerebral hemisphere.

Nominal Aphasia   NOMINAL APHASIA is difficulty in naming objects or in finding words, although the person may be able to choose the correct name from several offered. Nominal aphasia may be caused by generalized cerebral dysfunction or damage to specific language areas. (See also APRAXIA.)

aplysia   A sea slug (more accurately, sea hare) about the size of a human fist used in the study of memory and learning because of its relatively simple nervous system. This marine invertebrate contains fewer than 2×10^4 neurons; many of them are very large and can be seen with the naked eye. Sea slugs have no brain in the traditional sense; a collection of ganglia (or "subbrains") controls their functions.

apolipoprotein E (ApoE)   A protein whose main function is to transport cholesterol; one form of this protein has been linked to late-onset ALZHEIMER'S DISEASE. The gene for this protein is found on chromosome 19.

There are three forms of ApoE: e2, e3 and e4; ApoE-4 is associated with about 60 percent of late-onset Alzheimer's cases and is considered a risk factor for the disease. A person can have two ApoE-4 genes (one inherited from each parent), one ApoE-4 gene (inherited from one parent, but not the other) or no ApoE-4 variants at all. It seems that the ApoE-4 gene doesn't guarantee who will get Alzheimer's disease, but is an indication of who is more vulnerable.

It appears that the more ApoE-4 variants a person has, the quicker he or she will get Alzheimer's (if the person gets it at all). Research suggests that those with two E-4 varieties experience onset by age 80 to 85; those with one experiences onset by age 90 to 95; those with none of the E-4 varieties don't get the disease until age 95 to 100—if at all.

But not everyone with the gene goes on to develop Alzheimer's. Experts think that other factors, such as diseases like diabetes or atherosclerosis, boost the chance that the gene carrier will develop Alzheimer's. In one study of 6,000 healthy people over age 65, those who carried the ApoE-4 gene and who also had diabetes, atherosclerosis, or a circulation problem in hands, feet or legs, had a much higher risk of memory and thinking problems than those without the gene or the illnesses. Those with both atherosclerosis and ApoE-4 had more than an eightfold increased risk for problems in learning and memory. (And atherosclerosis alone also increased the risk for memory problems.)

Experts believe that people who have the gene should modify their lifestyle in order to prevent diabetes or heart disease. By watching diet and getting plenty of exercise, it is still possible to head off possible causes of dementia.

It is possible to be tested for the ApoE gene variant, but the test is a strong predictor of risk only for those younger than age 70.

apraxia Loss of previous ability to perform skilled motor acts that can't be explained by weakness, abnormal muscle tone or uncoordination. In this neurological condition patients fail to carry out skilled voluntary movements in the absence of paralysis or any defect in the peripheral muscles.

Apraxia is caused by damage to nerve tracts within the main mass of the brain (cerebrum) that translates the *idea* for a movement *into* that movement. While most patients with apraxia seem to know what they want to do, they seem to have lost the ability to recall from memory the sequence of actions they need to do to achieve the movement. A direct head injury, infection, stroke or brain tumor may have caused the damaged cerebrum.

There are several different types of apraxia, depending on which part of the brain has been damaged. A patient suffering from *ideomotor apraxia* can't carry out a spoken command to make a particular movement but at another time can be observed making those very same movements unconsciously. Other special forms of apraxia include AGRAPHIA (difficulty writing) and expressive APHASIA (severe difficulty in speaking).

Because recovery after stroke or brain injury differs widely from one patient to another, it is difficult to predict the recovery from any accompanying apraxia. In general, however, some deficit remains and the patient may need considerable patience and effort to relearn past skills. (See also ALEXIA; DYSPHASIA.)

Aquinas, St. Thomas (1225?–1274) The patron saint of MNEMONICS, this Italian scholastic philosopher was instrumental in making the trained memory a devotional and ethical art. During the Middle Ages, monks and philosophers were the only people who used trained-memory techniques, which were basic to some religions as a way to reach heaven and avoid hell.

Aquinas was truly talented at the art. As a boy, he could remember word for word everything his priests taught him, and as a young man he confounded Pope Urban by compiling a compendium of writing by church fathers from memory.

Today the memory system he used has been lost, but his belief in the value of images has survived.

Most people in the Middle Ages believed that images and everything else connected with the senses, the body and the natural world were dangerous and evil. But St. Thomas stood alone in praising the senses, explaining that people needed imagery to solidify their memories and discharge their ethical duty of keeping alive the memory of heaven, hell and church teachings. In fact, not only did he permit images—he advised his flock to cultivate them.

Aristotle (384 B.C.–321 B.C.) Author of a lost book on MNEMOTECHNICS, this Greek scientist and philosopher believed that thinking takes place in the head, but memory resides in the heart. Although his teacher, Plato, believed that the mind was separate from the body, Aristotle was convinced that both thought and memory resided somewhere within the body. In fact, he was echoing a Chinese belief already thousands of years old at that point—the Chinese ideograph for "remember" and "memory" are the same as "heart."

The key to his belief lay in the fact that he did not feel it was possible to think without mental images. He advocated the construction of complex "memory palaces" as a way of remembering everything that had to be learned by heart. Aristotle is credited with formulating the idea of association—that if one imagines a house and associates a piece of information with a part of that house, one can start in any room and move in either direction, effortlessly calling up more and more information.

Aristotle believed that imagination and memory occupy the same place in the mind, and their strength to hold on to sense impressions is very important—because he believed that the only way we learn is through the senses. He taught that memory could be divided into two parts. One type, common to all animals, he called memory, and a second, superior action peculiar to humans he called recall or reminiscence. This "reminiscence" involved a sense of time, deliberation and the relationship of a chain of experiences to a present experience.

Aristotle went on to explain the mechanics of memory, coming up with four kinds of association he thought would stimulate memory: things near each other (such as sky and horizon), things that happen at the same time (birth and pain), things that are similar (snow and water skis) and things in contrast (young and old).

He drilled his students in the art of memory for one primary reason: to win debates. He knew that linked images will come to mind automatically in a forceful progression as an argument progresses. Therefore, he taught his students to create memory palaces and people the rooms of these imaginary edifices with all the thoughts and information they needed to memorize.

Aristotle also had a theory about memory problems. He believed that a person who is in a state of rapid transition cannot store memories. "It is like a seal stamped on running water," he asserted, noting that this was the basis for memory problems in the very young and the very old: The first are growing, and the latter are decaying.

artificial memory   The synthesis and training of innate memory powers first developed in the Greek and Roman empires in order to run their large bureaucracies in the absence of paper or books. While the empires depended on "white-collar" workers, there was little way for the officials to keep records. Everything had to be memorized, and the bureaucrats needed a disciplined, well-trained and practiced memory.

Because a well-trained memory was such an integral part of the Roman culture, memory training was included as a standard part of education. The Romans called this memory training artificial memory and distinguished it from the inborn "natural memory" with which we remember normally. While the Romans sometimes used their artificial memory to dazzle their friends, its primary requirement was to preserve their own work—for use by lawyers, politicians and preachers. The ancients believed that artificial memory was a way to link themselves with whatever they had to remember.

The standard text on artificial memory was the Roman *AD HERENNIUM*, a book for rhetoric students written about 80 B.C. Rhetoric students learned effective means of communicating, especially effective public speaking. Since paper was scarce, rhetoric students had to learn how to memorize their speeches without referring to notes. The *Ad Herennium* provided the answer, outlining an amazing system of remembering facts by arranging them into scenes in a place that had been committed to memory.

This principle, called the method of loci, became an established part of ancient education and philosophy. (Indeed, the English word *topic* comes from the Greek *topoi*, for "place.") In the Greek and Roman systems, a "topic" was a place in the space where a memory image appeared.

As Rome's importance faded, along with the need for a well-trained memory, so did interest in artificial memory. Artificial memory was reborn during the Middle Ages, when religious leaders revived it as a way to form a personal bond between one's mind and religion. They did this by coming up with personally meaningful images of doctrine and then walking among those images, providing a means of private and intense devotion.

In 1491 the Italian author PETER OF RAVENNA published a book on how to improve memory *(The Phoenix)*, which became wildly popular—yet artificial memory was nowhere as popular as it had been. The availability of paper ended the necessity for extensive use of artificial memory.

The most radical opponents of artificial memory were the Puritans, who preferred impersonal rote memorization over the personal excitement of artificial memory. In the late 1500s and early 1600s, rising scientists such as Galileo, Descartes and Kepler understood the excitement of learning but rejected the vivid imagery, personal meaning and arbitrary order of artificial memory. The revolt was so powerful and so complete that the practice of artificial memory faded forever from the world.

Today we think of memorization exclusively as rote and we praise the ideal of scientific reasoning, forgetting completely that there had ever been any other way to understand memory and thought.

assessment of memory disorders   The assessment, study and treatment of memory disorders is part of neuropsychology, the subdiscipline of psychology concerned with the relationship between brain damage and psychological processes.

The first step in assessing a patient with a memory disorder is to determine whether the disorder is organic or psychogenic by studying the patient's medical record. Disorders caused by brain dysfunction are called organic, and those with no apparent physical cause are called functional or psychogenic. While determining the origin of a memory problem may seem simple, the reason is not always clearcut; sometimes psychogenic factors may overlay an organic impairment. At other times a psychogenic disorder may be complicated by a disorder such as epilepsy.

Second, it is important to determine how extensive the deficit is. While there exist many tests and procedures for evaluating a patient's memory deficit, certain basic tests should be done first. All patients should receive a preliminary screening for memory impairment using the WECHSLER MEMORY SCALE (WMS), developed by David Wechsler in 1945. The WMS is the most widely used clinical memory test today, although its value has been questioned because all but one of its subtests involve verbal memory. Because of this bias, the test may overestimate memory disorders in patients whose deficits are primarily verbal or underestimate memory impairment in those who have problems with nonverbal information.

Next, the RIVERMEAD BEHAVIORAL MEMORY TEST should be administered to obtain a more general impression of the patient's problems. Results of the WMS and the Rivermead test can give a qualitative indication of the patient's memory disorder and can then be backed up with more detailed tests aimed at specific memory functions.

These might include the Williams Scale for the Measurement of Memory (1968), which places more emphasis on nonverbal memory and past personal events. A more recent battery devised to detect minor deficits in the retention of verbal and visual information is the Recognition Memory Test (1985). It is especially useful in pinpointing right- or left-hemisphere damage.

Other memory tests could include the WISCONSIN CARD SORTING TEST, one of the most common ways to assess frontal lobe brain damage. The subject is given a deck of cards marked by a pattern with various symbol shapes, numbers and colors and asked to sort them by a particular order, such as placing all the cards with red squares in one pile. After ten correct tries, the subject must devise a new way to sort the cards. Patients with frontal lobe damage or

KORSAKOFF'S SYNDROME tend to make a perseveration error when asked to change sorting styles and continue to sort the cards by the first rule. Patients with MEDIAL TEMPORAL LOBE damage usually do not exhibit the perseveration error on this test.

Questionnaires also may be useful in evaluating the impact of the disorder on patients and their families. (See also MEMORY, DISORDERS OF; ORGANIC AMNESIA; PSYCHOGENIC AMNESIA.)

association The connection of one item to be remembered with others a person already knows. For example, the easiest way to tell the difference between *stationery* and *stationary* is that you use stationery to write a letter; to remember how to spell *believe*, never believe a lie. Association can be used consciously to remember information; but it also can occur unconsciously. The experience of hearing or seeing something that reminds one of something else occurs because such sounds or sights somehow were linked together in the past, so that remembering one bit of information automatically drew the other bit of information with it.

association, theories of A psychological theory that states that when any past event or experience is recalled, the act of recollection tends to bring forth other events and experiences related to this event in one or more specified ways. This general theory has been expanded to include almost everything that could happen in mental life (except for feeling an original sensation).

While the first theory of association generally is attributed to ARISTOTLE, who had proposed that there were three forms of association (similarity, contrast and contiguity), the philosophy of ASSOCIATIONISM is normally considered to be a British doctrine.

The association of ideas was first developed by John Locke in *An Essay Concerning Human Understanding* (1690), and David Hume expanded on these theories in *A Treatise of Human Nature* in 1739. Others who held various views of association included David Hartley in the 18th century and James and John Stuart Mill, Alexander Bain and Herbert Spencer in the 19th century.

In general, however, association says that knowledge is acquired through one or more of the senses, and by repetitions throughout life the original sensory data are interconnected and can be revived or reinstated as representative images or ideas.

But in 1890 the American philosopher William James suggested in *The Principles of Psychology* that the association of ideas should be replaced by an association of central nervous processes set up by overlapping (or successive) stimuli.

Thirteen years later Russian physiologist Ivan Pavlov studied what had been called association, eventually arriving at a complete description of all behavior, which he believed was derived from original and conditioned reflexes. For the next decades, various schools of thought debated the varieties of association; the Gestalt psychologists called for a total rejection of associationism as far as higher mental processes were concerned. Today very few psychologists support these theories completely, although most agree that association is an important and effective principle that affects all instances of learning through accumulated experience. (See also LOCKE, JOHN; PAVLOV, IVAN PETROVICH.)

associationism   The concept that very complex ideas can be built up from extremely simple ones. This philosophy was propounded by the 19th-century English philosopher John Locke, who was deeply interested in the study of memory and its laws.

association word lists   A type of common mnemonic device similar to the loci system of Simonides, in which a list of associated words are first memorized; information to be memorized is then linked to this already learned list. (See MNEMONIC STRATEGIES.)

Here is a typical association list, showing how one word is associated with the next

green light
car
garage
house
shag rug
lamp
chair

bed
pillow
goose feather
chicken

Associations between these words are established next; the power of this method depends on the cleverness of the associations between consecutive words.

For this list, the "green light" is a good way to begin, since "green light" means go. The green light means a car can go; cars use a garage; a garage is attached to a house; a house is carpeted in shag rugs; a rug is under a lamp; a lamp is beside the chair; the chair is beside the bed; and so on.

It's a good idea to try to make every fifth or tenth word stand out, so that the items to be remembered in sequence can be kept track of. In addition, both the base word list and the information to be remembered by association must be translated into striking visual images.

attention and memory   *Noticing,* or paying attention, is the first fully conscious step in the formation of a memory. It involves deciding which stimuli are worth remembering and which can be discarded and forgotten.

While some 19th-century psychologists, such as William James, focused on attention and the mind, others—such as Russian physiologist Ivan Pavlov—concentrated on attention and behavior. In his well-known experiments on dogs and bells, he noted the signs of attention in dogs and the role attention plays in the activation of conditioned reflexes in the animals.

Today researchers and psychologists consider attention against a background of unfocused awareness that can be focused if necessary. For example, while a person learns how to crochet she must devote all of her attention to the project; once the skill has been mastered, she can carry on conversations or watch TV, attending to her crocheting only if a problem occurs. This suggests that once learned, a skill is carried out in a state of unfocused awareness.

Usually the only way to tell if someone is paying attention is by studying the brain. If a person is given a signal that indicates a second signal will be coming, the electroencephalogram (EEG) shows a slow change in the negative charge of the brain's cortex. This is called the contingent negative variation (CNV) and is considered to be the clearest physical sign of attention.

With the development of computers, scientists have tried to compare attention and the way computers handle information. Called information theory, this approach focuses on the brain systems that may organize the flood of incoming data, allowing it to be attended to. These highly complex mechanisms, which appear to be located at different spots in the brain, must deal with a wide variety of information using different criteria of selection. In addition, attention also appears to be under at least partial voluntary control. (See also JAMES, WILLIAM; PAVLOV, IVAN PETROVICH.)

The most important thing to remember about attention is its fragility. For example, the attention span of the average audience is just 20 minutes, which is why public speakers are urged to convey the essential part of their message immediately. Once past an audience's maximum attention span, the good public speaker will resort to other ways to maintain attention—pauses, differences in tone or speed of delivery, good examples, anecdotes, humor or activity.

Attention can be measured in two ways—how well we avoid distraction and how well we can sustain concentration over a period of time. While humans are usually good at directing their attention to one source, there is evidence that information that is not attended to is still being analyzed to a considerable degree. In the "cocktail party effect," for example, a person who is concentrating on one conversation at a party will nonetheless likely notice if a nearby conversation suddenly switches to the same topic.

It is possible for humans to do more than one thing at a time—we can eat dinner and watch television, or talk and drive a car. It appears that as long as the tasks do not depend on the same mental processes, both can be handled at the same time. But if two tasks depend on the same type of mental process (such as listening to a story and reading a book), neither task can be accomplished very well.

The capacity for any one individual to pay attention to more than one stimulus at the same time varies from person to person and can be affected by alertness, age and motivation. In addition, certain brain lesions can cause severe impairments in the attentional mechanism.

There are also a number of situations in which it is difficult to sustain attention—when a person's attention is most vulnerable: when one is distracted, interrupted, tired, rushed or under stress; when one feels strong emotions, doesn't understand the material or is absorbed in an activity. People also have trouble paying attention if they are under the influence of drugs or alcohol, in familiar surroundings or doing something while on "automatic pilot."

Still, even if people are paying attention, it doesn't mean that they are going to be able to recall everything they are listening to on demand. Attention is required in order to record information, but people also must store that data along with cues for later recall, because recall is the most difficult of the three memory processes.

auditory memory The memory for sound. This type of sense memory is particularly strong among great musicians; the great conductor Arturo Toscanini, for example, could remember a score after hearing it one or two times and could write it out from memory 40 years later.

Augustine, St. (354–430) The bishop of Hippo in Roman Africa from 396 to 430 and the dominant personality in the Catholic church at the time. Recognized as the greatest thinker of Christian antiquity, Augustine pondered deeply on the problem of memory and the soul.

In the famous *Confessions*, which he wrote when he was middle-aged, Augustine told the story of his own restless youth and his eventual journey to the Catholic church. He appeared to be aware at some level of the art of ARTIFICIAL MEMORY, describing in a meditation on memory a series of spacious palaces stored in the "vast court" of memory. As a Christian, Augustine sought God in memory, believing that knowledge of the divine is naturally present there.

In *Confessions,* he summarized the paradox of memory when he wrote:

> When, therefore, the memory loses something—and this is what happens when we forget something and try to remember it—where are we to look for it except in the memory itself? And if the memory offers something else instead, as may happen, we reject what this offers until the one thing we want is presented. When it is presented to us we say "this is it," but we could not say this unless we recognized it and we could not recognize it unless we remembered it.

autistic savants   Individuals who lack normal intelligence but who possess one outstanding mental ability, such as a so-called photographic memory or the ability to do complex mathematical calculations in their heads. Autistic savants were formerly called idiot savants (meaning "wise idiot"), a term invented in 1887 by J. Langdon Down, a pioneer in the study of mental retardation. Autistic savants are usually incapable of activities of daily living other than their one ability and are often unable to reason or to comprehend meaning.

The savant syndrome is six times more likely to appear in males than females. Although it is considered rare, almost 10 percent of children diagnosed with autism may exhibit this syndrome.

No matter what their particular talent, all savants share a prodigious memory; their skills may appear in a range of areas, including calendar calculating, music, rapid calculating and mathematics, art or mechanical ability.

One of the more common patterns that can be found among savants is a triad of mental retardation, blindness and musical ability.

In 1988 the movie *Rain Man* won an Academy Award for Best Picture for its portrayal of a prodigious autistic savant; the feats of this savant were based on actual clinical literature.

autobiographical memory   A uniquely human function of early memories that begins at a certain point in childhood. It depends on a child's ability to speak, since it requires linguistic representations of events. The phenomenon of infantile amnesia was first identified by Sigmund Freud, but since Freud's time, scientists have learned that as children grow older they learn to share memories with others and acquire the narrative forms of memory recounting. Such recountings are effective in reinstating experienced memories only after the children can use another's representation of an experience in language as a reinstatement of their own experience. This requires an ability to understand language that appears in the mid- to late preschool years. (See also AMNESIA, CHILDHOOD; FREUD, SIGMUND; MEMORY IN INFANCY.)

automatic gestures   Habitual routines (such as locking your front door) that, because they are performed without any conscious thinking or awareness, may not be recorded in memory and therefore may not be recalled at a later date.

automatic processing   Memory functions are carried out with a minimum amount of conscious attention. While it is often argued that processing activities (such as ENCODING and RETRIEVAL) require different levels of attention, automatic processing tasks are disrupted only slightly by the simultaneous performance of other more demanding tasks regardless of their precise nature—and automatic processing disrupts only minimally the performance of these other tasks. In contrast, EFFORTFUL PROCESSING is disrupted by and disrupts other demanding tasks performed at the same time.

background context   When someone pays attention to episodic or semantic information, that information falls within a spacetime framework known as background context. This context includes not only the precise characteristics of events and facts but also other features of the background in which they occur; for example, colors or the objects present. Background context usually falls on the periphery of attention and may be processed automatically.

barbiturates   A group of sedative drugs that have been found to facilitate the recall of emotionally disturbing memories. Scientists believe that these drugs reduce anxiety so that the patient can tolerate the recollection of experiences that are too painful to recall in the normal conscious state. The most common barbiturates are SODIUM AMYTAL and SODIUM PENTOTHAL.

Bartlett, Sir Frederic C. (1896–1969)   An English psychologist who believed that the brain stores information by using what it already knows and placing a new pattern over a similar old one.

Bartlett's work was a departure from the popular theories and style of psychologist Hermann Ebbinghaus, who tested his own ability to memorize nonsense syllables. This memorization could be called rote learning, but modern researchers understand that what Ebbinghaus was really studying was rote learning without arousal—in other words, factual memory for events that have no emotional importance. And because rote learning without arousal is a poor way to construct memory, it is not surprising that Ebbinghaus and his colleagues concluded that memory doesn't work very well or endure for a very long time.

While Bartlett developed his technique as a way of sidestepping problems in memory study, it limited his ability to understand memory. He believed that memory was simply a storage bin for objective items that were either retained or not—a point of view that eventually was challenged by psychologists who believed that subjective factors also are vital to memory systems.

Bartlett did not believe that only objective factors should be studied; his work during the 1930s was designed to test the way people usually use their memories. As he described in his book *Remembering: A Study in Experimental and Social Psychology* (1967), Bartlett believed that remembering is active; it is not the reactivation of memory traces that have been filed away but an imaginative reconstruction built out of the relationship of the attitude toward a mass of organized past reactions and to little details. Therefore, he noted, memory is hardly ever exact, and he agreed with Sigmund Freud that personal view greatly affects memory.

In one of his most famous studies, he told an American Indian war story filled with unusual details; when it was over, subjects were asked to repeat the story after 15 minutes and then after four and six months. As time passed, the story grew shorter and shorter, and its Indian point of view disappeared. What Bartlett's study revealed was that memory alters information, omitting and distorting facts depending on personal prejudices and turning a puzzling but emotionally rich story into something that is dull but understandable.

Bartlett believed that what was going on was the operation of something he called a schema—an underlying subjective organizing principle. A person's memory of the Indian tale changed over time to conform with that person's underlying personal schema.

In *Remembering:* Bartlett explained that memory was based on the general impression that results from combining recalled details with the overall sense an individual forms of what has occurred. That overall sense, in turn, is affected by a person's general knowledge and the expectations that result from that knowledge. (See also EBBINGHAUS, HERMANN E.)

basal ganglia   The group of large paired nerve cell clusters buried deep in the forebrain and including the CAUDATE NUCLEUS, putamen and globus pallidus. These nerve cells lie above the brain stem and under the cerebrum.

The basal ganglia play an important role in control of movement and may help mediate the development of skills and habits. Diseases or degeneration of the basal ganglia and their connections may lead to the appearance of involuntary movements, trembling and weakness such as those found in PARKINSON'S DISEASE. (See also BRAIN DAMAGE; CARBON MONOXIDE POISONING; HUNTINGTON'S DISEASE.)

behavioral treatments of memory disorders
Techniques to improve memory that include chaining (breaking up a task into smaller units taught one at a time), flooding or modeling. Behavioral treatments of memory problems work well because they are adaptable to a wide range of patients, the goals are small and specific and treatment can be tested continually and easily.

The theoretical approaches underlying behavioral therapy draw upon a number of fields within psychology. While behavioral treatments have been used in rehabilitation for years, only recently have they been tried to ease acquired cognitive impairments.

A behavior program for patients with memory problems should specify the behavior to be changed, state the goals of treatment, measure deficit to obtain a baseline, plan/begin treatment, monitor progress and change the procedure if needed.

Bender-Gestalt test   One of the most widely used components of the typical psychological examination of adults and children. Dr. Lauretta Bender developed the test in 1938 to help tell the difference between ENDOGENOUS BRAIN DAMAGE and EXOGENOUS BRAIN DAMAGE.

The test requires subjects to copy nine geometric figures. There are several scoring systems for children and adults; the results provide an estimate of the person's ability to draw what they see. The test also provides a way of gauging the ability to transfer an image from SENSORY MEMORY to SHORT-TERM MEMORY.

benzodiazepines   A class of psychoactive drugs which includes diazepam (Valium) and lorazepam (Ativan) that can be used to promote sleep or reduce anxiety—but that also can impair memory and other aspects of mental function. For example, when Ativan is taken at night for sleep, patients experience a small memory impairment the next morning.

Under certain circumstances, benzodiazepines can induce a temporary amnesic state with a marked ANTEROGRADE AMNESIA. But since neither Valium nor Ativan has any effect on the recall of information presented shortly before giving the drug, researchers believe that memory impairment following the drug administration is caused by some aspect of acquisition.

The ability of the benzodiazepines to induce this type of amnesia can be used to the patient's advantage in a medical setting; some dentists use intravenous Valium for their patients who fear dental surgery, for example. Not only does the drug reduce anxiety, but patients have difficulty recalling the surgery itself, which is helpful if they need to face further surgery at a later date.

besipirdine   An acetylcholine-boosting drug currently being studied as a possible treatment for ALZHEIMER'S DISEASE. The drug mimics acetylcholine, a chemical necessary for brain cell communication, which is severely depleted in Alzheimer's.

beta-amyloid protein   A normally harmless protein found in the brain that, in ALZHEIMER'S DISEASE, is triggered by an unknown stimulus to fold and twist into a different shape. As it changes, the protein begins forming abnormal strands that build up on brain cells, forming plaques and killing them.

These plaques appear to be made, in part, from protein molecules called AMYLOID PRECURSOR PROTEIN (APP)—that normally are essential components of the brain. Plaques occur when an enzyme snips APP apart at a specific place and then leaves the fragments (beta-amyloid) in brain tissue, where they come together in abnormal plaque deposits.

It appears that beta-amyloid also induces another harmless brain protein, tau, to become a killer as well. (See TAU PROTEIN.) Together, the two destroy the brain cells of people with Alzheimer's, forming the plaques and tangles that have been the hallmarks of the disease since it was first described in 1907 by Alois Alzheimer. Scientists disagree about whether it's the sticky plaques of beta-amyloid in the brain or the tangles of tau protein inside brain nerve fibers that play a more central role in the destruction of brain cells. Most Alzheimer's researchers have focused attention on amyloid as the substance that kills brain cells. They believe excessive amounts of beta-amyloid are toxic to neurons in the same way that too much cholesterol is toxic to the cells in blood vessel walls.

What is known is that increases of beta-amyloid in brain tissue are associated with increasing severity of mental decline, with the highest levels of beta-amyloid found in the brains of patients with the greatest degree of dementia. See also DEMENTIA; PRESENILINS.

Binet, Alfred (1857–1911) This noted French psychologist and co-developer of the Binet-Simon standardized intelligence test that bears his name also was interested in children's memory. It was Binet who suggested that children remember the basic idea or the underlying message of long passages. The popularity of the behavioral viewpoint during the first part of the 20th century diminished the impact of Binet's work.

Binswanger's disease An extremely rare form of dementia characterized by lesions in the white matter deep inside the brain, resulting in loss of memory, thinking and learning. The disease is a slowly progressive condition for which there is no cure, often marked by strokes and partial recovery. Patients with this disorder usually die within five years after its onset.

Symptoms
In addition to memory and learning problems, patients usually show signs of abnormal blood pressure, stroke, blood problems, mood disorders, disease of the large blood vessels in the neck and disease of the heart valves. Other prominent features of the disease include urinary incontinence, difficulty walking, Parkinson-like tremors and depression. These symptoms, which tend to begin after the age of 60, are not always present in all patients and may sometimes appear only as a passing phase. Seizures may also be present.

Treatment
There is no specific treatment for Binswanger's disease. Medications can be used to control high blood pressure, depression, abnormal heart rhythms and low blood pressure.

biofeedback A technique in which a person uses information about a normally unconscious body function such as blood pressure, to gain conscious control over that function. Biofeedback may help in the treatment of stress-related conditions such as hypertension or migraine.

The subject is connected to a recording instrument that can measure one of the unconscious body activities—blood pressure, pulse rate, body temperature, muscle tensions, sweat on the skin, brain waves or stomach acidity. The subject receives the information (feedback) on the changing levels of the body activities from alterations in the instrument's signals (flashing lights, fluctuating needle, changing sounds).

With practice, the person starts to become aware of how he or she is feeling whenever there is a change in the recording instrument's signal. Relaxation techniques also may be used to bring about a change in the signal; the instrument's response may indicate which methods of relaxation work best.

Eventually the subject learns to change the signal by consciously controlling the body function being tested. Once learned, control can be exerted without the equipment.

Many at-home versions of biofeedback machines are now available, including a home blood pressure monitoring kit for measuring blood pressure with the fingertip.

blackouts, alcoholic   Blackouts are a common phenomenon among alcoholics and normal drinkers who overindulge, involving a loss of memory during the drunken state. During a blackout, the individual is not unconscious or incapacitated, and usually possesses most of his or her faculties.

In one form of alcoholic blackout, called en bloc, the person experiences AMNESIA that has a clear beginning and end; in this form, the patient knows there has been a "lost period." In a second form of blackout, the person is not aware of any amnesia and also may have exhibited memory problems while drinking without any recollection of them.

Experts once believed that blackouts were a form of state-dependent forgetting, that is, a person can remember information learned in a state only when in that state. In other words, a person who commits a crime while drunk would only remember that crime while drunk. However, at least one research study did not support this theory. In a study of five convicted murderers who had committed their crimes while drunk and claimed amnesia for their activities, the murderers were allowed to become drunk. None recalled their crimes while drunk, and when they were sober again all had varying degrees of amnesia for the experiment.

The researchers believe that alcoholic blackouts occur because the original level of alcohol intoxication was enough to disrupt the physiological processes involved in forming memories.

Boston remote memory battery   The most extensive test for RETROGRADE AMNESIA, devised by Marilyn Albert in 1979. Its three components each have "easy" and "hard" questions; the easy questions reflect information that might be answered on the basis of general knowledge, while the hard questions reflect information whose recollection relies much more on remembering a particular time period.

Unfortunately, the test is considered to be culture-specific and cannot be used with patients outside the United States. (See also ASSESSMENT OF MEMORY DISORDERS.)

brain abscess   A collection of pus inside inflamed brain tissue that is almost always caused by the spread of infection elsewhere in the body; about 40 percent of abscesses are caused by middle ear or sinus infections. Among other symptoms, brain abscesses can cause memory problems due to raised pressure and local damage to nerve tracts. The most common sites of brain abscesses are the FRONTAL and TEMPORAL LOBES of the cerebrum. Other causes of brain abscess include infection following a penetrating brain injury and multiple abscesses from blood-borne infections, such as endocarditis and some immunodeficiency disorders.

Besides memory problems, the most common symptoms are headache, drowsiness and vomiting, together with vision problems, fever, epileptic seizures and symptoms caused by local brain damage (partial paralysis and speech problems).

A brain scan (computerized tomography or magnetic resonance imaging) may suggest a diagnosis. Abscesses are treated with high doses of intravenous antibiotics, but because antibiotics alone may not cure an abscess, surgery may be required. After the operation, antibiotics are usually given for one or two months.

In the surgery, a section of the skull is opened to provide access to the abscess and to facilitate drainage. If the abscess has penetrated any area of the skull, some of the affected bone may be removed. Locating and removing all traces of infection is sometimes difficult, and recovery may be complicated by reinfection.

Brain abscesses are fatal in about 10 percent of cases, and surviving patients often suffer some residual brain dysfunction. Because many patients experience epilepsy after brain abscesses, anticonvulsant drugs are often administered after removal or drainage of the abscess.

Brain abscesses are relatively rare today because the widespread use of antibiotics controls many infections in the early stages.

brain damage Degeneration or death of nerve cells and tracts within the brain, which may be localized in particular areas (causing specific defects) or more diffuse, causing mental problems or severe physical handicap. Memory is very sensitive to brain damage, since it is dependent on such a wide range of interacting processes; even limited brain damage may affect some of these processes. Many brain structures seem to be involved in the process of memory, including the HIPPOCAMPUS, hypothalamus, THALAMUS and TEMPORAL LOBE. Damage to any of them can cause memory problems.

Most people with organic amnesia will have experienced one of the following: HEAD INJURY, cerebral vascular accident, progressive DEMENTIA, BRAIN TUMOR, toxic disorder, brain surgery or nutritional disorder. (See CEREBROVASCULAR ACCIDENT [CVA].)

Memory deficits may be a lifelong handicap for brain-damaged patients and their families. Such patients are liable to a greater risk of personal danger (by forgetting a lighted cigarette or a pot on the stove), increased annoyance from others by repeatedly failing to remember and social isolation.

Localized Brain Damage This form of brain damage can occur as a result of a head injury (especially those that penetrate the skull) or from a STROKE, brain tumor or BRAIN ABSCESS. It also may be caused by damage to the brain at birth from jaundice (excess bilirubin levels). The BASAL GANGLIA also may be damaged by CARBON MONOXIDE POISONING.

Diffuse Brain Damage This more severe type of brain damage may result from hypoxia (lack of oxygen in the brain) that may occur during birth; from cardiac or respiratory arrest; or from poisoning, drowning, electric shock or prolonged convulsions. It also may be caused by the accumulation of toxic substances in the brain, as occurs in phenylketonuria or galactosemia, or of environmental poisons (such as lead or mercury). Other possible causes include brain infections (such as encephalitis) or, rarely, a reaction after immunization. In addition, there is some evidence that the tips and undersurface of the temporal lobes may be more susceptible to traumatic damage than other parts of the brain; if so, then memory problems following diffuse brain damage may in fact indicate hippocampal damage. Encephalitic patients, too, may suffer extensive temporal lobe lesions (although the virus does not always attack this area).

Patients who have suffered head injury or stroke are likely to experience memory problems in addition to other symptoms. Unlike nerves in the limbs or trunk, nerve cells and tracts in the brain and spinal cord do not recover their function if they have been destroyed. However, patients may improve somewhat after brain damage as they learn to use other parts of the brain to compensate for the loss.

The ability to store and recall memories following brain injury may be affected in quite different ways from one patient to the next. This is because there is not just one kind of memory, but many—verbal and nonverbal memory, visual and auditory memory, short-term and long-term memory, episodic and semantic memory. Moreover, even in the same patient, some memory functions may work fine while others show more disruption.

There are three main ways to improve memory performance for brain-damaged patients—physical treatment (such as medication) and internal and external aids.

Internal aids include mnemonics, rehearsal strategies or anything a patient does mentally to the information to be remembered. External aids include diaries, notebooks and calendars, alarm clocks, gadgets and computers. Environmental aids also may be used to help mold behavior in patients with severe memory problems, for example, lines may be painted on the ground to help them find their way around. One hospital geriatric unit reduced its incontinency problem among patients by painting all the lavatory doors a different color from other doors.

The effectiveness of external aids is related to the attitude toward their use; in some cases patients need counseling before they will accept the aids. One of the most effective aids is the combination of a digital alarm watch and a notebook with the day's activities; whenever the alarm goes off, the patient consults the notebook.

The ability of a brain-damaged patient to recover memory depends on the cause and site of the damage, the individual's personality and how motivated he or she is to recover. Indeed, researchers agree there is little evidence that practice by itself will significantly improve a brain-damaged person's memory. (See also MEMORY FOR FACES; VISUAL IMAGERY METHOD.)

brain scans   A group of specialized tests that chart brain function using a variety of chemical, electrical or magnetic technologies ranging from positron emission tomography (PET) to SQUID (superconducting quantum interference devices). Each type of brain scan has its pros and cons; some are so precise they can distinguish structures as small as a millimeter but are so slow they can't differentiate between neurons. Others can track brain function but can't resolve structures less than half an inch apart.

The computerized scanning equipment introduced over the past 15 years has revolutionized diagnostic neurology. The two most commonly used scans are computerized tomographic (CT) scanning (see COMPUTERIZED [CT] SCAN) and MAGNETIC RESONANCE IMAGING (MRI), also known as NMR or nuclear magnetic resonance.

While the computerized scanning techniques of CT and MRI are similar and noninvasive, they rely on two distinct methods of producing an image. CT scans use an ultra-thin X-ray beam; MRI uses a very strong magnetic field. During CT scans, an X-ray beam passes through the body; various tissues absorb different amounts of the beam, and the intensity of the beam that emerges from the body is measured by an X-ray detector. On the scan, tissues appear as various shades of gray; bone—appearing white—is at one end of this spectrum, and air is at the opposite end (appearing black).

During an MRI scan, each hydrogen atom in the body responds to the magnetic field produced by the device; a magnetic field detector measures the responses of the atom. The degree of response depends on the type of tissue or its water content. There is no radiation in an MRI scan, but the magnetic field may affect heart pacemakers, inner ear implants, brain aneurysm clips or embedded shrapnel.

Both CT and MRI scans are done by taking detector measurements from thousands of angles all over the body while the patient lies on a special table; these data are then processed by computer to create a composite three-dimensional representation of the body. Any particular slice can be selected from this representation and displayed on a TV screen for examination, and still photos also can be produced.

CT scans show internal structures much better than conventional X rays. They are particularly useful for brain disorders such as strokes, hemorrhages, injuries, tumors, abscesses, cysts, swelling, fluid accumulation and dead tissue.

MRI scans are especially useful for imaging areas where soft and hard tissue meet and areas affected by stroke that can't be seen well on a CT scan. They also are used to diagnose nerve fiber disorders (such as multiple sclerosis).

Other brain scan technology includes ELECTROENCEPHALOGRAM (EEGs) and SPECT (single-photon emission computerized tomography).

brain surgery and memory   Operations on one TEMPORAL LOBE (when there has been unsuspected damage in the other lobe) can cause a severe and persistent general memory defect very similar to postencephalitic amnesia. This memory loss is especially pervasive for SHORT-TERM MEMORY and in learning with a RETROGRADE AMNESIA involving at least the past several years of a patient's life before surgery.

It's also possible, during open brain surgery, to stimulate the temporal lobes with an electrode and produce hallucinogeniclike memories. This was first discovered in the 1950s by Canadian neurosurgeon Wilder Penfield, whose patients reported meaningful, integrated experiences including sound, movement and color while Penfield held the electrode in certain parts of their brain. Sometimes his patients did not recall the memories after the operation; often the memories were far more detailed, specific and accurate than normal recall. Stimulating one particular part of the brain brought back the memory of a mother calling her child or a certain song. Stimulating the same point brought back the same memory every time. (See also AMNESIA; ANESTHESIA AND MEMORY; ENCEPHALITIS AND MEMORY; MEDIAL TEMPORAL LOBE; PENFIELD, WILDER.)

brain tissue transplants   Initial research with rats has suggested the possibility of restoring some types of memory using fetal brain tissue transplants. However, the moral and philosophical issues surrounding their use in humans presents many problems. Moreover, the fact that successful transplants depend on the availability of fetal brain tissue adds to the ethical and legal dilemma.

One of the greatest problems in treating BRAIN DAMAGE is the fact that the brain cannot regenerate very well. And when particular areas of the brain are damaged, other regions do not always take over the function of the disabled sections.

Scientists destroyed connections in the septo-hippocampal region of young rats who had already learned several mazes. Following the damage, the rats' performance was impaired. After being given grafts of septo-hippocampal tissue taken from rat fetuses, the rats went on to show improvement in their maze-learning tasks. This suggests that the grafts had become effective parts of the animals' memory system. Other studies showed that the neutral tissue taken from the same region in rat fetuses could improve the age-related learning impairments in rats.

Scientists are already transplanting fetal brain cells into the brains of Parkinson's disease patients, hoping that the new cells will begin to churn out dopamine, a key brain chemical that is deficient in the disease. Early results have been encouraging, and some patients have shown some improvement, although not total health.

Someday soon scientists hope they will be able to tackle some of the most intractable diseases of the brain, including ALZHEIMER'S DISEASE, that short-circuit brain cells and destroy memory and personality—and with it, the essence that makes us human.

Genetically altered cells, and genes themselves, can be injected into the brain to combat or reverse damage caused by degenerative diseases. The new approaches rely on the same basic strategy: using living tissue instead of drugs to supply chemicals crucial to brain function. Scientists at Brown University, for example, are developing a way to encapsulate small clumps of cells that produce desired chemicals, letting out the substances through holes in the plastic capsule that are too small to let anti-

bodies in. In that way, the body's immune systems can't reject the cells when the capsule is implanted. The technique has been used to reverse memory impairment and Parkinson-like damage in rats.

In other studies, Harvard scientists have put new genes in rat brains by linking the new DNA to a weakened herpes virus; the virus splices in the new genes when it infects neurons. While scientists aren't sure whether the genes can be "turned on" to work effectively, the number of potential uses could be limitless.

brain tumor   An abnormal growth that destroys brain tissue and puts pressure on neighboring brain structures. Tumors causing particular memory problems are often found on the floor of the third ventricle, adjacent to diencephalic structures; tumors in this area produce amnesia resembling KORSAKOFF'S SYNDROME. In fact, in a study of 180 cerebral tumors, more than half the patients with marked memory impairment had tumors involving the third ventricle.

Patients suffering from a wide variety of tumors are likely to exhibit memory deficits. For example, frontal lobe tumor patients have memory problems comparable to patients with Korsakoff's syndrome and other diencephalic amnesias. Patients with corpus callosum tumors also are likely to show a severe memory impairment, which rapidly progresses to general intellectual deficits. This type of general impairment is often seen in patients with temporal lobe tumors, but parietal tumors are less likely to result in memory problems. Occipital tumors, however, can lead to memory problems.

Tumors of the parietal lobe of the cerebral hemispheres also frequently cause AGNOSIA (loss of the ability to recognize objects or people), while tumors of the parietal lobe of the dominant cerebral hemisphere can cause AGRAPHIA (loss of ability to write, a form of aphasia).

Fifty-seven percent of patients with temporal lobe lesions exhibit memory problems; 50 percent of patients with frontal lobe lesions, 45 percent of patients with occipital lobe lesions and 25 percent of patients with parietal lobe lesions do so.

Tumors of the posterior fossa (that is, the cerebellum, cerebellopontine angle and brain stem) are less likely to cause cognitive deficits than tumors just described, unless the increase in intracranial pressure causes hydrocephalus.

Estimates suggest that 15 percent of all patients suffering from brain tumors were initially diagnosed with dementia, which gradually interfered with writing, reading and calculations. In fact, frontal lobe tumors are the most likely to be confused with dementia, especially when both lobes are involved and the tumor develops in the midline. In addition, slow-growing tumors often mimic the symptoms of Alzheimer's disease, but a cancer spreading from another area of the body (such as the lung or breast) may cause memory impairment as well.

In the United States, about six new cases of primary brain tumor per 100,000 are diagnosed each year, occurring most often around the age of 50.

Symptoms

In addition to memory problems, compression of brain tissue or nerve tracts near the tumor may cause muscle weakness, vision loss, sensory disturbances, speech problems and epileptic seizures. An expanding tumor can raise pressure inside the skull, causing headaches, vomiting, visual disturbances and impaired mental function.

Diagnosis

Common diagnostic tests for brain tumors may include a myelogram, angiogram (or arteriogram), pneumoencephalogram, brain scans, spinal tap or electroencephalogram (EEG). The most accurate diagnostic procedure, however, is a biopsy of tumor tissue.

Treatment

While any surgical operation carries risk, a skilled surgeon can operate on many parts of the brain without destroying important functions. However, surgery in the temporal lobes is extremely difficult because intellectual functions (memory, speech, ability to comprehend abstractions) can be profoundly reduced by cutting into this center. Other treatments besides surgery include radiation and chemotherapy with anticancer or corticosteroid drugs.

If a tumor is inaccessible or too large to be removed, as much of it as possible is cut away to relieve pressure on the brain, but the outlook in these cases is poor; fewer than 20 percent of such patients survive for one year.

BRAT battery   A nickname for the basic psychological examination group of intelligence test, achievement test and visual-motor integration test given to children with learning and behavioral problems. The designation originally was derived loosely from the names of the typical tests used in the basic group, including the BENDER-GESTALT TEST, WISC (Wechsler Intelligence Scale for Children), and Wide Range Achievement Test (whose acronym WRAT is pronounced "rat").

Breuer, Josef (1842–1925)   An Austrian physician and physiologist who was acknowledged by Sigmund Freud and others as the principal developer of psychoanalysis. In 1880 Breuer was able to relieve the symptoms of hysteria in "Anna O" after he had induced her to recall unpleasant past experiences under HYPNOSIS. Breuer concluded that neurotic symptoms result from unconscious processes and disappear when those processes become conscious.

He later described his methods and results to Freud, and referred patients to him; together the two wrote *Studien uber Hysterie* (1895), in which Breuer described his treatment of hysteria. Breuer and Freud eventually became enemies, however, over disagreements on basic theories of therapy. (See also ANNA O; FREUD, SIGMUND.)

Broca, Paul (1824–1880)   A French surgeon whose study of brain lesions contributed significantly to the understanding of the origins of APHASIA (the loss or impairment of the ability to form or articulate words).

Broca founded the anthropology lab at the École des Hautes Études in Paris in 1858 and the Société d'Anthropologie de Paris in 1859, where he developed his research into the comparative study of the craniums of the races of mankind, studying the form, structure and topography of the brain.

In 1861 he announced his discovery of the seat of articulate speech, located in the left frontal region of the brain, since known as the convolution of Broca. With this discovery, Broca provided the first anatomical proof of the localization of brain function. (See also BROCA'S APHASIA.)

Broca's aphasia   An expressive disorder that affects both written and spoken speech, producing nonfluent, slow, labored and arrhythmic speech. Patients usually retain reasonably good comprehension of some words, such as nouns, and the few words they can utter tend to be meaningful.

Broca's aphasia is caused by a lesion in the left frontal cortex, although a lesion serious enough to produce a permanent disorder probably also affects parts of the BASAL GANGLIA. (See also APHASIA; BROCA, PAUL; WERNICKE'S [RECEPTIVE] APHASIA.)

Brown-Peterson task   This commonly used test of recall over delays of a few seconds features items presented to subjects (usually in threes), after which the subject engages in some interfering activity (such as counting backward) until the end of the retention interval. At that point subjects are asked to recall the items just presented.

Although recall usually declines steeply after a 30-second delay, researchers believe that the interfering task makes recall more difficult but does not completely prevent it. Patients with ALZHEIMER'S DISEASE and some with AMNESIA usually perform badly on this test.

caffeine and memory   While the amount of caffeine in coffee or tea is a mild stimulant and may keep one awake enough to pay attention, it also may make one too jittery to learn, and is just as likely to have a negative effect on memory as a positive one.

Studies have shown that a person who is already wide awake and rested will not find much of a memory boost from caffeine. But too much coffee (and the exact amount varies from person to person) can bring on the jitters, insomnia and memory problems. For a habitual user, however, omitting this stimulant will have the same negative effect.

Effects

Caffeine acts on the brain, affecting coordination, concentration, sleep patterns and behavior. The gastrointestinal tract absorbs almost all the caffeine and distributes it to all tissues and organs within minutes of consumption; maximum blood levels are reached within 45 minutes. While it may improve simple motor tasks, it may disrupt more complex tasks involving fine motor coordination and quick reactions. Of course, any drug's effect depends on the amount consumed, how often, how much the body absorbs and how quickly it is metabolized.

Some research has shown that administering small amounts (two or more cups of regular coffee) did not affect performance when compared with subjects drinking the same amount of decaffeinated coffee. In addition, one study suggests that caffeine may interfere with memory only in women. No information is available about possible memory-enhancement possibilities of non-prescription caffeine-based stimulants.

A separate study of healthy college students found that their ability to remember lists of words they had just heard was diminished following the administration of caffeine. Combining caffeine and alcohol actually slowed the reaction time of eight subjects in one study, making subjects more drunk than the alcohol alone.

In any case, caffeine may be hard to avoid. A staggeringly large number of products in the United States contain caffeine; in addition to food and beverages, caffeine is found in over-the-counter stimulants, analgesics, cold preparations, antihistamines and prescription drugs. In fact, more than 2,000 nonprescription drugs and 1,000 prescription drugs contain caffeine or caffeine-type stimulants.

calcium   The most abundant mineral in the body, this substance has been implicated as both a possible cause of mental decline and as (through its release of CALPAIN) a memory enhancer. Calcium is essential for proper cell function, muscle contraction, nerve impulse transmission and blood clotting.

The drug NIMODIPINE, which blocks excess calcium in the part of the brain associated with memory and learning, has been used successfully to improve memory loss in STROKE victims. In addition, conditions that result in a flood of calcium in the brain lead to memory problems, which some researchers believe is caused by a release of too *much* protein-eating calpain. At the same time, normal levels of calcium release calpain, which seems to improve memory by improving cell-to-cell communication.

The main dietary sources of calcium are milk and dairy products, eggs, fish, green vegetables and fruit. The amount of calcium in the body is controlled by the action of two hormones, parathyroid hormone and calcitonin. When the level of calcium drops, the parathyroid glands release more parathyroid hormone, raising blood calcium levels by helping to release calcium from reservoirs in bones.

calendar calculators   See AUTISTIC SAVANTS.

calpain   One of several brain chemicals called neurotransmitters currently being studied for their role in memory. (See NEUROTRANSMITTERS AND MEMORY.) Released by CALCIUM in the cells, calpain can digest protein and appears to clean up blocked receptors and let neurons communicate more easily with each other. Some researchers suspect that reduced calcium levels in older patients may be one reason that senior citizens so often experience memory loss.

To test this hypothesis, researchers used a calpain blocker called leupeptin to interfere with the level of calpain in rats and then tested the animals' ability to solve an eight-sided maze. In the experiment, a rat is placed in the middle of a maze with eight tunnels; at the end of each is food. Rats quickly learn to run to the end of one tunnel, get the food and move on to the next alley without returning to the chambers where they had already eaten the reward. While the rats appeared to be normal and clearly recognized their surroundings, they had a hard time actually remembering which paths they had visited, especially if they were removed in the middle of the experiment and returned a few moments later. The calpain blocker seemed to be interfering directly with their ability to form memories. But other researchers have disagreed with these findings, since not a great deal is known about leupeptin.

Capgras, Jean Marie Joseph (1873–1950)   A well-known French psychopathologist who first identified the delusional syndrome called reduplicative paramnesia (or CAPGRAS SYNDROME) that today bears his name.

Capgras and J. Reboul-Lachaux first noted the syndrome in 1923 in a female patient with a chronic paranoid psychosis who also insisted that various individuals involved in her life had been replaced by doubles. Capgras and Reboul-Lachaux called the condition *l'illusion des sosies* (the illusion of doubles).

Capgras syndrome   One form of reduplicative paramnesia, this is a delusional condition also called the syndrome of "doubles," in which a patient fails to recognize well-known people or places, believing that doubles have replaced them. The delusion is often quite strong and can be deeply disturbing to family and friends whose identity is constantly denied. Generally, the person accused as an "imposter" also is believed to have harmful intentions toward the patient.

The effect can be induced by showing patients a picture and then, a few minutes later, producing the same picture again. The patients will probably say they have seen a similar picture, but insist it is definitely not the one they are now looking at. This disorder is believed to have a psychological origin, although more recent research suggests there may be an organic cause. It is typically associated with CONFABULATION, speech disorders and denial of illness.

It was first described by Jean Marie Capgras and J. Reboul-Lachaux in 1923, who discussed a female patient with a chronic paranoid psychosis who also insisted that various individuals involved in her life had been replaced by doubles. Capgras and Reboul-Lachaux called the condition *l'illusion des sosies* (the illusion of doubles).

Capgras syndrome is one of a group of MISIDENTIFICATION SYNDROMES that can occur in psychotic patients. It also may occur as a result of brain injury. Although the precise cause of this unusual syndrome is uncertain, it may involve extensive cerebral damage, probably with extensive frontal lesions.

Frontal lesions may cause problems in the integration of different kinds of information, and when these problems are combined with perceptual and memory deficits from other brain lesions, reduplicative paramnesia or Capgras syndrome may result. (See also CAPGRAS, JEAN MARIE JOSEPH.)

carbon monoxide poisoning   Poisoning with carbon monoxide, a tasteless, colorless, odorless gas, can lead to profound cognitive impairment (including memory loss).

Anoxia (lack of oxygen to the brain) causes brain damage, particularly to the BASAL GANGLIA. Common sources of exposure to carbon monoxide include smoke inhalation in fires, automobile exhaust fumes, faulty or poorly ventilated charcoal, kerosene or gas stoves, cigarette smoke and methylene chloride. Several minutes of exposure to 1,000 parts per million (0.1 percent) may cause fatal poisoning.

People exposed to carbon monoxide complain of headache, dizziness and nausea; patients with heart problems may experience angina or myocardial infarction. More severe exposures bring on impaired thinking, coma and convulsions. Survivors may suffer numerous neurological problems, such as Parkinsonism and personality and memory disorders.

LEVELS OF CARBON MONOXIDE POISONING

Carbon Monoxide Concentration	Symptoms
Less than 35 ppm (cigarette smoke)	None, or mild headache
0.005% (50 ppm)	Slight headache
0.01% (100 ppm)	Throbbing headache
0.02% (200 ppm)	Severe headache, irritability, fatigue
0.03%–0.05% (300–500 ppm)	Headache, confusion, lethargy, collapse
0.08%–0.12% (800–1,200 ppm)	Coma, convulsions
0.19% (1,900 ppm)	Rapidly fatal

Treatment includes the administration of oxygen in the highest possible concentration (100 percent); some experts support the use of hyperbaric chambers, which can enhance the elimination of carbon monoxide. Such treatment may be useful to patients exposed to very high levels of carbon monoxide and who are reasonably close to a chamber. (See also CHEMICALS AND MEMORY LOSS.)

CAT scans   See COMPUTERIZED TOMOGRAPHY SCAN.

catharsis   The therapeutic release of ideas through talking about conscious material, accompanied by an appropriate emotional reaction. Catharsis also refers to the release into awareness of repressed material from the unconscious. (See also REPRESSED MEMORIES; REPRESSION.)

caudate nucleus   A part of the BASAL GANGLIA often referred to as the enostriatum. The deterioration of this part of the brain results in HUNTINGTON'S DISEASE.

cell phones and memory   Some studies suggest that the microwaves emanating from cell phones may impair long-term memory. Seattle scientists tested rats trained to remember the location of a platform, and found that rats exposed to microwaves took longer to find the platforms.

Other human studies in England found that people performed worse on tests of word and picture recall, spatial memory and reaction time after exposing their heads to the same amount of microwave energy found in active mobile phones.

Studies on cell phones and health continue. No link to specific brain dysfunction in humans has yet been proven.

centrophenoxine (Lucidril)   A drug that may improve various aspects of memory function. It is believed to remove LIPOFUSCIN deposits, the material of which "age spots" are made. Lipofuscin buildup in heart, skin and brain cells appears with age; decreased deposits have been correlated with improved learning ability.

In some studies centrophenoxine appears to remove these deposits and repair synapses. In the bloodstream, centrophenoxine breaks down into dimethylaminoethanol (DMAE), a naturally occurring nutrient found in seafood that is normally present in the brain in small amounts. DMAE also is believed to enhance brain function.

Scientists have shown that centrophenoxine can protect the brains of animals against lack of oxygen and may be of value in treating diseases in which tissue oxygenation is lowered (such as DEMENTIA or STROKE). While centrophenoxine does not seem effective in the treatment of ALZHEIMER'S DISEASE, it may help in cases where the brain is not getting enough oxygen.

Centrophenoxine should not be used by patients who are easily excitable, hypertensive or subject to convulsions or involuntary musculoskeletal movements.

cerebrovascular accident (CVA)   Sudden rupture or blockage of a blood vessel within the brain (also called stroke) resulting in serious bleeding or local obstruction to blood circulation. Several researchers have reported AMNESIA after a blockage in the posterior cerebral artery (a blood vessel that supplies the HIPPOCAMPUS); less often, CVAs may cause amnesia by damaging the diencephalic structures.

Cause

Blockage may be due to a clot formation (thrombosis) or an embolism, and rupture of different blood vessels may cause different patterns of bleeding.

About 8 percent of cerebral vascular accidents are due to a SUBARACHNOID HEMORRHAGE, which usually affects younger people who are less likely to suffer from widespread cerebral vascular disease. The usual cause of such a hemorrhage is the rupture of a brain aneurysm (ballooning of an artery), which bleeds into the subarachnoid space surrounding the brain.

The anterior communicating artery (located between the frontal lobes) often is associated with ruptured aneurysms. Other common sites are the middle cerebral artery and the posterior communicating artery.

While a hemorrhage sometimes may be caused by a ruptured benign tumor, in about 20 percent of cases no structural cause is known. Shortly after the hemorrhage, symptoms similar to those found in KORSAKOFF'S SYNDROME may occur, including disorientation, CONFABULATION and impaired memory. Memory impairment following a subarachnoid hemorrhage may be temporary or permanent.

Finally, TRANSIENT GLOBAL AMNESIA almost always is due to a cerebral vascular cause, with a sudden onset of symptoms in an otherwise normal patient. The episode may begin with a brief clouding of consciousness, and the amnesia usually lasts for several hours, ending in complete recovery.

cerebropathia psychica toxemica   The original term for KORSAKOFF'S SYNDROME used by Russian psychiatrist Sergey Sergeyevich Korsakoff, who first described it in 1887. (See also KORSAKOFF, SERGEY SERGEYEVICH.)

cerebrum   The largest area of the brain, the cerebrum is arranged in two hemispheres (or halves), called the right and left cerebral hemisphere. It is the part of the brain responsible for higher-order thinking and decision making. The right side of the cerebrum controls the left side of the body, and the left side of the cerebrum controls the right side of the body.

The outer layer of the cerebrum is called the CORTEX (or "gray matter"); the inner portion is the white matter. Indentations (called fissures) divide each cerebral hemisphere into four lobes: the frontal lobe, parietal lobe, TEMPORAL LOBE and occipital lobe. Functions involving memory are thought to take place within the frontal lobe, the parietal lobe and the temporal lobe.

chaining   A behavioral method for helping patients with memory problems handle everyday tasks. In this method, a particular task is broken down into a series of smaller units and taught one at a time. (See also BEHAVIORAL TREATMENTS OF MEMORY DISORDERS.)

chemicals and memory loss   A wide variety of drugs and chemicals have been implicated in memory problems.

Calcium   CALCIUM has been implicated as a possible cause of mental decline over time. The drug nimodipine, which blocks excess calcium in the part of the brain associated with memory and learning, has been used successfully to improve memory loss in stroke victims.

Choline Acetyltransferase   Choline acetyltransferase is deficient in the brains of Alzheimer's patients and is believed to be the primary reason behind their deficiency of ACETYLCHOLINE.

Carbon Monoxide Poisoning   Survivors of CARBON MONOXIDE POISONING can be left with profound cognitive impairment; carbon monoxide poisoning may also damage the BASAL GANGLIA.

Lipofuscin   Buildup of lipofuscin, of which "age spots" are made, has been linked to decreased learning ability.

chess and memory   When it comes to memory for the game of chess, studies have shown that chess masters don't have superior memories, but they have better memories for meaningful, properly structured information in their particular knowledge domain. Experts perceive board positions in terms of relations between groups of pieces. Whereas amateur players must memorize the position of each individual piece, experts only have to remember the group. Experts organize information into chunks in accordance with the patterns resulting from the attacking and defensive moves that occur in the game.

child abuse, memory of   Most people who were abused as children remember all or part of what happened to them, although they may not fully understand or disclose it, according to most psychologists and memory experts. This does not mean, however, that it's impossible for a memory to be forgotten and then remembered—or that a false "memory" can't be suggested and then remembered as true.

These two possibilities lie at the heart of controversy about the memory of childhood abuse and recovered memories. While experts agree more research is needed, most leaders in the field do agree that although it is a rare occurrence, a memory of early childhood abuse that has been forgotten can be remembered later. However, these experts also agree that it is possible to construct convincing pseudomemories (false memories) for events that never occurred. At this point, experts say it is impossible (without other backup evidence) to distinguish a true memory from a false one.

Experienced clinical psychologists believe that the phenomenon of a recovered memory is rare. For example, one experienced practitioner reported having a patient recover a buried memory only once in 20 years of practice. And while studies have shown that memory is often inaccurate and can be influenced by outside factors, memory research usually takes place in a lab—for ethical reasons, researchers can't subject people

to a traumatic event in order to test their memory of it.

Therefore, because the issue hasn't been studied directly, it's not possible to know whether a traumatic event is encoded and stored differently from a memory of a nontraumatic event.

Some clinicians suspect that children understand and respond to trauma differently from adults, and some believe that childhood trauma may lead to problems in memory storage and retrieval. These clinicians believe that dissociation is a likely explanation for a memory that was forgotten and later recalled. (Dissociation means that a memory isn't really lost, but it can't be retrieved for a period of time.) Some experts suspect that severe forms of child sexual abuse are especially likely to lead to dissociation or delayed memory. Many clinicians who work with trauma victims believe that this dissociation is a coping mechanism to protect against a painful memory. On the other hand, critics argue that there is little or no empirical support for such a theory.

The controversy over the validity of memories of childhood abuse has raised many critical issues for the psychological community, leaving many questions unanswered. The American Psychological Association has outlined a number of areas of controversy that should be pursued, such as:

- how accurate or inaccurate recollections of events may be created
- which techniques are most likely to lead to the creation of pseudomemories
- which techniques work best in creating the conditions under which actual events of childhood abuse can be remembered with accuracy
- how trauma and traumatic response affect the memory process
- are some people more susceptible than others to memory suggestion and if so, why

The issue of repressed or suggested memories has been sensationalized by the news media to the point that the idea of a total amnesia of a childhood event is portrayed as the most common occurrence, when in fact it is extremely rare. In fact, most people who are victims of childhood sexual abuse remember all or part of what happened to them.

childhood memories   See AMNESIA, CHILDHOOD.

choline   This dietary substance is an essential part of ACETYLCHOLINE (a brain compound necessary for transmitting nerve impulses) and has been implicated as a possible aid to improving memory by increasing the amount of acetylcholine in the brain.

In one federal study, a single 10-gram dose of choline significantly improved both memory and recall in healthy subjects; those with the worst memory were the ones most helped by the choline. Other tests suggest that choline may improve thinking ability, muscle control and the nervous system.

However, repeated studies of administering choline to treat the memory problems of ALZHEIMER'S DISEASE patients have resulted in conflicting evidence, although the majority found that giving choline was not helpful.

The major dietary source of choline is LECITHIN; foods rich in lecithin include eggs (average size), salmon and lean beef. While researchers dismiss the idea that eating these foods can significantly improve memory, other scientists believe that a "normal" level of lecithin in the diet may not be enough as people age.

The body uses phosphatidyl choline to make cell membranes, where most of the important electrochemical activities arise. Nerve and brain cells especially repair and maintain themselves with large quantities of this substance.

In research at the University of Ohio, scientists noted that levels of choline drop as a person ages and that levels are especially low in people with Alzheimer's disease.

choline acetyltransferase (ChAT)   An enzyme in the brain that is a crucial ingredient of the chemical process that produces ACETYLCHOLINE, a neurotransmitter involved in both learning and memory.

cholinergic basal forebrain   Nuclei in the deep regions of the forebrain containing neurons that release the neurotransmitter ACETYLCHOLINE. The cholinergic basal forebrain includes the medial septum, which projects to the HIPPOCAMPUS; the band of Broca, which projects to the hippocampus and amygdala; and the nucleus basalis of Meynert, which projects to the neocortex and AMYGDALA. Damage to these structures of the brain is believed to contribute to organic amnesia.

cholinergic hypothesis of Alzheimer's disease   There is a link between memory loss and the decrease in the activity of the enzyme CHOLINE ACETYLTRANSFERASE (CHAT) in the brain of Alzheimer's patients. (See ALZHEIMER'S DISEASE.)

ChAT is a crucial ingredient in the chemical process that produces ACETYLCHOLINE, a neurotransmitter involved in learning and memory. There has been a link between this decrease in neurochemical activity and changes in memory loss and disorientation and the physical appearance of Alzheimer brains (especially in the number of plaques).

Researchers have found a marked loss of nerve cells among Alzheimer's patients in a part of the base of the brain called the nucleus basalis; some patients with classical Alzheimer's disease have been shown to lose as many as 90 percent of these cells. The nucleus basalis produces acetylcholine, and uses it and its enzymes to communicate with the brain's cortex.

cholinomimetic agents   Drugs that mimic the activity of the neurotransmitter ACETYLCHOLINE, which is important in both learning and memory. The cholinomimetic agents include arecoline, which enhances learning in normal humans and aging primates. Researchers have found that clonidine, a substance that promotes the activity of catecholamines, improves the learning capability of aging monkeys and a few KORSAKOFF'S SYNDROME patients. Still, treatment aimed at replacing or stimulating cholinergic activity has had little success in improving memory in Alzheimer's disease patients.

chunking, process of   Grouping several separate bits of information into larger chunks in order to better remember them; often organizing them in a particular way, such as according to sound, rules of grammar, rhythm and so on, helps a person to recall them. For example, it's easier to remember a phone number broken up into chunks of three,

three and four digits (215-555-1328) than to remember a ten-digit number: 2155551328.

Cicero (106 B.C.–43 B.C.) One of the greatest of the Roman orators and a devoted mnemonist and teacher of memory systems and rhetoric, Cicero also believed (as did PLATO) that humans possess divine memory. He wrote that the memories of the lawyers and orators of his time were aided by systems and training that he used himself.

Oratory was an important career in Cicero's time, and the ancient Greeks and Romans realized that memory training could help the thinking process itself. In fact, a papyrus fragment dated to 400 B.C. extols the value of a trained memory.

In addition to the classical memory method of loci (building memory palaces), Cicero also learned how to make mental notes and remember words verbatim, but this memory system of Cicero's is lost; the AD HERENNIUM considered it to be too hard to use—and Cicero agreed. However, Cicero did borrow from his system to introduce to Rome a new way of writing called shorthand, which the church of the Middle Ages believed was grievous heresy and condemned as springing from the devil.

cigarettes and memory See SMOKING AND MEMORY.

circadian rhythm and memory A person's strength for memory tasks is cyclical, rising and falling during certain times of the day and of the week. Although most people experience a period of "peak" efficiency somewhere between 11 A.M. and 4 P.M., every person's internal body clock is different. As the day progresses, a person gets more involved in activities, but by lunchtime tiredness sets in. The daily biological cycles (body temperature, respiration and pulse rate) vary the power of attention and, therefore, of memory ability.

People who go to bed and wake up early learn more readily at the beginning of the day, while those who have a later schedule experience the opposite. Those who work a night shift probably experience different cyclical peak times from those who work a nine-to-five schedule.

In addition, research has shown that for some reason, memory ability tends to be at its best on Friday and Saturday, probably because the anticipation of the weekend improves a person's outlook and mood.

Disruptions to a person's normal cycle interfere with learning and memory ability. A new parent whose baby wakes every few hours all night long will experience memory problems due to chronic sleep interruption. Jet lag also can affect memory efficiency.

circulation and memory The proper function of memory requires a steady supply of blood and oxygen to the brain. Excess antihypertensive medication can lower the blood pressure to the point where it isn't sufficient to pump the blood to the brain, especially when a patient stands up. This causes a lack of blood supply in the brain that can produce a loss of memory. However, this memory loss only occurs when the brain has been subjected to low blood pressure repeatedly for several months. It usually affects patients over age 70.

classical conditioning A type of learning in which a previously neutral stimulus elicits a response. The most famous example of classical conditioning is Ivan Pavlov's dogs, which were trained to salivate (an existing response) when hearing the sound of a bell (neutral stimulus) because it had previously been associated with food. (See also PAVLOV, IVAN PETROVICH.)

Amnesic patients can learn through classical conditioning; when two amnesic patients acquired a conditioned eye-blink response to a buzzer and puff of air, the patients showed no recollection of the conditioning procedure but maintained the conditioned response.

Classical conditioning is the type of learning most often studied by scientists trying to locate the source of memory in the brain.

clioquinol An active component of many antidiarrhea drugs until it was banned, clioquinol also may cause memory problems. In 1966 clioquinol was distributed in Japan to treat dysentery after widespread flooding; soon thereafter more than 100 people reported a TRANSIENT GLOBAL AMNE-SIA. Other sporadic cases have occurred in Europe.

Clioquinol is still contained in creams, lotions and ointments as an antibacterial and antifungal, but it should not be taken internally.

Coenzyme Q10   Coenzyme Q10 (or ubiquinone) is an antioxidant that occurs naturally in the body and is needed for normal cell reactions to occur. Although this compound has not been researched to determine its effectiveness in treating ALZ-HEIMER'S DISEASE, some people believe it may be effective as an alternative treatment.

A synthetic version of this compound, called IDEBENONE, was tested for Alzheimer's, but was found not to be effective. Little is known about what dosage of coenzyme Q10 is considered safe, and there could be harmful effects in overdose.

coexistence hypothesis   A theory about eyewitness memory that explains why people report incorrect facts after witnessing an event. According to the hypothesis, both the original memory and the false postevent memory exist in the brain, as two competing alternatives. When a witness is asked about the event, he or she usually responds with the false version because it is the more recent memory and is therefore more accessible. However, even if a person produces a false memory, the original is recoverable, according to the coexistence hypothesis. (See also EYEWITNESS TESTIMONY; MEMORY FOR EVENTS.)

Cognex   See TACRINE.

cognition   The processing of information by the brain; specifically, perception, reasoning and memory.

cognitive development   The acquisition of intelligence, conscious thought and problem-solving skills beginning in infancy and progressing throughout life. (See also MEMORY IN INFANCY; PIAGET, JEAN.)

Cognitive Failures Questionnaire   A test that assesses a person's susceptibility to slips of action and other failures of memory and perception. On the test, subjects are asked to assess the frequency with which they experienced specific examples of cognitive failure, such as: "Do you forget whether you've turned off the stove?" The test then gives a five-point scale ranging from "never" to "very often."

Scores from this test are not related to performance on tests of immediate and delayed memory or to perception as measured by performance on a word-identification test. The test scores are related to a person's ability to perform two tasks at the same time; the inability to pay attention and allocate processing resources effectively is associated with frequent slips of action as well as other forms of memory deficits.

Test scores are also related to forward digit span (ability to repeat back a sequence of digits in the correct order), which is involved in carrying out action sequences, such as remembering to turn off the stove. (See also ASSESSMENT OF MEMORY DISORDERS.)

cognitive map   A person's internal method of remembering how to find directions in unknown locations.

cognitive triage   The tendency to recall hard-to-remember items first in a series of lists of items. Scientists speculate that cognitive triage may be an unconscious adaptive strategy for getting weakly remembered items to surface first.

Previously, psychologists believed that when people try to recall several items, they remember easily recalled items first. But new research by scientists at the University of Arizona at Tucson suggest that by as early as age six, people asked on memory tests to recall lists of items in any order first remember items they previously had trouble recalling.

If the theory of cognitive triage is correct, researchers say, police officers interrogating children who have witnessed crimes might obtain more information by asking questions about critical and disturbing events first rather than starting out with easy questions in order to relax the children.

collective unconscious A term coined by Swiss psychiatrist Carl Jung (1875–1961) to indicate a portion of shared ideas in the unconscious common to all people; also called racial unconscious or racial memory. Jung regarded the foundation of such mythical images as positive and creative (compared to Sigmund Freud's more negative view of mythology).

As part of his theory on the collective unconscious, Jung postulated a theory of archetypes—broadly similar images and symbols that occur in myths, fairy tales and dreams around the world. Jung believed these archetypes were inherited from experiences in our distant past, and that they are present in each person's unconscious, controlling the way he or she views the world. Jung believed the human psyche has an inbuilt tendency to dwell on certain inherited motifs, and that the basic pattern of these archetypes persists, however much details may vary.

While Jung also believed that every person had a personal unconscious of life experiences, he felt that the collective unconscious was superior. His aim in therapy was to put the patient in touch with the profound insight of the collective unconscious, particularly through dream interpretation.

combat amnesia Once called combat fatigue, this is a type of traumatic AMNESIA occurring after combat in which the amnesia has a straightforward origin—a distressing event during war. One method of treating combat amnesia is by the SODIUM PENTOTHAL interview, in which a slow intravenous injection of the drug relieves the patient's anxiety to the point of drowsiness. Then the injection is stopped, and the therapist can begin to question the patient about the traumatic incident. The recall at this point is often profoundly disturbing to the patient, who reaches the height of the reaction and then collapses, then often is able to pick up the story at a less traumatic point. One interpretation of this type of treatment is that the narcosis allows the patient to reinstate the extreme emotion felt during combat itself, unlocking the forgotten event.

A range of BARBITURATES, including sodium pentothal, have been used to facilitate the recall of emotionally disturbing memories; the most com-

mon alternative to sodium pentothal is SODIUM AMYTAL (amylbarbitone).

compensation neurosis See AMNESIA, SIMULATED.

computerized tomography (CT) scan Commonly known as a CAT (computerized axial tomography) scan, this is a quick and accurate diagnostic technique utilizing a computer and X rays passed through the brain at different angles to produce clear cross-sectional pictures of the tissue being examined. The CT scan provides a clearer and more detailed picture of the brain than X rays alone, and it tends to minimize the amount of radiation exposure.

Before the scan is performed, a contrast dye may be injected to make blood vessels or abnormalities show up more clearly. A number of low-dose X-ray beams are passed through the brain at different angles as the scanner rotates around the patient.

Using the information produced by the scanner, a computer constructs cross-sectional pictures of the brain, which are then displayed on a TV screen and can reveal soft tissue, including tumors, more clearly than normal X rays. CT scans are particularly useful in scanning the brain because they sharply define the ventricles (fluid-filled spaces).

The first scanner was developed as a brain research tool and was used clinically in 1972. Since then CT brain scans have improved the diagnosis and treatment of strokes, head injuries, tumors, abscesses and brain hemorrhages.

computer use and memory Because of the computer's ability to focus attention without distraction, recent research suggests that playing computer games and using computers may influence memory and cognition, especially in the elderly. In a preliminary study in Rockville, Maryland, 50 nursing home residents in their 70s, 80s and 90s were introduced to video games modified so they would have a greater chance of success. Other than those with severe mental impairment, residents—even those with Alzheimer's or Parkinson's disease—were able to participate and sharpen their memory skills.

concealing memories   See SCREEN MEMORIES.

concussion   Brief unconsciousness (usually for only a few seconds) following a severe blow to the head or neck caused by a disturbance of the electrical activity in the brain. The impact creates a sudden movement of the brain within the skull, which can produce a wide range of injuries including a loss of memory for experiences just before and during the accident that caused the concussion. However, memory loss may encompass a few weeks or, rarely, months before the accident. The recovery of memory usually progresses from the more distant past to the recent experience. (See RIBOT'S LAW.)

There may be no evident structural damage to the brain with a concussion, although there may be cuts or bruises on the skin outside the skull.

About a third of all those with concussion have a combination of symptoms called postconcussion syndrome for some time after a HEAD INJURY. Recent research has suggested that postconcussion syndrome can include significant memory problems, dizziness and behavioral changes that can disturb patients for as long as six months to a year following the head injury. Precisely why these symptoms occur in some people is not known.

Concussions usually are caused by traffic or industrial accidents, falls and physical assaults. Accidents are the leading cause of death from men under age 35, and more than 70 percent involve head injuries.

Symptoms

Common symptoms immediately following a concussion include confusion, inability to remember events immediately before the injury, dizziness, blurred vision and vomiting. Partial paralysis and shock are also possible. The longer the period of unconsciousness, the more serious and persistent symptoms tend to be. During the 24 hours after the injury, symptoms may include headache, vomiting, increased pulse rate and anxiety. Initial symptoms usually begin to fade within a few days, but if they fail to do so a physician should be consulted.

A physician should be seen after any loss of consciousness, since the possibility of serious bleeding within the skull could require emergency surgery.

Symptoms of serious damage may be immediately obvious or may not appear for some time.

Diagnosis

Diagnosis could include X rays or CT scans. A patient who has experienced concussion should be confined to bed for 24 hours in a hospital or at home under observation, and should not drive a car or play sports. If new symptoms develop (drowsiness, breathing problems, repeated vomiting or visual disturbances), they should be reported to a physician immediately since they indicate potential damage to the brain or bleeding between the skull and the outside of the brain.

Treatment

While generally no treatment is needed, acetaminophen or a stronger painkiller may be prescribed for headache. Aspirin is not generally recommended because it can contribute to bleeding. Rest and relaxation with no activities requiring concentration or vigorous movement will speed recovery within a few days.

Repeated concussions such as the blows boxers experience can damage the brain, impair concentration, slow thinking and slur speech. Initial symptoms usually begin to fade within a few days, although it is not uncommon for symptoms to last up to six months to a year. Concussed athletes should have a medical evaluation before returning to their sport. (See also PARKINSON'S DISEASE; "PUNCH DRUNK" SYNDROME.)

conditioning   The formation of a specific type of response or behavior to a specific stimulus in the environment. Conditioning theories have been advanced in part by the psychologists Ivan Pavlov and B. F. Skinner, whose names are associated with classical conditioning.

If a stimulus that is known consistently to produce a response is paired consistently with a second "neutral" stimulus, eventually the second stimulus alone will produce the response. The most famous example of this type of conditioning was devised by Pavlov; each time food was presented to a dog, making it salivate, a bell was rung. Eventually the dog would salivate in response to the bell alone. Pavlov noted that the response would generalize to similar stimuli; thus, a dog conditioned to salivate when shown a round object also would salivate (although not as much) when shown an elliptical one. Pavlov also discovered that the conditioned response would fade if not reinforced occasionally with the original neutral stimulus.

In *operant conditioning,* behavior is determined by rewards and punishments. Skinner placed a hungry rat in a box; it moved randomly about the cage, but once in a while it accidentally pawed a lever that released a pellet of food. Eventually the rat learned to press the lever whenever it wanted food; thus, it became conditioned.

Behavioral psychologists believe that all behavior is learned this way, and they regard psychiatric problems as learned behavior patterns. They base treatment for psychiatric disorders on the same principles, since a behavior that has been learned can be unlearned by reinforcing a more appropriate form of behavior. (See also CLASSICAL CONDITIONING; PAVLOV, IVAN PETROVICH.)

confabulation The production of false recollections. Confabulation is very common in psychiatric disorders and occurs especially in memories with a tinge of grandiosity. Confabulation memories also may borrow from fantasy or dream.

This problem was once thought to be a product of a person's embarrassment at losing memories, but many patients with severe AMNESIA do not confabulate. There appears to be no relationship between the severity of the amnesia and the tendency to confabulate; instead, the tendency may be related to personality traits in force before the onset of amnesia. People who are outwardly sociable but inwardly secretive are particularly prone to produce these false memories. Patients with the greatest tendency toward confabulation, however, are those with the least insight into their own memory disorder and who deny that a problem exists.

consciousness and memory The consciousness or awareness of self shows most clearly the intimate relationship between memory and consciousness. In order to be perceived as continuous, the self requires continuity of memories.

Some researchers, including neurological expert Endel Tulving, have postulated that there are three varieties of consciousness: noetic, autonomous and anoetic. Noetic consciousness implies a semantic memory, since it involves thinking about objects and events and relationships among them in their absence. Autonomous consciousness is self-knowing; it is related to episodic memory that recognizes events as in the personal past. Anoetic consciousness is the state of nonknowing, but it is still consciousness because it allows appropriate behavioral responses to aspects of the environment.

Some scientists believe that the perception of consciousness occurs when nerve cells fire at similar frequencies, which imposes a "global unity" on nerve cells in different brain areas.

consolidation A change in the structure of memory, other than the forgetting that occurs with the passage of time after learning.

Modern theories of consolidation can be traced to the work of Donald Hebb (1904–85), who believed that new information is first represented by a temporary trace, a specific pattern of activity within a group of interconnected neurons (which Hebb called a cell assembly). At this stage, any disruption in the pattern of activity will cause the information to be lost completely. But if the activity is maintained for enough time, structural changes in the cell will occur, causing a permanent memory trace. Once this trace is formed, there is no more need to maintain the initial pattern of activity, and the information is then in "passive storage."

Many scientists believe that the structural change underlying consolidation involves an altered pattern of synapse activity. It has been estimated that the brain has many synapses that could handle the levels of information storage in memory.

The exact way that synapses change is not known, although scientists speculate that it may involve how much neurotransmitter is released at the synapses.

context The placement of information under consideration. There are three types: semantic context, which determines the meaning of the information; situational context—details of the physical setting in which the information was received; personal context—emotions, state of health and levels of arousal at the time the information was received.

continuous amnesia   A type of PSYCHOGENIC AMNESIA in which the patient cannot recall events subsequent to a specific time up to and including the present. (See also HYSTERICAL AMNESIA.)

contrecoup effects   Damage to the side of the brain opposite the point of impact following a closed HEAD INJURY. Contrecoup effects are especially likely to occur in the temporal and orbital regions of the brain and may destroy neurons which later results in subcortical demyelination. Lesions in the corpus callosum following head injury also have been reported.

conversion   An unconscious defense mechanism by which conflicts that would otherwise cause anxiety are instead given symbolic external expression. The repressed impulses and the defenses against them are converted into a variety of symptoms involving the nervous system, which may include paralysis, pain or loss of sensory function.

cortex   The home of the most lofty abilities in the brain, the cortex is a quarter-inch-thick pad of grooved tissue running from the eyebrows to the ears, with a right and left hemisphere, each of which has four distinct lobes. The lobes are connected by a pathway of fibers called the corpus callosum.

Research studies have pinpointed scores of regions within the cortex that seem to specialize in different jobs, especially in the diffuse storing of memories. The cortex stores a person's abstract memory, a huge jumble of events and objects. Damage to the temporal, parietal or occipital cortex affects abstract memory in different ways. For example, damage to the left temporal or parietal lobe produces problems in reading, writing, speaking and simple arithmetic skills, but other mental abilities and memory remain intact. However,

damage to the right temporal or parietal lobe causes subjects to become lost easily even in familiar surroundings; they cannot negotiate simple mazes, use or draw maps, match or copy the slant of a line, copy simple shapes or arrange blocks to form required patterns, or judge size, distance and direction of objects.

The sensory and motor areas of the cortex take up relatively little space, compared with the huge areas occupied by the association parts of the brain. The sensory areas of the cortex receive sensations of the muscles, skin and organs, such as temperature or touch. These sensory areas are responsible for locating the area in the body from which feelings are coming. Motor areas of the cortex send out messages that control muscles or muscle groups, which make the body move. The association areas of the cortex link the sensory areas with motor areas; these association areas are the true seat of the personality, intelligence, language, judgment, emotions and memory. In essence, the association areas of the brain allow the brain to think.

Creutzfeldt-Jakob disease   A very rare infectious disease of the nervous system caused by a transmissible infectious organism called a PRION that leads to a progressive dementia. It is usually distinguished from other dementias by its rapid course; it takes only months from onset of symptoms until death. CJD is much more common than its cousin, bovine spongiform encephalopathy (MAD COW DISEASE), but it gets much less attention from the media. It strikes about 250 Americans each year, usually over age 58, with a usually swift and inevitably fatal course. Although scientists believe that the disease incubates over many years, patients typically live a few months to a year after symptoms appear.

The disease is considered infectious, but not contagious—it can't be passed from one human to another in casual contact, by hugging, kissing or sexual intercourse. But scientists have found in laboratory tests that healthy mice contract the disease when they are injected with brain fluid from a sick mouse. Infected patients can transmit the disease to monkeys, cats and guinea pigs. In addition, infection has been linked to brain surgery with contaminated instruments or transplantation of an infected cornea. There are also indications that there may be a genetic link.

By contrast, the much-publicized mad cow disease, which scientists call "new-variant CJD" is actually much rarer. As of January 1, 1999, this disease has killed 39 people in Britain and one in France; no known cases of new-variant CJD in cattle or humans have been found in the United States.

Types

There are three types of CJD: sporadic, acquired and hereditary. *Sporadic CJD* accounts for at least 85 percent of the cases, in which patients usually have no known risk for the disease, which seems to appear out of nowhere. *Acquired CJD* includes both new-variant CJD ("mad cow disease") and medically-induced CJD, which is transmitted through exposure to brain or nervous system tissue, including eye tissue and spinal cord fluid. *Hereditary CJD* occurs in people who have a family history of the disease and test positive for the genetic mutation in their prion proteins. This version accounts for 10 to 15 percent of cases.

Cause

CJD and related diseases are caused not by viruses, bacteria or toxins, but by a progressive malformation of certain proteins in the brain called prions, according to Stanley Prusiner, M.D., a neurologist from the University of California-San Francisco. Proteins are made of long chains of amino acids folded in specific patterns. Prusiner theorizes that in CJD, an amino-acid chain in a protein folds abnormally, forming a prion; a single prion has the ability to force other proteins directly around it to misfold similarly. The prions bunch together, changing the formation of the brain cells, leaving behind soft holes in the patient's brain. When the brain is examined after death, it is honeycombed with holes in disease-specific formations called plaques.

Symptoms

The first symptoms involve a sudden progressive memory loss, insomnia, personality changes, bizarre behavior, visual distortions, hallucinations and problems in judgment and thinking. As the disease progresses, patients soon lose the ability to communicate and control their muscles, often developing involuntary spasms. Mental deterioration becomes pronounced, and the patient lapses into a coma.

Diagnosis

There is no single test for CJD; doctors rely on a series of tests, including a very specific pattern on EEG (electroencephalogram) and MRI scans, and a spinal fluid screen showing trauma to the brain. Still, the diagnosis can't be confirmed without a doubt until pathologists see the patient's brain after death.

Treatment

There is no treatment other than easing symptoms. There are medications for the spasms, for seizures and for stiffness.

cross-racial witness identification People are better at recognizing faces of those of their own race than those of a different race, even if subjects have had extensive contact with other races. But this cross-racial identification problem is not related to the fact that people have greater prejudices or less experience with members of the other race. All studies, which include ones of black and white subjects as well as Asians and students from India, report the same findings.

Researchers suspect that members of a different race often have distinctive features in common. For example, most Asians have distinctive eyes; when a non-Asian sees an Asian for a few seconds, the distinctive eyes stand out, attract the viewer's attention and take up most of the processing time. When later asked to pick an Asian out of a group of Asians, the one feature that was attended to—the eyes—aren't helpful in distinguishing one Asian from another. (See also AGE AND EYEWITNESS ABILITY; EYEWITNESS TESTIMONY.)

cryptomnesia A phenomenon in which experiences that originally make little conscious impression are nonetheless filed away in the brain and only later are remembered suddenly in graphic detail as "hidden memories." Some brain experts believe that irregular or "supernatural" experiences such as alien abductions, satanic kidnappings, channeling of spirits and recall of past lives are all evidence of cryptomnesia.

One well-known example of this occurred to a young Helen Keller, who—at the age of 11—wrote a short story entitled "The Frost King" as a birthday present to the president of the Perkins School for the Blind. The story was so delightful and so packed with visual imagery that the educator published it in one of the school's reports; it was then reprinted in a weekly magazine.

Eventually, however, it became clear that Keller's story was closely patterned after the short story "The Frost Fairies," written by Margaret Canby before Keller's birth. The theme and some of the passages of the two stories were so close that it was clear Keller's story was derived from the earlier work, but both Keller and her teacher, Anne Sullivan, denied that Sullivan had "read" her the story.

Eventually Sullivan stated that a family friend whom Keller had visited three years earlier had a copy of Canby's book and had indeed "read" it to the girl, although Keller had no memory of having "heard" it. (In a separate account, the young Helen was alleged to have confided that Sullivan did, in fact, "read" her the story.)

In any case, recent research has suggested that people can retrieve recently acquired information from memory without experiencing the information as the recall of a memory. This suggests that there is an important distinction to be made between something remembered and the experience of remembering something. In fact, the experience of remembering when there is nothing to remember is a problem called CONFABULATION, or false memories.

CT scan   See COMPUTERIZED TOMOGRAPHY (CT) SCAN.

cue-dependent forgetting   An explanation of forgetting that centers on problems in retrieval. With cue-dependent forgetting, the memory does not fade away, nor is it displaced by other information; instead, it merely depends on using the right cue to retrieve it.

With the right cue, the information can be retrieved from memory; if the item is "forgotten," it is because the wrong cue has been used. An example of cue-dependent forgetting is when a person can't remember a fact until something "jogs" his or her memory.

Cushing's syndrome   A hormonal disorder caused by an abnormally high circulating level of corticosteroid hormones. The abnormal level of hormones may be produced directly by an adrenal gland tumor, by prolonged administration of corticosteroid drugs or by enlarged adrenal glands resulting from a pituitary tumor. Sometimes a malignant tumor of the lung or other organ will cause Cushing's syndrome. While possible at any age, it is most common during middle years.

Symptoms
Named for Harvey Cushing, an early 20th-century American surgeon, the disease often produces multiple abnormalities, including memory loss, agitation, depression and delusions. Patients have a humped upper back, wasted limbs, an obese trunk and the face has a characteristic round, reddened appearance. Frequent or spontaneous bruising on the arms and legs is another symptom; acne develops and purple stretch marks may appear on abdomen, thighs and breasts. Women may become more hairy, and patients may be more susceptible to infection and experience ulcers.

Diagnosis
An endocrinologist may order tests including examination of blood and urine for the presence of higher-than-normal amounts of steroid hormones; a computerized tomography (CT) scan of the pituitary and adrenal glands may also be ordered.

Treatment
The successful removal of a benign pituitary or adrenal tumor will probably cure the disorder, although long-term hormone therapy may be necessary. If left untreated, this syndrome eventually may end in death. If the symptoms are caused by excess steroids, the medication is decreased and then stopped; *sudden discontinuation of steroids may aggravate the underlying disorder.*

If Cushing's syndrome is caused by a tumor, removal of the tumor or the entire gland may be necessary. Radiation therapy may be an option if the tumor is located in the pituitary gland. If the treatment inactivates the adrenal glands, oral drugs must be taken to replace the missing hormones.

CVAs See CEREBROVASCULAR ACCIDENT (CVA).

decay One of many theories of FORGETTING that suggests memories leave a physical trace in the brain that gradually fades away with time after a period of nonuse. (See also TRACE DECAY.)

declarative memory The type of memory network responsible for memory of facts, as opposed to PROCEDURAL MEMORY, the memory for procedures—learning *what* versus learning *how*. Scientists believe that the HIPPOCAMPUS is critical to storing facts but not procedures. An amnesiac with a damaged hippocampus can still learn simple skills (such as reading reversed print in a mirror), but she can't remember anything about the training session.

Likewise, riding a bicycle involves *procedural* memory; after learning to ride the bike, people can't articulate the knowledge they have learned; all the micromovements that go into riding a bike are stored implicitly throughout the central nervous system as processes, not fact. (See also HM.)

defense mechanism The unconscious process that provides relief from emotional conflict and anxiety. Conscious efforts often are made for the same reasons, but the true defense mechanism is unconscious. Some of the common defense mechanisms include compensation, CONVERSION, denial, displacement, DISSOCIATION, idealization, identification, incorporation, introjection, projection, rationalization, reaction formation, regression, sublimation, substitution, symbolization and undoing.

dehydroepiandrosterone (DHEA) A natural steroid hormone produced in the adrenal glands from the metabolism of cholesterol. Proponents believe that DHEA, the most common steroid in the human body, may be an important part of cognitive enhancement, but there has not yet been conclusive proof.

Proponents believe that taking DHEA supplements beginning at middle age could improve quality of life, but evidence has been inconclusive. Critics point out that taking any type of hormones on a regular basis without medical supervision could cause problems, especially in women with a history of breast cancer. DHEA is a steroid that the body converts into estrogens and androgens. Side effects can include acne, facial-hair growth in women, deepening of the voice and mood changes.

déjà vu French for "already seen," this is the haunting sense or illusion that one is seeing what one has seen before. Almost all people at some point in their lives have had the sense of recognition and familiarity when they come upon a new landscape and feel sure they have been there before. The sense of familiarity is sometimes so vivid that it almost seems like a hallucination.

Examples of déjà vu have been recorded for millennia; but while descriptions of the experience have been traced as far back as St. Augustine, no one has yet come up with the definitive theory about what causes it. Plato argued that déjà vu is a real memory of events that took place in a previous existence and that prove the theory of reincarnation. Nineteenth-century Romantic poets also believed the déjà vu experience supported the idea of reincarnation, but modern scientists believe it is a disturbance of the temporal lobe of the brain.

Other scientists suggest déjà vu is really a false memory, triggered by a current experience that has some features in common with an earlier one. They believe that memories are stored in the brain in the form of holograms and that any part of the hologram has enough information stored in it to reproduce the whole picture.

This theory helps explain how memories can be brought forward by stimulating a section of the brain and why the memory may remain even after that section is surgically removed. This fact implies that—just as with a hologram—there is enough information in any one cluster of brain cells to evoke the entire memory.

In cases of déjà vu, then, while clumps of holographic data may form entirely different memories, portions of them may be identical. This could fool us momentarily into thinking we are reexperiencing something.

Freud expressed the idea of déjà vu in relationship to consciousness and unconsciousness; a conscious experience touching on a repressed memory, he said, would set off the feeling of déjà vu. More modern psychoanalysts believe that feelings of déjà vu occur during moments of anxiety, as a means of reassurance.

delayed matching to sample   A task developed to test memory in nonhuman primates. The animal sees an object and then, after a delay, sees two objects—the one already shown and a new one. The animal receives a reward by choosing the familiar object.

delayed nonmatching to sample   A task developed to test memory in nonhuman primates. Animals see a single object and then, after a delay, see both the recently presented object and a new one. The animal earns a reward by choosing the second, new object.

delayed recall task   A part of the MENTAL STATUS EXAMINATION in which a patient is given a sentence, a series of numbers, or a group of unrelated words, and told to remember them and repeat them later. After a certain amount of time, the subject is asked to repeat the information. Such a task can provide one way of testing a person's short-term memory.

delirium   Acute mental confusion, usually brought on by a physical disease. Symptoms mimic those of disordered brain function, and include the failure to understand events or remember what has been happening, mood swings and physical restlessness. Delirious patients may experience hallucinations or panic attacks and resort to violence or shouting. Symptoms are usually worse at night because of sleep disturbance and the fact that darkness and quiet make visual disturbances more likely.

While delirium may be caused by any severe illness, high fever and disturbances of body chemistry are usually the prime factors. Children and older people are most prone to delirium, especially after major surgery or in the presence of a preexisting brain disturbance such as DEMENTIA. Drugs, poisons and alcohol also may cause delirium.

Delirium is treated by easing the underlying disorder and appropriate care to relieve anxiety, together with calm environment, seclusion, clear communication and trusted attendants. The patient must get enough fluids and good nutrition, but tranquilizers (such as chlorpromazine, haloperidol or thioridazine) often are necessary to ease restlessness. Antibiotic treatment to control infection has made delirium less of a problem than it was in the past.

delirium tremens (DTs)   An acute brain disorder characterized by a state of confusion together with trembling and vivid hallucinations usually experienced by chronic alcoholics after withdrawal or abstinence from alcohol. DTs often occur after hospital admission and are fatal in 10 to 15 percent of untreated cases.

Symptoms, which usually develop within 24 to 96 hours after stopping drinking, include restlessness, agitation, trembling and sleeplessness, with rapid heartbeat, fever, widened pupils, profuse sweating, confusion, visual or auditory hallucinations, illusions, delusions, paranoia terror and convulsions. Symptoms usually subside within three days.

The condition often is accompanied by nutritional deficiencies. Treatment includes rest, rehydration and sedation (chlorpromazine or chlordiazepoxide) with vitamin injections (especially thiamine), since some of the features of delirium tremens seem linked with thiamine deficiency.

DTs are caused by the withdrawal of alcohol after the brain and other organs have become accustomed to tolerating elevated levels.

demand characteristics hypothesis A theory about eyewitness memory that explains why people report incorrect facts after an event they have witnessed. The theory, similar to the COEXISTENCE HYPOTHESIS, says that when false information is provided about an event, both incorrect and correct memories about an event exist and both are equally accessible. Supposedly people produce the false memory because they think it is the one that is demanded of them, not because it is more accessible. When eyewitness expert Elizabeth Loftus tested this theory by asking subjects who witnessed an event to recall both the original and the false memory versions, very few subjects could produce both. (See also EYEWITNESS TESTIMONY; MEMORY FOR EVENTS; SUBSTITUTION HYPOTHESIS.)

dementia The loss of intellectual functions such as thinking and memory that interferes with daily function. It is not a disease in itself, but a group of symptoms that may accompany a condition, all of which produce a gradual decline in intellectual function and almost always a significant deterioration of memory.

Loss of memory is usually the first sign, with patients asking the same question, forgetting to turn off the stove and so on. As dementia continues, symptoms worsen, including more and more confused episodes, and more drastic impairments (such as language problems) begin to appear. Because of similar symptoms, it is often difficult to diagnose particular forms of dementia, but a number of distinct forms have been recognized.

The term *dementia* is not used to indicate a particular loss of mental function, such as occurs in amnesia, aphasia, agnosia or apraxia; in dementia, the decline usually involves memory, other cognitive capacities and adaptive behavior without any major change in consciousness.

For centuries dementia was dismissed as SENILITY and considered an inevitable fact of aging. In fact, it is *not* a part of normal aging, but a symptom of an underlying condition.

The patient may or may not be aware of the condition, but in almost all cases the loss of memory is accompanied by defects in one or more areas of intellectual function, such as language, spatial or temporal orientation, judgment and abstract thought. While some criteria for dementia require defects in one or more of the components of intellect, others require that the defect involve all components of intellectual function.

Cause

Dementia is a result of dysfunction of the brain, especially in those parts of the cerebrum known as the association areas, which combine perception, purposeful action and thought to enable a person to adjust and survive in his or her environment. Dementia is not the same thing as mental retardation, although a person with mental retardation may become demented upon losing intellectual abilities he or she once had. Dementia is also not the same thing as psychosis; a demented patient may or may not be psychotic, and a patient with psychosis may or may not be demented.

Although it occurs at all ages, the chance of dementia increases with advancing age; its highest rate is in the population over age 75. According to recent estimates, dementia costs the United States more than $40 billion.

Symptoms

The onset of dementia is usually gradual; it begins with mild forgetfulness, restlessness or apathy followed by an increasing tendency to misplace things and small inconsistencies in some of the ordinary daily living tasks. Words or actions may begin to be repeated. As the dementia worsens, the cognitive dysfunction worsens and patients may begin to have problems at work, lose their way in their own neighborhoods, fail to recognize friends or family and reverse sleep cycles.

These symptoms may be followed by hallucinations, delusions, paranoia, or inappropriate or antisocial behavior. Depending on the cause of the dementia, there may or may not be indications of organic brain disease in addition to the intellectual or behavioral changes, such as problems with balance, senses or vision.

Diagnosis

Proper identification of the cause of dementia is critical to treatment, since some diseases that produce dementia can be treated or reversed. (These include benign brain lesions, intoxication, infections and metabolic and nutritional disorders.) It is likewise important to differentiate the early stages of dementia from nonprogressive cognitive changes found in normal aging—but it's not always possible. The best way to tell the difference is through a series of observations over a period of time; still, diagnoses of many of the most common dementing diseases can be confirmed only upon autopsy.

The patient's history is the most important component of the initial evaluation, and should be obtained from the patient and the family. Family members most often in contact with the patient should be interviewed first, followed by other family members, friends and neighbors. Important objective information also can be provided by community health workers, social workers and nurses. Previous medical records should be reviewed. A chronological account of the patient's current problems—symptoms, duration of disease and specific intellectual and behavioral changes—should be noted. The medical history should include inquiries about relevant systemic diseases, trauma, surgery, psychiatric disorders, nutrition, alcohol and substance abuse.

The two most common forms of dementia in old age are MULTI-INFARCT DEMENTIA and ALZHEIMER'S DISEASE, but the many different diseases capable of producing dementia can be divided into two main groups. The first group includes those disorders that appear to originate in the brain and that inevitably produce dementia. The second group includes those that begin outside the brain and affect it secondarily, and may or may not produce dementia depending on how the brain is affected—liver disease, certain metabolic disorders and infectious disorders such as syphilis or AIDS.

Parkinson's Disease

As many as 30 percent to 40 percent of people with PARKINSON'S DISEASE (a progressive, neurodegenerative condition) will develop dementia during the later course of the disease. Some Alzheimer patients develop symptoms of Parkinson's disease.

Lewy Body Dementia

LEWY BODY DEMENTIA is a type of dementia similar to both Parkinson's disease and Alzheimer's disease—but also unique. Lewy bodies are protein deposits found in deteriorating nerve cells that often appear in the brains of people with Parkinson's disease. When Lewy bodies disperse throughout the brain, it causes a dementia with symptoms much like Alzheimer's disease. However, Lewy body dementia progresses differently from Alzheimer's, involving hallucinations and fluctuations in cognitive impairment.

Huntington's Disease

HUNTINGTON'S DISEASE is a progressive, degenerative disease that affects the body and mind. It stems from a disorder within the brain that causes certain nerve cells to waste away. As the disease progresses, changes in personality and declines in intellect, memory, speech and judgment occur. Dementia may develop in the later stages of the disease. Huntington's is known to be caused by a genetic disorder, and the gene that causes this disease has been identified.

Creutzfeldt-Jakob Disease

Dementias may occur in young or middle-aged people. CREUTZFELDT-JAKOB DISEASE is a rare and fatal brain disorder thought to be caused by a PRION. The earliest symptom of the disease may be memory impairment and behavior changes. The disease progresses rapidly with mental deterioration, involuntary movements (muscle jerks), weakness in the limbs, blindness and eventually coma.

Pick's Disease

PICK'S DISEASE is a rare brain disorder characterized by disturbances in behavior, personality and eventually memory. The disease is relentless in its progression, which may ultimately include language impairment, erratic behavior and dementia. Because of the strange behavior associated with Pick's, people are often seen first by psychiatrists. Like Alzheimer's disease, a diagnosis is usually confirmed at autopsy.

In addition, there are a great number of reversible causes of dementia:

Drug-Related Dementia Overdose of medication or chemicals is capable of causing a dementia. Neuroactive and psychoactive drugs, opiate painkillers and the adrenocortical steroids are the most common causes. About 5 percent of dementia cases are drug-related. However, some often-used drugs may cause or aggravate dementia, including anticholinergic medicines used in the treatment of movement disorders, allergic reactions or gastrointestinal disorders; and drugs used to treat heart problems, such as high blood pressure. Almost all street drugs (from heroin to glue) can cause dementia, as can a range of common chemicals such as carbon monoxide, carbon disulfide, lead, mercury and manganese. While all these chemicals may have irreversible or fatal effects, they are often the cause of reversible dementia.

Many medications taken by older people can cause subtle cognitive impairment, but when several drugs are taken at the same time—as often happens among the elderly—significant Alzheimer's-like problems appear: memory loss, absentmindedness, confusion, disorientation and emotional outbursts. Alcohol use aggravates drug-related dementia.

Infections Any infection that involves the brain is capable of producing dementia. Dementia from infections such as leptomeningitis and encephalitis, if they are treated early, can be prevented. Chronic infectious diseases such as syphilis, Whipple's disease or cryptococcus affect the brain, but the dementia can still be stopped—and sometimes reversed—at least to a degree. Chronic viral illnesses such as AIDS often produce dementia, but it is not known whether drugs that retard the AIDS process can stop or reverse changes in the nervous system that lead to dementia. The agents responsible for diseases such as Creutzfeldt-Jakob disease and progressive multifocal leukoencephalopathy do not respond to any kind of treatment. Postinfectious encephalomyelitis sometimes can result in dementia.

Metabolic Diseases Chronic diseases of the thyroid, parathyroid and adrenal glands and the pituitary are easily diagnosed and the resulting dementia can be reversed. A number of inherited metabolic diseases that appear in adult life, including Wilson's disease, metachromatic leukodystrophy and neuronal storage diseases, also cause a reversible dementia.

Nutritional Disorders Poor nutrition can lead to dementia in about 5 percent of cognitive deterioration cases. Nutrient deficiencies most closely associated with dementia include the B vitamins: thiamine (B_1), niacin (B_3), folate (folic acid), and vitamin B_{12}. Of these, folate and B_{12} deficiencies are most common. Blood tests to assess their levels are a standard part of the clinical assessment for Alzheimer's disease. The hallmark of B-vitamin deficiency dementia is memory loss with possible coordination problems (ataxia).

Although patients who have thinking problems may not eat well and could therefore have a vitamin deficiency as a result of their dementia, several studies have shown that people with both dementia and B_{12} deficiencies recover when given the vitamin by injection. Other studies have shown mental improvement when people with folate and niacin deficiencies have received supplemental vitamins. Unfortunately, only about 25 percent of those with dementia due to thiamine deficiency recover completely when given supplements; another 50 percent show partial recovery. Wernicke-Korsakoff's encephalopathy is caused by a loss of thiamine, which can lead to the irreversible Korsakoff's dementia. Thiamine deficiency is usually seen in alcoholic patients, but it also can be found among depressed people and pregnant women suffering with chronic vomiting.

Cardiovascular Disorders High blood pressure is one of the most frequent causes of MULTI-INFARCT DEMENTIA, by causing frequent blood clots in the brain. Other causes are some forms of arteriosclerosis (a group of disorders causing thickening of artery walls), vasculitis (inflammation of blood vessels) and blood clots. The inability of the heart to pump blood efficiently also can produce dementia by single or repeated episodes of ischemia (insufficient supply of blood to the brain), which cuts off oxygen to the brain. Chronic blockage of arteries leading to the brain does not cause dementia if brain tissue has not been damaged by loss of oxygen.

Lesions A chronic subdural hematoma (large blood clot in the space between the dura, the tough outer layer of covering of the brain [meninges] and the middle meningeal layer) can produce dementia, a not-uncommon cause of dementia in older patients. Benign tumors of the brain, especially those on the orbital surface of the frontal lobe or on the medial surface of the temporal lobe, also can cause dementia, depending on their size and location. Brain tumors cause about 3 percent of the cases of dementia. Obstructive hydrocephalus (spinal fluid on the brain) may produce dementia when certain benign lesions such as some neurofibromas press on the brain. Malignant tumors of the brain also often produce dementia; only rarely does this type of dementia respond to treatment.

Normal-Pressure Hydrocephalus   This uncommon disorder is characterized by a blocked flow of cerebrospinal fluid that causes a buildup of this fluid on the brain. Symptoms include dementia, urinary incontinence and difficulty in walking. The condition may be caused by meningitis, encephalitis or head injury. If diagnosed early in the disease, normal-pressure hydrocephalus is treatable by surgery in which a shunt is inserted to divert the fluid away from the brain.

Depression   Depressed adults are often mistakenly diagnosed as demented. Symptoms of depression include sadness, difficulty thinking and concentrating, feelings of despair and inactivity, poor concentration and inattention. When dementia and depression occur together, (which can often happen), the intellectual deterioration may be more extreme. Depression is treatable.

Delirium   This state of temporary mental confusion is common in older people who have lung or heart disease, long-term infections, poor nutrition, medication interactions or hormone disorders. Emergency treatment of delirium is vital since a serious medical illness such as bacterial meningitis may be the underlying cause. Symptoms of delirium are sometimes confused with dementia, but a person who suddenly seems to have impaired thinking, who becomes disoriented or loses consciousness is more likely to be delirious rather than demented.

Progressive Degenerative Diseases   Most of the progressive degenerative diseases that cause dementia are not treatable; they originate primarily in the brain and may or may not cause other neurological signs. Alzheimer's disease is the most common of these diseases. Progressive degenerative diseases causing dementia that appear with other prominent neurological signs include diseases of the BASAL GANGLIA (Parkinson's and Huntington's diseases), cerebellar and spinocerebellar degenerations, and amyotrophic lateral sclerosis (Lou Gehrig's disease).

Treatment

If there is a diagnosis of a curable cause of dementia, the doctor will be able to recommend the best treatment. Even if the diagnosis is one of the irreversible disorders, much can be done to help the patient and family. Careful use of drugs can lessen agitation, anxiety and depression and improve sleeping patterns, if needed. Proper nutrition is particularly important, although special diets or supplements usually are not necessary.

Daily routines, physical activities and social contacts are all important. Often, stimulating the individual by supplying information about time of day, place and what's going on in the world encourages the use of remaining skills and information. This keeps brain activity from failing at a faster rate. In the same way, providing memory cues helps people help themselves—these cues might include a visible calendar, a list of daily activities, written notes about simple safety measures and directions to and labeling of commonly used items.

Prevention

Developing interests or hobbies and becoming involved in activities that keep the mind and body active are among the best ways to avoid problems that can mimic irreversible brain disorders. Certain physical and mental changes seem to occur with age even in healthy people, but senility is by no means inevitable after age 65.

The purpose of testing a patient for dementia is to rule out treatable causes of the impairment; therefore, an accurate diagnosis is important. There are a wide range of treatable causes of dementia, including depression, drug reactions, vitamin B_{12} deficiency, thyroid abnormalities, alcoholism, drug abuse or systemic disease.

Evaluation of the patient begins with a detailed history of symptoms with physical and neurological examinations together with a battery of lab tests. A mental status exam is often part of the neurological evaluation; this is not a test of sanity, but assesses various mental functions such as memory, attention, language and perception.

In particular, memory may be tested exhaustively, since memory problems are a prominent feature of dementia. Tests should include an assessment of a person's ability to learn both verbal and nonverbal information and the ability to recall items from the remote past. The patient may be asked to construct objects by drawing or recall these drawings later.

In addition, an assessment usually will include a battery of standardized tests of intelligence (such as the Wechsler Adult Intelligence Scale, or WAIS), memory (the Wechsler Memory Scale), language (Boston Diagnostic Aphasia Examination) and prior academic achievement (the Wide Range Achievement Test).

Lab tests may help rule out diseases with certain brain disorders, such as tumors, abscesses, strokes, fluid accumulation, heart and lung disorders, liver disease, kidney disease, infections such as AIDS or SYPHILIS. Other tests that look for these disorders might include a brain scan (magnetic resonance imaging or computerized tomography), electrocardiogram, chest X ray, blood chemistry and urine tests and drug screening, electroencephalography (EEG), lumbar puncture or radioisotope studies.

If all other diseases and injuries are ruled out, the patient may be suffering from ALZHEIMER'S DISEASE; there is no specific test that can uncover Alzheimer's, which is diagnosed only after all other possibilities have been exhausted. An absolute diagnosis can be made only at autopsy.

dementia praecocissiima A form of DEMENTIA PRAECOX diagnosed before puberty. The term was first used in 1905 by Italian psychiatrist Sante De Sanctis.

dementia praecox This term refers to a markedly rapid mental disintegration into senility in younger patients, which usually occurs only in very old or brain-damaged individuals.

The term *demence precoce* was first used in 1852 by Benedict Augustin Morel in his book *Etudes cliniques*. It was used 46 years later by noted psychiatrist Emil Kraepelin in his textbook *Psychiatrie* to describe the progressively degenerative mental disorder accompanied by acute or subacute mental disturbance. Kraepelin noted that dementia praecox began in late adolescence or early adulthood and that half his cases began between ages 16 and 22. He believed that the disease might be caused not only by heredity but by an organic brain disease that was degenerative and not reversible.

denial An unconscious defense mechanism used to resolve emotional conflict and allay anxiety by disavowing thoughts, feelings, wishes and needs that are consciously intolerable. This behavior is often seen in those with psychotic disorders; in its extreme form, denial can appear to have an almost delusional quality.

deprenyl A substance also known as selegiline (trade names: Eldepryl, Jumex) that has been used as a treatment for PARKINSON'S DISEASE and is currently being studied for the treatment of ALZHEIMER'S DISEASE. Some researchers also are studying the drug as a life span extender and a memory enhancer.

The treatment of choice in Parkinson's disease, deprenyl also has been said to improve cognition in some patients, improving attention, memory and reaction times. The disease has a much slower progression in newly diagnosed Parkinson patients who receive deprenyl.

Deprenyl is chemically related to phenylethylamine, a substance found in chocolate, and to amphetamine. A monoamine oxidase (MAO) inhibitor, deprenyl can correct the age-related decrease in neurotransmitters. Deprenyl is the only drug that researchers know that stimulates the substantia nigra, a tiny brain region rich in dopamine-using brain cells. (A deficiency of dopamine can result in Parkinson's symptoms.) But degeneration of the neurons in the substantia nigra also has been associated with the aging process.

Therefore, deprenyl protects against the age-related degeneration of the substantia nigra and the nervous system.

In an Italian study, administration of the drug to ten Alzheimer's patients improved memory, attention and language ability compared to those who received a placebo. Another study of 20 Alzheimer's patients for six months also showed significant improvements in memory and attention. A third study of verbal memory and deprenyl in Alzheimer's disease showed a significant improvement in verbal memory and improved information-processing abilities and learning strategies at the moment of acquisition.

Deprenyl was more effective than OXIRACETAM, another drug being tested for use with Alzheimer's patients, at improving higher cognitive functions and reducing impairment in daily living, and better short- and long-term memory and attention. Other studies also found deprenyl to be slightly more effective than ACETYL-L-CARNITINE and more effective than PHOSPHATIDYLSERINE in measures of cognition in Alzheimer's disease patients.

depression and memory   Severe depression is accompanied by physical symptoms, such as sleep disturbances and loss of interest in food and sex— but it is also associated with a memory deficit that is in some ways similar to the loss shown by some patients with schizophrenia and by those with lesions in the frontal lobe. Depression alters brain chemistry in a way that slows absorption and emergence of information, lowering the level of attention and reducing the capacity to concentrate.

Depressed individuals have trouble remembering recent and sometimes past events. Other memory processes most impaired by depression include recall of positive words (that are incongruent with the subjects' mood), immediate recall and recognition of verbal stimuli. One day a depressed person's memory may work well, and the next day the person can't remember anything. Depressed people can't concentrate, and they feel confused and bewildered. Some depressed patients may ramble, finding it hard to keep to one topic.

Studies have shown that depressed subjects can remember incidental information, but they are not so good at storing information that requires more focused attention. In a study testing the memory of 32 depressed patients, 32 normals and 32 diabetics (with a mean age of 66 to 68), Palo Alto Veterans Hospital researchers found that depressed patients tended to use more passive approaches to remembering. They did not use semantic clustering as often as did the other subjects. (Semantic clustering involves remembering similar words together.)

Especially among older subjects, there was a correlation between poorer performance on memory tests and the physical symptoms of depression (sleepiness, appetite loss, problems in getting started in the morning). Those who reported negative feelings during the memory test also tended to do more poorly.

Depression so closely mimics SENILE DEMENTIA (characterized by forgetfulness, confusion and behavioral changes) that it is often diagnosed as PSEUDODEMENTIA.

However, depression usually is caused by some sort of loss—a spouse, self-esteem, status, job or health. One report indicates that depression is so prevalent among those aged 65 and over that 13 percent need intervention. Still, although depressive illness is serious, it is no bigger a problem in later life than in earlier stages.

Depression, whether present alone or in combination with dementia, can be reversed with proper treatment, which usually includes some type of cognitive therapy. Therefore, a good diagnosis is important. Unfortunately, many physicians still don't know what signs to look for and, as a result, often diagnose senile dementia instead of depression. The difference between the two diagnoses are important: A depressed person will anguish over forgetfulness, whereas a senile person will try to hide it; a depressed person makes little effort to perform tasks, whereas a senile person will struggle to perform well.

depth of processing   Mental processes and strategies such as IMAGE ASSOCIATION, visualization, verbal elaboration, review and summarization that are indispensable to the recording of a good memory trace.

detail salience   How memorable a detail is. When a person sees a complex event, not all the details are equally memorable. Some things catch a person's attention more quickly than others: Colorful, extraordinary, novel and interesting scenes attract our attention and hold our interest. Both attention and interest are important in the encoding of memories. Boring, routine, common or insignificant circumstances are rarely remembered as specific incidents.

Interestingly, witness estimates of time, speed and distance are often inaccurate, and speed is especially difficult to estimate. In one study administered to air force personnel who knew beforehand that they would be questioned about the speed of a moving auto, estimates ranged from 10 to 50 miles an hour. The car actually had been going only 12 miles an hour. In estimates of time, most witnesses overestimate the amount of time an event took. (See also AGE AND EYEWITNESS ABILITY; MEMORY FOR EVENTS.)

DHEA   See DEHYDROEPIANDROSTERONE (DHEA).

diabetes and memory   Older people with diabetes may have more problems with memory and concentration than those without the disease. In fact, one study showed that not only do diabetic women over age 65 have twice the risk for a decline in memory and thinking abilities, they lose these abilities more quickly than do healthy women of the same age.

Scientists aren't sure how diabetes affects mental acuity. It may be linked to the fact that diabetics also tend to have a higher risk for stroke and vascular disease, which can have an impact on how well the brain functions.

diencephalic amnesia   A type of permanent, global AMNESIA caused by lesions in the DIENCEPHALON caused by accident or illness. It usually appears as a result of KORSAKOFF'S SYNDROME.

This type of memory loss selectively impairs some aspects of memory while leaving others alone. Patients will score normally on IQ tests but will not do nearly so well on clinical memory tests. They have particular problems in remembering new information, buy they can understand sentences—they just can't repeat them after a certain period of time. Skills that were learned before the lesions appeared are unaffected.

Controversy continues as to whether this type of amnesia and MEDIAL TEMPORAL AMNESIA are separate syndromes or the same type of amnesic syndrome. (See also AMNESIC SYNDROME.)

diencephalon   An area in the uppermost part of the brain stem that includes the THALAMUS; it connects via the FORNIX to the TEMPORAL LOBES. The diencephalon and the MEDIAL TEMPORAL LOBE are the two structures that are crucially concerned with memory. The diencephalon is one of the structures most commonly involved in KORSAKOFF'S SYNDROME, and tumors found on the third ventricle (a part of the diencephalon) usually cause memory disorders. In fact, AMNESIA following damage to the diencephalon (from disease, neurosurgery, head injury, stroke or the deprivation of oxygen) is quite common.

diet and memory   While much research linking diet and memory is still inconclusive, there have been some studies that suggest a link between certain foods and memory.

Since medieval times, memory experts believed a good diet could enhance memory performance, although it was not always understood what constituted a good "memory diet." For example, 15th-century nutritionists advised citizens to eat hearty food for a good memory—roasted fowl, apples, nuts and red wine. Today, scientists have a different perspective on the role that nutrition plays in health and memory.

Scientists do know, for example, that imbalances in the diet can cause problems; a child's ability to remember is affected by iron, mineral and vitamin deficiencies, food additives, too much sugar and too little protein. And deficiencies of almost any nutrient can cause impaired nervous system function. Imbalances in certain vitamins and minerals also appear to play a part in problems with memory.

Water is also important in maintaining memory systems, especially in the elderly. Lack of water in the body has a direct and profound effect on memory, and dehydration leads to confusion and thinking problems.

Although researchers don't know exactly how nutrition affects memory, they do know that essential nutrients are important for enhancing chemical processes (such as registering, retaining and remembering information). These essential nutrients include protein, carbohydrates, lecithin and vitamin B_1.

Still, experts aren't sure if some of these foods are better at boosting memory than others. As a result, physicians advise that the best memory insurance is to eat "a good, balanced diet": a variety of dairy products, bread and cereals, vegetable and fruit, seafood, poultry or meat. Without sufficient levels of thiamine, folate and vitamin B_{12}, the brain cannot function properly, and this may lead to memory and concentration problems.

In addition, it's not a good idea to eat large amounts of food right before beginning a thinking task; loading up the stomach impairs performance and distracts the mind during the critical registration and remembering phase. For this reason, memory experts advise eating only a light meal before giving a speech, taking a test or attending class.

Some experts advocate the use of "memory nutrients" (CHOLINE, B-complex vitamins, iodine, manganese and folic acid), although other researchers argue that studies have not yet proven their efficacy.

When foods rich in choline (liver, soybeans, lecithin, eggs and fish) were fed to subjects in one study, the diet sparked an increase in ACETYL-CHOLINE, the brain neurotransmitter crucial to the memory process. When the subjects then took 10 grams of choline, they were able to recall a list of unrelated words more quickly than those who did not take choline. In other studies, ALZHEIMER'S DISEASE patients showed improved memories when treated with choline.

Vitamins Texas researchers found that rats deprived of B_6 and copper showed evidence of deteriorating dendrites (branchlike extensions that carry electrical impulses from one brain cell to the next). Researchers speculate that a mild deficiency of these nutrients over the course of years could have the same devastating effects on humans.

When researchers in New Mexico tested a group of normal subjects 60 years old and older on memory and problem-solving ability, they found that those with the lowest vitamin B_{12} and C levels did poorly on the memory test. Those with the lowest

levels of vitamins B_{12} and C, riboflavin and folate scored the worst on problem-solving tests. And common deficiencies of vitamins B_{12} and B_6 and folic acid in the elderly can impair some of the body's enzymes, which may be responsible for at least some of the memory impairment observed in older patients.

Zinc is another substance that seems to affect memory. When researchers studied more than 1,200 patients over age 55, the 220 senile people in the group had significantly lower zinc levels than those who were not senile.

Dieting At the same time, decreasing the amount of nutrients to the brain by going on a diet may affect the memory, too. Experts warn that any diet providing fewer than 2,100 calories a day for an adult is likely to be deficient in some vitamin, mineral or trace element unless the diet is carefully monitored by a physician. When a person diets, the brain (like the rest of the organs in the body) must make up a shortage of dietary nutrients by drawing on its own reserves. When those reserves are depleted, the dieter can become nervous, easily upset, clumsy, and experience memory problems.

In fact, one recent Mayo Clinic study found that healthy patients on a low-calorie diet for three months became quarrelsome, hostile and anxious, felt persecuted, had nightmares and panic attacks, experienced attention deficits and had memory problems.

digit span A technique to measure MEMORY SPAN by noting the number of randomly arranged digits that a person can repeat in the correct order immediately after hearing or seeing them. Normal subjects can recall about seven digits (plus or minus two).

Dilantin (phenytoin) This well-known treatment for epilepsy also is reputed to have a wide range of other pharmacologic effects beyond its anticonvulsant benefits. More than 8,000 studies have examined the drug in a wide variety of uses, reporting that it may improve intelligence, concentration and learning. Studies have suggested that, given twice daily, it can improve long-term memory and verbal performance in young and old alike. However, excess amounts of the drug have the opposite effect on memory, intelligence and reaction time.

In the United States, Dilantin's only approved use is to control various types of seizures, since it works by stabilizing electrical activity in cell membranes.

dimethylaminoethanol (DMAE) This naturally occurring nutrient found in some types of seafood (such as sardines) also is normally found in human brains in small amounts. According to some research, DMAE has been found to improve memory and learning, elevate mood and increase physical energy in studies of lab animals. It is said to be both a mild stimulant and a sleep enhancer.

DMAE is believed to work by speeding up the brain's production of ACETYLCHOLINE, which plays an important part in memory and maintaining memory ability in the elderly.

There are reports that overdoses of DMAE may cause insomnia, headache or muscle tension, but no serious adverse effects have been reported. It has been found, however, to deepen the depression phase in manic-depressive patients.

DMAE is considered to be a nutritional supplement and can be found under a variety of trade names in health food stores in bulk powder, capsules or liquid form.

direct priming When amnesic patients are shown a list of words and later tested on recall, they perform very poorly on "yes/no" direct recognition tests. But by providing a portion of each word that had been on the list, subjects are able to fill in the blanks and come up with the word. This effect is called *direct priming*.

Scientists believe that direct priming results from some temporary activation of information in semantic memory, which is not affected by AMNESIA. Scientists assume that everyone has an individual representation for every word we know, and exposure of a word in a learning list leads to that representation becoming more active. Therefore, it is more easily recalled than comparable words that have not been preexposed.

However, direct priming appears to be restricted to preexisting associations and has only limited value in a therapeutic setting.

dissociation An unconscious defense mechanism through which emotional significance and affect are separated and detached from an idea, situation or object. Dissociation may defer or postpone experience with some emotional impact, as in selective AMNESIA.

This splitting of the normally integrated functions of consciousness (especially identity and memory) is the defining characteristic of the DISSOCIATIVE DISORDERS, which include MULTIPLE PERSONALITY DISORDER, PSYCHOGENIC AMNESIA, psychogenic FUGUE, and depersonalization disorder.

Dissociation was first mentioned by French *alieniste* (psychiatrist) Jacques Joseph Moreau de Tours in 1845 in his book about ALTERED STATES OF CONSCIOUSNESS. The first psychological elaboration of the concept of dissociation was written in 1889 by Pierre Janet (1859–1947) in *L'Automatisme Psychologique*.

In this book, Janet describes a syndrome he calls *desegregation*, in which associated ideas split off from consciousness and exist in a parallel with the dominant stream of consciousness. Janet believed this was a pathological psychological process that occurred in HYPNOSIS, hysteria and instances of multiple personality.

The syndrome was further discussed in *Studies on Hysteria* (1895) by Sigmund Freud (1856–1939) and Josef Breuer (1842–1925), who interpreted the famous case of ANNA O. Anna, who suffered from psychosomatic problems and dissociation, had been treated for two years by Breuer. But Breuer and Freud disagreed about the nature of Anna's absences; Breuer thought they represented a form of autohypnosis, while Freud interpreted Anna's symptoms as a defense mechanism.

Freud's theory won acceptance by clinicians over the years, although Breuer's autohypnotic explanation has won converts for its explanation of early childhood creation of multiple personality. (See also BREUER, JOSEF; FREUD, SIGMUND; JANET, PIERRE.)

dissociative disorders A category of psychological disorders in which there is a sudden, temporary alteration in normally integrated function of consciousness, identity or motor behavior so that some part of one or more of these functions is lost. While the process of dissociation is common in everyday life (for example, when a person is concentrating intensely on a task and doesn't hear what is being said), in extreme cases the behavior can lead to serious problems.

The disorders were first grouped together in 1987 in the *Diagnostic and Statistical Manual of Mental Disorders,* 3rd edition, revised (DSM-III-R), with the primary symptom of DISSOCIATION. The amnesia found in these disorders is a repression of disturbing memories; once the memories are repressed, access to them is cut off temporarily. The disorders include PSYCHOGENIC AMNESIA, FUGUE, MULTIPLE PERSONALITY and depersonalization disorder.

The dissociative disorders may often be misdiagnosed as more serious disorders such as schizophrenia, but because patients do not exhibit a significant break with reality, they are not considered psychotic. The dissociative disorders also may be referred to as hysterical neuroses, dissociative type. (See also CHILD ABUSE, MEMORY OF.)

distortions, memory   Memory can be affected by a person's interests or values so that an experience is remembered the way a person *wants* to remember it. In other words, memories can be changed to fit what we want them to be or how we think they ought to be.

This theory can be tested by asking someone to repeat as many as possible of the following words that are read aloud: dream, awake, tired, bed, night, rest, sound, slumber, snore. Most people will also recall the word *sleep,* although that particular word does not appear on the list. People recall that word because most of the words on the list are related to sleep, and it seems as if that word *ought* to be on the list.

Distortion is of particular importance in the courtroom, where a leading question may cause a witness to "remember" something that did not exist. For example, asking "What color was the victim's sweater?" may cause a witness to remember a sweater that was not even worn. Statements that imply a conclusion may cause a person to remember the conclusion as if it had happened. Madison Avenue ad agencies often use this aspect of distortion to promote products without directly making false claims.

DMAE   See DIMETHYLAMINOETHANOL.

domain-specific knowledge   Information relating to a particular setting in which a patient currently experiences difficulty.

donepezil (Aricept)   One of only three drugs approved for the treatment of ALZHEIMER'S DISEASE (the other two are TACRINE and RIVASTIGMINE), donepezil is available in 5 mg or 10 mg tablets and is usually given at bedtime with or without food. Individuals with Alzheimer's have generally responded well to this drug, showing improvement in cognition, general function and behavior.

The drug works by blocking an enzyme that destroys acetylcholine. Animal tests suggest that it might also make a difference in less serious memory disorders; the National Institute on Aging is embarking on a study to determine if Aricept can help people with mild cognitive impairment. Fifty percent of people over age 65 with MCI will develop Alzheimer's within five years.

Side Effects
Although many patients can better tolerate Aricept, it can cause diarrhea and vomiting, nausea, insomnia, fatigue and anorexia. These effects are mild in most cases and usually last from one to three weeks, declining with continued use of the drug.

dopamine   A chemical messenger in the brain and a member of the class of catecholamines. Dopamine is a neurotransmitter that appears to play some role in memory and thinking. (See NEUROTRANSMITTERS AND MEMORY.) Dopamine receptors decrease by 6 percent for each decade of life, beginning at age 20. As dopamine receptors decrease, so does brain activity. Compensating for this loss might help restore mental sharpness, some experts believe.

dreams and memory   While all humans dream, the ability to remember dreams varies a great deal from one person to the next. Some people have such poor memories for their dreams that they insist they never dream. In fact, however, research has revealed that every human being dreams during regular periods of each night, as evidenced by rapid eye movement (REM) when the eyelids flicker and the entire body may move.

People can be taught to recall their dreams. The first step is actually retrieving the dream itself. This can be done by "setting" the mind before sleep by one saying gently and firmly, "I will remember my dream." This prompts the brain to give priority to the recall of the dream on awakening. It may take up to three weeks of such training before dreams can be remembered with regularity.

Studies suggest that older subjects dream less than younger people do and therefore have fewer dreams to report. This may be due in part to the decline of spontaneous mental imagery related to old age; however, the ability to form mental images is a skill that can be improved with practice at any age.

drugs and memory   There are a number of drugs that interfere with memory. Any medication that causes drowsiness is capable of affecting memory. Almost all psychotropic drugs can interfere with certain components of memory, including the benzodiazepines, neuroleptics, antidepressants and lithium, although these different drug classes may not cause the same type of memory deficit. In fact, all drugs in the same class don't all cause the same type or amount of memory loss. For example, one type of antidepressant that interferes with serotonin reuptake may improve memory, compared to the tricyclic antidepressants that interfere with memory.

Neurological drugs have been less extensively studied. All the older anti-epileptic drugs are considered harmful, unlike the novel compounds Vigabatrin and Lamotrigine. Drugs used in the treatment of PARKINSON'S DISEASE should be considered as memory-enhancing, unlike the atropine derivatives, which typically induce AMNESIA.

Many substances not used in neuropsychiatry also may cause memory problems, including quinidine, naproxen, opiates, antibiotics like clioquinol or the quinolones, antihistamines and interferons.

The best-known of all drugs that affect memory is ethanol (the alcohol contained in alcoholic beverages). Ethanol interferes with the capacity to learn, and slows down mental functions that create defective recording and storing of memory.

Other drugs that can affect memory include antihypertensives (blood pressure drugs), painkillers, insulin, beta blockers (especially those used to control glaucoma), methyldopa, seasickness patches and certain anti-epileptic drugs.

duplex theory of memory   The idea that short-term and long-term memory are fundamentally different systems.

dyslexia and memory   A specific reading disability characterized by poor verbal memory and problems in coping with written symbols. Research suggests that problems in encoding are the cause of a dyslexic person's problems with verbal memory. Other theories have pointed to a specific, sometimes inherited, neurological disorder, emotional disturbance, minor visual defects or a lack of attention. Some scientists using clinical tests of many more memory measures have challenged the long-held view that verbal memory problems of dyslexic children are related to their attention span, memory strategy use or ability to retrieve memories. But the relationship between verbal memory and reading problems is still unclear.

In a Nova University study of 122 children eight to ten years old, the dyslexic subjects differed from normals only in their ability to encode words—to store the word in memory when they hear it. Both dyslexic and normal children had the same attention spans.

While some researchers had believed that dyslexic subjects' memory problems are actually a retrieval problem (they encode the words, but then can't recall them), researchers found that both normal and dyslexic children improved at the same rate when given memory cues, indicating that retrieval is not a problem.

Symptoms
Some 90 percent of dyslexics are male; most of the time, their intelligence is normal but the attainment of reading skills lags far behind other abilities and overall IQ. Usually dyslexic children can read musical notes or numbers much more easily than letters. While many children in the first two ele-

mentary grades make common mistakes in reversing letters or words, dyslexic children continue to make these errors. Letters are transposed ("saw" for "was") and spelling errors are common. Writing from dictation may be hard, although most can copy sentences.

Treatment

Early diagnosis is critical in maintaining a child's self-esteem and to avoid any added frustrations. Specific remedial methods can help the child develop tricks to cope with the disorder, and praise for success is crucial. With the right support and training, dyslexics can usually overcome their problems.

dysmnesia/dysmnesic syndrome General intellectual impairment secondary to defects of memory and orientation.

dysphasia A disturbance in the ability to select the words with which to speak and write, comprehend and read. Dysphasia is caused by damage to regions of the brain concerned with speech and comprehension. (See also AGRAPHIA; ALEXIA; APHASIA; APRAXIA.)

Ebbinghaus, Hermann E. (1850–1909) The father of the psychological study of memory, this German pioneer proposed three basic questions: How much information can we store, how fast can we acquire it and how long can we keep it? To this day, many psychology labs still use his basic method of testing memory for lists.

Ebbinghaus began the first modern systematic study of memory in 1879, using himself as his subject in research designed to test the above questions by first inventing a string of nonsense syllables (two consonants with a verb in between) and then reciting them in sequence to see how many repeats he needed before he could memorize them. Ebbinghaus assumed that memory involved the storage of items somewhere in the brain and that remembering required a person to reproduce the information using accurate recall. In his studies, Ebbinghaus refused to use any methods (he called them tricks) to make recall easier, hoping to study natural (not artificial) memory.

Ebbinghaus discovered that he learned at a constant rate, and the more often he repeated the syllables to himself, the better he could remember them. He also discovered that he could remember much better if he studied first thing in the morning than if he studied at 4 P.M., and he concluded that fatigue affected memory. Moreover, after mastering lists of these nonsense syllables, the number of syllables he could remember fell off in a predictable way. This enabled Ebbinghaus to fit a logarithmic curve to the retention as a function of time.

His studies led him to describe three possible ways we forget:

1. INTERFERENCE THEORY: Early memories basically get buried by later-memorized ones.

2. TRACE DECAY: Memories undergo changes over time that affect their nature.

3. Forgetting occurs when memories "fall apart" and crumble into parts, where separate components are lost.

Ebbinghaus's work led to the publication in 1885 of his classic book, *On Memory*, which opened up the study of memory as an experimental problem. In the book he charted the decay of memories and suggested that a great deal of information is forgotten immediately after it is acquired. If the information is remembered for as long as a day or two, he wrote, it is likely to be retained for a much longer period.

The basic style of learning that Ebbinghaus described could be called rote learning, or verbal list learning. Modern researchers understand, however, that what Ebbinghaus was really studying was rote learning *without arousal;* in other words, factual memory for events that have no emotional importance. And because rote learning without arousal is a poor way to construct memory, it is not surprising that Ebbinghaus and his colleagues concluded that memory doesn't work very well or endure for a very long time.

While Ebbinghaus developed his technique as a way of sidestepping problems in memory study, the technique limited his ability to understand memory. He believed that memory was simply a storage bin for objective items that were either retained or not—a point of view that eventually was challenged by psychologists who believed that subjective factors are also vital to memory systems. (See also BARTLETT, SIR FREDERIC C.)

Eccles, Sir John Carew (1903–1997) The Nobel Prize-winning Australian scientist who was one of the 20th century's pioneers in discovering and exploring how messages are transmitted in the brain and nervous system. Eccles showed that the excitement of a nerve cell causes one kind of SYNAPSE to release a neurotransmitter into the next cell that expands the pores in nerve membranes. (See NEUROTRANSMITTERS.) These expanded pores allow sodium ions to pass into the neighboring cell, reversing the polarity of electric charge, which is conducted from one cell to another as a nerve impulse.

Sir John, an Australian-born former college pole-vaulter, pursued scientific study and research in Australia, Britain, New Zealand and the State University of New York at Buffalo, before moving to Switzerland. Sir John, who shared the 1963 Nobel Prize in physiology or medicine, tackled some of the most fundamental problems of his time, working toward an ultimate understanding of the mind and consciousness. His Nobel Prize was awarded for his discovery of the chemical means by which impulses are communicated or suppressed by nerve cells.

Sir John was born Jan. 27, 1903, in Melbourne, the son of teachers. By age 18, he had acquired an interest in the link between the action of the brain and the nature of consciousness. After graduating in medicine from Melbourne University, he went on a Rhodes Scholarship to Oxford University to study under one of the great figures in brain research, Sir Charles Sherrington, who is credited with coining the term *synapse*. After research in the 1930s with Sir Charles on switching on and off of nerve impulses, Sir John returned home. During World War II, he was involved in medical work in behalf of his country's military effort. His early work focused on cells in the spinal cord that control the action of muscles; later he moved closer to the centers of consciousness in the brain.

Sir John stood out among the scientists who produced the growing modern appreciation of the chemical mechanisms underlying the action of the brain and nervous system. He did not consider the brain and the mind to be the same thing. He believed he could explain his own body and brain, he once said, but he could not explain his own existence. The complexity of the brain so impressed Eccles that he called the mind the so-called ghost in the machine, an incorporeal essence in the body.

Sir John was knighted by Queen Elizabeth II in 1958 and held many other honors. His marriage to Irene Frances Miller, with whom he had nine children, ended in divorce after 40 years. He later married scientist Helena Taborikova.

echoic memory   The registration of sounds. This form of memory lasts up to four seconds. The long-term form of echoic memory is called AUDITORY MEMORY.

EEG   See ELECTROENCEPHALOGRAM.

effortful processing   Effortful encoding and retrieval of memory. This effortful processing uses a great deal of attentional capacity and therefore disrupts—and is disrupted by—the simultaneous performance of another attention-demanding task. Effortful processing probably always requires planning, therefore it is likely to be damaged by frontal cortex lesions that disrupt the ability to plan.

ego   One of the three major divisions in the psychoanalyst's model of the psychic apparatus; the others are the id and the superego. The ego represents the sum of certain mental mechanisms, including memory, and specific defense mechanisms. It mediates between the demands of primitive instinct (the id) and of internalized parental and social prohibitions (the superego).

eidetic memory   Similar to the idea of "photographic memory," an eidetic ("identical" or "duplicative") image is a very strong afterimage that allows a person to duplicate a picture mentally and describe it in detail after looking at it. Among children the ability to form eidetic images is rare (no more than 10 percent of children have the ability), and it is even rarer after adolescence. An eidetic image may be a MEMORY, FANTASY or dream.

An eidetic person not only can imagine an object that isn't there, but behaves as if it really can be seen, either with closed eyes or while looking at some surface that serves as a convenient background for the image. While a particular object can be recalled eidetically immediately after its disappearance or after a lapse of minutes, days or years, spontaneously appearing eidetic images also have been reported. Sometimes eidetic images and the objects they represent have different colors, forms, size, position and richness of detail, or the objects may be reproduced in almost photographic detail and fidelity.

Most experts suspect that eidetic imagery is not a different kind of visual memory, but just a greater skill in the ability to form visual images that everyone has to some degree.

While eidetic imagery is most likely the source of the concept of a photographic memory, there are differences in the two concepts. An eidetic image fades soon after one sees the original image and does not stay with a person over time. The image is subjective, and the details of greatest interest to the person are the ones most easily reproduced. Moreover, a person can't form an eidetic image in one second, as a camera can snap a photo; several seconds are required to scan the picture. Once the picture has faded away, eidetic images cannot be retrieved. Those who can form eidetic images don't seem to be able to use their special ability to improve long-term memory.

Phenomena corresponding to visual eidetic images are believed to exist in other sense fields as well, but research has not uncovered much about their nature, causes and significance.

elaboration The formation of a more richly encoded memory trace or ENGRAM that is more easily accessible because there are many different ways of contacting it in the process of retrieving a memory. Elaboration is an unconscious process of expansion and embellishment of detail, especially with reference to a symbol or representation in a dream. To consolidate a memory trace for long-term storage, a person needs to observe, analyze and judge.

electrical stimulation of the brain Stimulating various areas of the cortex produces a range of responses from patients; however, only stimulation of the temporal lobes elicits meaningful, integrated experiences, including sound, movement and color, far more detailed, accurate and specific than normal recall.

Stimulating one side of the brain may bring back a certain song to one patient, the memory of a moment in a garden listening to a mother calling her child to another. Interestingly, stimulating the same point in the brain elicits the same memory every time. (See also EMOTIONS AND MEMORY; PENFIELD, WILDER.)

electroconvulsive therapy (ECT) and memory
ECT therapy is a controversial therapy still used in psychiatric treatment to induce a seizure, most often in cases of severe depression; it also can cause a temporary memory loss. The question of whether ECT affects memory permanently is still debated.

In ECT therapy, patients are given an anesthetic and a muscle relaxant before two padded electrodes are applied to the temples. A controlled electric pulse is delivered to the electrodes until the patients experience a brain seizure. Treatment usually consists of six to 12 seizures (two or three a week).

After the treatment, patients usually experience a period of confusion, which they do not remember afterward; there is usually also a brief period of AMNESIA covering the time right before the treatment. On regaining consciousness, patients who have received ECT are similar in many ways to those who have experienced posttraumatic amnesia. Typically, patients first regain their personal identity followed by the knowledge of where they are; orientation in time occurs last of all.

Tests of memory after ECT reveal a substantial memory impairment in addition to a clear ANTEROGRADE AMNESIA. However, after a number of treatments some patients say they experience a more serious memory loss, involving everyday forgetfulness, which usually disappears within a few weeks after treatment. Critics of ECT claim, however, that it produces more substantial effects on memory.

New research suggests that ECT administered to only one side of the head produces equally beneficial results to the more standard method without any accompanying memory loss.

The origins of ECT are thought to lie in the ancient Roman tradition of applying electric eels to the head as a cure for madness; mild electric shocks have been used since the late 1700s to treat illness. A machine using weak electric currents was used in Middlesex Hospital in England in 1767 to treat a range of illnesses, and at the same time London brain surgeon John Birch used a machine to shock the brain of depressed patients.

At about the same time, American inventor and patriot Benjamin Franklin was shocked into unconsciousness—and suffered a RETROGRADE AMNESIA—during one of his electricity experiments; he is said to have recommended electric shock for the treatment of mental illness.

However, the modern practice of electric shock treatment for the treatment of depression and mental illness is less than 65 years old. A Hungarian psychiatrist noted a number of studies reporting that schizophrenia and epilepsy did not occur in the same patient and wondered if an artificially induced seizure might cure schizophrenia. While the seizures were originally induced through the use of camphor and other drugs, Italian psychiatrist Ugo Cerletti and colleagues explored the possibility of using electric shock to achieve similar results. Cerletti's idea was considered an improvement over the drug-induced seizures, which were associated with toxic side effects.

The first patient to receive ECT to treat schizophrenia received it on April 15, 1938. Because it was simple and inexpensive, the use of ECT spread, and by the 1950s it was the primary method of treatment for schizophrenia and depression. The discovery of neuroleptic drugs led to a substantial decline in its use.

The controversy surrounding ETC is likely to continue for some time, and the question of whether ECT affects permanent memory remains unclear. Many studies that have examined long-term experience with ECT and controlled for influence of other factors indicate that ECT doesn't have any extensive effect on permanent memory function. All patients show some amount of retrograde amnesia for events immediately before ECT itself.

Some scientists believe that some patients may falsely conclude that their memory is impaired. In one study, scientists found significant differences between patients who reported memory problems and those who didn't. Those who complained tended to believe the ECT hadn't helped their depression, which could mean that their own assessment of memory might be the result of their continuing illness. Three years after treatment, this group insisted their memory problems, which they believed were of an amnesic type, remained—even though there was no objective proof of this. Researchers believe that these patients' initial experience of true amnesia immediately following ECT might have caused them to question whether their memory function had really recovered.

Still, in elderly depressive patients ECT can worsen their decline in the presence of DEMENTIA, and ECT can be abused as a treatment. Even ECT proponents admit adverse reactions to the treatment are possible, although estimates of how great a risk exists vary.

electroencephalogram (EEG)   One of the first brain-monitoring techniques, EEGs chart the electrical activity of the brain through electrodes attached to the scalp. An EEG can uncover brain abnormalities because each brain region has its own characteristic pattern of electrophysiological activity. An EEG averages the electrical activity from a large area of the brain and is a valuable means of diagnosing epilepsy. However, the test is of limited use in locating specific areas of brain damage.

A more recent addition to the EEG arsenal is the quantitative EEG (qEEG). A quantitative EEG is different from an EEG in that the signals from the brain are played into a computer, digitized and stored. This type of EEG can measure the time delay between two regions of the cortex, for example, and the amount of time it takes for information to be transmitted from one region to another. (See also BRAIN SCANS; COMPUTERIZED TOMOGRAPHY (CT) SCAN; MAGNETIC RESONANCE IMAGING; PET.)

emotions and memory   Emotions play a complex negative and positive role in the formation of memory. Emotions are so powerful that they can seal a memory trace, protecting it from the passing years. It is for this reason that we remember most vividly what touches our heart and our spirit.

The idea that emotions and memory were intertwined has been a popular belief for centuries. Scientists as early as Sir Francis Bacon (1561–1626) believed that events associated with strong emotions (whether good or bad) were remembered more easily than those that aroused little emotion.

The idea appealed to Sigmund Freud, who blamed REPRESSION for the selective memory of some things. According to Freud, a person "forgets" (or represses) information or memories that would cause anxiety. Freud's ideas about repression usually were drawn from psychoanalytical interviews with the mentally ill, but he also believed that normal people repressed information.

Today scientists believe that emotions are essential for creating and filing memories away; in fact, both perception and recollection seem to require the aid of the limbic system (seat of the emotions). If the limbic area is damaged, thereby interfering with emotion and memory, the patient experiences confusion, automatism and AMNESIA. Of course, the activation of the limbic system alone is not enough to give a true sensation of memory.

Interestingly, some studies suggest that emotion exerts state-dependent effects on retrieval. That is, a person's mood experienced at the time of an event becomes a part of that memory of the event, and retrieving that memory is easier if the person's mood when trying to remember is similar to that associated with events he or she is trying to recall. In the study, scientists read stories to hypnotized subjects about a sad character and a happy character when half the subjects were in a happy mood and half in a sad mood. They found that most subjects remembered more facts about the character that was consistent with their mood while listening to the story. (See also FREUD, SIGMUND; HEDONIC SELECTIVITY; RESPONSE BIAS.)

encephalitis and memory   Encephalitis (inflammation of the brain) is an often-fatal viral disease that damages the brain on both sides, especially the MEDIAL TEMPORAL LOBE and the orbital frontal lobe, and often causes a form of AMNESIA resulting from brain damage. Encephalitis may be caused by several different viruses, but the herpes simplex virus is the most common cause.

The amnesia in patients with this disorder is probably caused by the destruction of the HIP-POCAMPUS and AMYGDALA, whereas the poor recall for previously well-established memories that these patients have been reported to show may be caused by destruction of the temporal association neocortex. Some patients also may suffer damage to the frontal lobes and in extreme cases show symptoms of the KLÜVER-BUCY SYNDROME, which causes a range of symptoms including amnesia, visual AGNOSIA and altered sexual behavior.

Another cause of postencephalic amnesia is a virus transmitted to humans by mosquitoes, which causes an illness called St. Louis encephalitis. In addition, an increasing number of cases are caused by infection with HIV (human immunodeficiency virus), the organism responsible for AIDS.

A form of brain inflammation called acute inclusion body encephalitis can cause a severe and persistent memory defect that resembles KORSAKOFF'S SYNDROME, except that the patient usually recognizes the memory problems and does not lie about the condition.

encoding   The process by which information is translated into electrical impulses in the brain. In order for a new memory trace (engram) to be formed, information must be translated into this code.

There are two main kinds of encoding—maintenance and elaborative encoding. *Maintenance encoding* consists of repeating word chunks over and over, which is good for recognition but usually is not enough for recall. *Elaborative encoding* may take several forms:

- Reorganizing chunks by classifying and categorizing them so that they can be associated more easily with ideas already held in long-term memory
- Associating chunks with images
- Changing chunks for easier repetition (for example, changing them into rhymes)
- Noting distinctive features of a chunk
- Rehearsing and self-testing

Encoding can be understood best by looking at how a person remembers words—visually, acoustically or semantically (having to do with meaning).

Because of the multifaceted nature of words, there is some flexibility in how they can be represented in memory. If a person wanted to memorize the word *chair*, for example, the brain could devise a code based on visual, acoustic or semantic properties (or a combination of any or all three).

encoding deficit theories   There are two general types of theories regarding encoding deficits: The problem is either a failure of effortful processing or a failure of automatic processing. Proponents of the first theory believe that AMNESIA resulting from "effortful processing" failures is caused by a failure to pay adequate attention to the meaningful aspects of stimuli and that amnesics encode at a shallow level.

encoding specificity   A theory stating that memory retrieval is enhanced when the original encoding situation is reinstated at the time of recall. Therefore, if the recall (or test situation) is similar to the situation present during the original learning, more information will be retrieved. (See also PQRST METHOD.)

endogenous brain damage   Brain damage that occurs as the result of a disease process, stroke, aneurysm and so on. A brain tumor, or ALZHEIMER'S DISEASE, would be considered endogenous brain damage.

It is the opposite of EXOGENOUS BRAIN DAMAGE, which might be caused by a head injury.

engram   Also known as a memory trace, an engram is the physical basis of memory, a unit of information encoded as a pattern of lowered resistance to electrical impulses or an increased readiness to respond to neurotransmitters. (See NEUROTRANSMITTERS AND MEMORY.) Engrams are presumed to persist in a network of nerve cells as the result of the consolidation of memory.

Memories seem to be encoded in the brain's cells (neurons), which convert chemical signals to electrical signals and then back to chemical signals again. Each neuron receives electrical impulses through dendrites, whose tiny branches direct signals into the body of the cell. When some of the arriving signals stimulate the neuron, others inhibit it; if there are enough stimulating signals, the neuron fires, sending its own pulse down its axon, which connects by a synapse into the dendrites of other cells.

Electrical pulses carry information inside a neuron; once the signal reaches the end of the axon, neurotransmitters carry it across the synaptic gap. On the other side of the synapse is another dendrite, containing "receptors," which recognize the neurotransmitters. If enough signals are registered, the second cell fires. A single neuron can receive signals from thousands of other neurons, and its axon can branch repeatedly, sending signals to thousands more.

While researchers have long understood the mechanism of neurons, only recently have they begun to understand how these cells might be able to store memories. Most agree that when a person experiences a new event (such as meeting a new person), a unique pattern of neurons (an engram) is activated in some way, and within the entire configuration of brain cells, certain ones light up.

In order to store this memory of the new person, there must be a way to save the memory—to forge connections between neurons to create a new circuit that acts as a symbol of something in the outside world. By reactivating the circuit, the brain can retrieve the memory—a replica of the original perception.

We would recognize the person again when we encountered something that evoked a neural pattern similar to one that was already stored in the brain. Seeing a picture of that person in a photo album might cause the lighting up of a pattern of neurons that resembled the patterns joined together during the initial introduction. The brain would detect the similarity and there would be a pleasant shock of recognition.

Unlike the wiring in appliances at home, the brain's circuits are not permanent but malleable; as knowledge is acquired, circuits break up and form new connections, constantly rewiring themselves and influencing our representations of the world. Scientists believe that ideas are formed in the same way. The neural circuit forming the concept of "table," for example, would preserve the overlapping features of each of the many different types of tables stored in memory.

For a memory as complex as a person's wedding day, the engram would not be stored in one tiny place in the brain, but would be encoded within the vast weblike structure of neurons sprawling throughout the brain.

Engrams are formed on tasks we must perform over and over again, such as threading a needle; to thread the needle, the person must activate the appropriate engram. The motor area of the brain then reads this engram, and the person threads the needle. When someone has trouble getting the thread through the eye, sensory signals from the fingers don't match the information stored in the engram; this triggers the brain to send out more signals so that the sensory signals sent back by the fingers now match the engram. This is how we store the ability to perform skills precisely over and over. Engrams are not constructed quickly; the more complex the activity, the more time and rehearsal it takes to form a reliable engram.

Not all memories are stored in the same way, so that not all memories are remembered equally well. Certain memories have left stronger or weaker traces, depending on how they were used. What remains in long-term memory has been used many times, recalled and stored differently with multiple references that allow the trace to be systematically integrated.

Every time a memory is recalled, it appears in a different context and is altered by the new recall; some elements have been expanded at the expense of others. The more time that has elapsed, the greater the chance that the memory trace has been manipulated.

Scientists weren't sure whether an original memory trace is overwritten or displaced, whether a new memory blends old and new attributes or whether the original memory and a memory of the new postevent information both exist at the same time. Recent research at Rutgers University has found that original memories can be overwritten, but only if new information is presented immediately afterward. Given the specificity of early memories and the strong contextual constraints on their retrieval, scientists think that early memories of unique events that were protected from modification are quite likely to be accurate reflections of events as the child originally perceived them.

From the time of Plato up to the 19th century, scientists believed that memories were stored permanently in the mind. In fact, for many years scientists thought that engrams were stored in a specific place in the brain. Neurological researcher Karl Lashley was searching for this specific area when he began a series of experiments in the 1920s. He trained rats to run mazes, cut out snippets of their brain tissue and then set the rats loose in the mazes again. After operating on hordes of rats, Lashley could not find one single place in the brain where the memory of the maze existed.

Not surprisingly, the more bits of brain he cut away, the more problems the rats had running a maze—but it didn't seem to matter *what* portion of the brain he cut out. Eventually Lashley gave up trying to map the location of memory in the brain, believing that memory existed everywhere, disseminating like smoke throughout the folds and fissures of the brain.

By the 1950s, neuroscientists turned to new metaphors in their search for an understanding of memory. Using laser beams, scientists created eerie three-dimensional photographs called holograms that, when cut apart, retained the entire image in each fragment. Neurologists began to wonder whether this might be the way the brain retained memories, with each tiny neuron containing the entire memory of the animal.

Into this ideological fray stepped Canadian surgeon Wilder Penfield, who stumbled upon evidence during open brain surgery that seemed to show that engrams could be activated and replayed like records on a stereo. What Penfield found amazing was that when he touched an electrode in a specific spot, the patient would instantly become aware of everything that was in his memory during an earlier time. Sometimes these memories were visual, sometimes aural—but the memory stopped when the electrode was removed and replayed if the electrode was replaced without delay. Some scientists argued that what Penfield was activating were not memories at all but hallucinations.

As the computer rose to popularity at the end of the 20th century, the idea that memories could be stored as engrams in specific locations became popular once more, since this is the way computers store memory. Other researchers began to wonder if—based on the double helix structure of DNA—memory might be stored within molecules in the brain. If molecules could encode genetic information, these scientists argued, it seemed logical that they could record memories in the same fashion. Scientists began studying the nucleic acids adenine, cytosine, thymine and guanine, molecules that carry the blueprint for making enzymes and proteins. Other scientists argued that memories might lie not in nucleic acids but in amino acids that make up protein chains.

Scientists believe that engrams (memory traces) are encoded in the neurons throughout the brain, a theory that encompasses both Lashley's and Penfield's ideas. And like any circuit, touching one part of it with an electrode could produce the entire memory. (See also NEURON; PENFIELD, WILDER.)

epilepsy   A disorder marked by recurrent seizures or temporary alteration in one or more brain functions. Temporal lobe epilepsy, which is a type of partial seizure of the brain, may result in uncontrollable flashbacks to distant memories.

Surgery to remove temporal lobe tissue that produces symptoms of epilepsy may cause a degree of memory defect. Operations on the dominant temporal lobe often interfere with the ability to learn verbal information by hearing or reading and may last for as long as three years after surgery.

In a series of operations during the mid-1950s, surgeons removed the medial temporal lobe in ten epileptic patients in order to lessen seizures. While the operations were successful, eight of the ten suffered pronounced memory deficits. The most famous of these patients was known as HM, whose AMNESIC SYNDROME is considered to be among the purest ever studied. After the operation, HM was unable to remember anything other than a handful of events since the time of his operation and was described as living in the "eternal present."

The study revealed that amnesia was present only in those who had lost both the HIPPOCAMPUS and the AMYGDALA; removal of the amygdala alone did not produce amnesia.

epinephrine   Also known as adrenaline, this naturally occurring hormone may be a primary piece of the puzzle involved in locking memories in place. Produced synthetically as a drug since 1900, it is released into the bloodstream by the adrenal gland in response to signals from the autonomic nervous system triggered by stress, exercise or fear. Epinephrine increases the speed and force of the heart, allowing it to do more work, and seems to be responsible for imprinting memories indelibly in the long-term memory. In other words, people seem to remember better when their bodies are flooded with adrenaline. Some scientists suggest that hormones such as epinephrine may act as a "fixative" to lock memories of stimulating or shocking events in the brain. This could allow the brain to discard unimportant information while maintaining the important impressions we experience. On the other hand, some memories are so unpleasant that although they are retained in long-term memory, they are not available to the conscious mind. It is believed that these memories are so potentially harmful to the psyche that the brain actually guards against their recall.

Additional research also suggests that adrenaline plays an important role in regulating memory storage; it enhances memory for many different kinds of tasks, including those that train animals using rewards as well as punishment.

Some researchers have discovered that rats not capable of producing epinephrine have a poorer recall ability than their normal rat relatives. And rats injected with additional epinephrine after a learning task appear to remember it better.

Some studies also suggest that injecting epinephrine into older rats after they had learned how to run a maze improved their performance in maze running, leading to the conclusion that older people with memory problems may be deficient in epinephrine.

Epinephrine may act directly on the brain, or it may alter brain chemistry that allows another substance to travel to the brain and "fix" the memory.

However, although epinephrine appears to regulate memory storage, it is clear that the hormone itself does not pass from blood into brain cells—at least not in amounts large enough to measure. Instead, research suggests that epinephrine's action outside the brain might be responsible for modulating memory storage. Findings indicate that epinephrine release results in an increase in plasma levels of glucose, which also has been implicated in memory improvement. It appears, then, that epinephrine release may in turn initiate the release of glucose, which crosses the blood-brain barrier and affects memory storage.

Unfortunately, because epinephrine has a variety of unpleasant side effects on the heart and other body systems—especially in older patients—more research needs to be completed before it can be used as some sort of "memory enhancement" drug.

episodic memory Memories for individual episodes in someone's personal life, such as the senior prom or a first date.

According to psychologist Endel Tulving, episodic memory is one of the five major human memory systems for which reasonable evidence is now available. (The others are semantic, procedural, perceptual representation and short-term memory.) Several of these systems, according to Tulving, usually interact to perform everyday tasks. It is episodic memory that enables a person to remember personal experiences, to be consciously aware of an earlier experience in a certain situation at a certain time.

Tulving believes that episodic memory has evolved out of semantic memory, the memory system that registers and stores knowledge about the world in the broadest sense and makes it available for retrieval. Episodic memory cannot operate independently of semantic memory, although it is not necessary for encoding and storing information into semantic memory.

event factors Factors that can reduce a witness's ability to report facts accurately. Event factors include how long and how often an event was viewed, salience and type of details and violence.

Exposure Time The less time a witness has to look at something, the less accurate the perception. When an event occurs over a long period of time, a witness should be better able to recall it.

Frequency Also, the number of times a witness has to observe particular details, the better memory he or she will have of those details.

Detail Salience When a person sees a complex event, not all the details are equally salient, or memorable. Some things (color, novelty, interest) catch a person's attention more quickly than others; interesting scenes attract our attention and hold our interest. And both attention and interest are important in the encoding of memories.

On the other hand, boring, routine, common or insignificant circumstances are rarely remembered as specific incidents.

Detail Type It's important to remember that details (a person's height, weight, speed, conversational details, colors) are not all remembered equally. The estimates of time, speed and distance—especially speed—are often inaccurate. And initial inaccuracies in these details can guarantee that they also will be recalled incorrectly. Interestingly, while most people have great trouble estimating how long an event takes, their mistakes are almost always *overestimates*.

Violence Research has found that testimony about an emotionally volatile incident may be more likely to be incorrect than testimony about a less emotional incident. It is suspected that viewing a violent scene is so emotionally stressful that an eyewitness's ability to recall the events accurately is negatively influenced. (See also AGE AND EYEWITNESS ABILITY; CROSS-RACIAL WITNESS IDENTIFICATION; EYEWITNESS TESTIMONY; GENDER AND EYEWITNESS ABILITY.)

event memory The limitless capacity for images of past events, centered in the HIPPOCAMPUS and the cortex of the frontal lobes.

exercise and memory Aerobic exercise may help maintain short-term memory, particularly as it applies to general memory and verbal memory tests. This type of memory is particularly important in recalling names, directions and telephone numbers, or pairing a name with a face.

While scientists are not yet sure why aerobic exercise seems to help, researchers believe it may be due to increased oxygen efficiency to the brain or a rise in GLUCOSE metabolism. Other research suggests that exercise boosts brain-derived neurotrophic factor (BDNF), a growth factor that makes brain cells healthier. In one study, a group of 30 volunteers took an in-pool aerobics program or simply socialized or did nothing for nine weeks. In the workout group, the three-times-a-week sessions included water aerobics and some resistance training exercises. After the nine weeks, general memory tests were given to all groups. The results of this study suggest that those who become actively involved in an aerobic exercise program may be able to improve general short-term memory.

In another study, Utah researchers studied out-of-shape subjects aged 55 to 70, putting them on a four-month program of brisk walking. All participants increased their short-term memory, ability to reason and reaction time.

Other good aerobic exercises are cycling, swimming, jogging and racquet sports. For best results, these activities should be done three times a week for 30 minutes each.

exogenous brain damage   Brain damage coming from outside a person, such as through injury, as opposed to ENDOGENOUS BRAIN DAMAGE. For example, brain damage due to a gunshot wound to the head would be considered exogenous brain damage.

explicit memory   Another name for intentional recollection or declarative memory, this is one of two types of memory—the other is its opposite, IMPLICIT MEMORY.

Explicit memory differs most importantly from implicit memory in the way memories are retrieved. A person uses explicit memory when struggling to recall information, such as a person's name. Implicit memory is being used if a person's name "pops into the head" effortlessly and automatically. Research studies indicate that explicit memory declines as a person ages, in contrast to implicit memory.

Within explicit memory are specific subsystems that handle faces, names, shapes, sounds, textures—even distinct systems that remember nouns as opposed to verbs.

All of these different types of memory are ultimately stored in the furrowed outer layer of the brain's cortex, a component of the brain more complex than comparable areas in other species. Experts in brain imaging are only beginning to understand how the areas work together as a coherent whole.

The two terms were invented in 1985 by psychologists Peter Graf and Daniel Schacter of the University of Arizona, although researchers recognized that two memory systems existed five years earlier. Traditionally, memory experts have tested only explicit memory by giving subjects lists of items to recall intentionally during a study period before a test. (A test of implicit memory would require subjects to respond to questions that don't require any sort of intentional recall, but only to respond with whatever comes to mind.)

Interestingly, techniques that improve explicit memory do not improve the implicit system, and vice versa. Studies also show that amnesic patients who have serious problems with explicit memory do not show problems with implicit memory.

Researchers suspect there are two separate biological systems for implicit and explicit memory and that the implicit memory system develops first; the explicit memory system is then built onto the implicit system and, being more vulnerable, suffers from life stress.

external memory aids   A variety of techniques to help a person remember, such as notebooks, signs, electronic devices and the like.

Diaries and daily timetables are very helpful to those with memory problems, since they can store information about what patients have to do at certain times. These types of aids can help patients remember appointments, recall routines and reduce daily life activity problems. *Lists and plans* can be displayed prominently so that patients can have easy access to general information.

For those patients with both retrograde and ANTEROGRADE AMNESIA, *photos and memorabilia* can be displayed to help jog memory.

To be most effective, external memory aids must be given as close as possible to the time at which a desired act is required; it is not helpful to remind someone with memory problems in the morning of a task that must be done after dinner. The aids also must be active rather than passive—they must alert the patient to the fact that something needs to be done. And they should specify as clearly as possible what needs to be done. Therefore, the best external memory aid is a timer that can be programmed to display specific messages at set times or a simple timing device with a timetable or diary. All the patient needs to know is to check the timetable when the alarm goes off. (See also RETROGRADE AMNESIA.)

extrinsic context   Also called independent context, this term comprises both background and format awareness; it does not affect the meaningful interpretation of target information. It is the opposite of INTRINSIC CONTEXT, which is recently perceived.

Priming can occur with items that already exist in well-established memories and with items not presented before. There is some evidence that both forms of priming may be preserved in organic AMNESIA.

eyewitness testimony   If 100 people saw the same auto accident, no two reports would be identical. People who are generally anxious, neurotic or preoccupied tend to make slightly worse eyewitnesses than those who generally are not, since high arousal apparently causes witnesses to concentrate on certain details and neglect others.

According to psychologist Elizabeth Loftus, witness accuracy may be affected by stress, arousal and attention. Other factors also may influence whether an eyewitness can accurately report an occurrence: sex, age, amount of general anxiety or happiness and amount of training.

When a witness sees a serious crime or traffic accident, a range of errors can interfere with accurate recall at different stages of the event. During the actual event, the witness is affected by the amount of time the event lasted and how much stress he or she experienced. Both factors can dramatically affect a witness's ability to perceive the events accurately.

People who are highly anxious and preoccupied tend to do worse on eyewitness tasks and aren't able to identify faces as well as those who aren't as anxious. This is because high-anxiety subjects don't use as much of the information as they could be using when they initially look at a face or a scene. Those who are experiencing great life stress also have a slight tendency to perform more poorly on a test of eyewitness ability. Neurotic individuals also fared worse on tests of eyewitness ability.

The time between a complex experience such as witnessing a crime and the recollection of that event is crucial to accurately remembering facts. It is well established that witnesses are less accurate and complete in their descriptions of an event after a long interval than after a short one. Classic research in this area was performed by Hermann Ebbinghaus, who tested how well he could remember a list of nonsense syllables after an elapse of time and then how well he could relearn them. His results, which he plotted on the famous FORGETTING CURVE, proved that people forget very rapidly after an event, but that forgetting becomes more and more gradual as time goes by.

Other researchers have shown that after a year, memory will be less accurate than after a month, and after a month it will be less accurate than after a week. But it is not just time that begins to erase information held in memory, it's what goes on during that time. For example, a witness sees a car accident, but later reads in the paper that the driver had been abusing drugs. Research suggests that such new information can dramatically affect the memory of the original event, changing a witness's memory and absorbing itself into a previously acquired memory.

When witnesses see an event and later hear information that conflicts with the original memory, many will compromise, consciously or unconsciously, what they have seen with what they have heard after the fact—particularly in estimating size or remembering color.

On the other hand, it is possible to introduce nonexistent objects into a witness's recall; casually mentioning a nonexistent object during the course of questioning can increase the likelihood that a person later will report having seen that nonexistent object. It's also possible to "remember" events from the past that never happened at all.

Psychologist Jean Piaget describes his vivid childhood memory from the age of two, when his nurse saved him from abduction by kidnappers. He remembered everything, from the scratches on his nurse's face to the size of the crowd and the appearance of the policeman. However, at the age of 15 his nurse (who had since joined the Salvation Army) confessed to having made up the entire story, and returned the watch she had been given as a reward. Apparently the young Piaget had heard discussions of this event as a child and projected the story into his past in the form of a visual memory.

Sex and Eyewitness Ability   Other research has found that both men and women pay more attention to items that catch their interest, and therefore store more or better information in memory about those items, according to Loftus. In a study of 50 subjects who were tested after looking at 24 slides of a wallet-snatching incident, women were only slightly more accurate overall. But women were far more accurate than men on questions dealing with women's clothing or actions, and men were far more accurate on questions concerning the thief's appearance and the surroundings.

Age and Witness Ability   In general, recall and recognition ability improves up to about age 15 or 20, and a decline may begin to occur about age 60. In numerous cross-sectional studies comparing eyewitness ability of children of different ages, older children outperformed younger ones in most. Often this increased ability is due to the fact that older children make many fewer false identifications, which may be because older children are less

likely to guess when they aren't certain. However, it also could represent a genuine improvement in the ability to discriminate what was seen from what was not.

However, eyewitness accuracy does not continue to improve forever. Eyewitnesses over age 60 perform more poorly than do somewhat younger people, and many tasks show some decrease in performance between ages 40 and 60. But although some tasks, such as memory for details, may weaken slightly with age, other cognitive skills are maintained as people age. In addition, there are great individual differences among people. Therefore, while performance on some tasks may decline somewhat, performance on others—memory for logical relationships or the ability to make complex inferences, for example—doesn't deteriorate.

In addition, age may affect whether a witness is susceptible to potential biases and misleading information. Researchers always have believed children were both highly suggestible and particularly inaccurate.

Training   While a witness's prior knowledge and expectations can influence perception and memory, researchers found there were no significant differences between the number of true detections of people and actions between the police and civilians. (See also AGE AND EYEWITNESS ABILITY; CROSS-RACIAL WITNESS IDENTIFICATION; GENDER AND EYEWITNESS ABILITY.)

face-name association method   A type of memory system relying on visual imagery for success. The technique includes four stages. First, the subject is asked to select a distinctive feature from the face of the person to be remembered (such as flaming red-orange hair) and, second, to transform the person's name into one or two common nouns (change "Carol" into "carrot"). Third, the distinctive feature and the transformed name must be linked in some way (imagine an orange carrot), and then recall the name. Research subjects with normal memories who followed all the steps in the procedure remembered names better than did those who only selected the distinctive feature or transformed the name into a noun.

familiarity   The more a person is familiar with a topic, the easier it is to learn, remember and understand new information about it. The reason is that if a person already knows something about a subject, the new information will be more meaningful and there will be something with which to associate the new information.

Familiarity also works by the concept of *exposure;* exposure to information may result in partial learning even if a person does not intend to learn it. Therefore, young children whose parents read to them may later learn to read more easily.

fantasy   An imagined sequence of events or mental images (such as daydreams) that serve to express unconscious conflicts, to gratify unconscious wishes or to prepare for anticipated future events.

"fat lady" syndrome   A phenomenon involving the ability of overweight anesthetized patients to be aware, on some level, of disparaging remarks made about their weight to the detriment of their recovery.

In several cases, unkind remarks made during surgery of obese women appeared to be linked to unexplained heart attacks shortly after surgery. At least one lawsuit was settled out of court regarding comments about a "beached whale" by surgeons around an anesthetized obese woman. In this case, the woman suffered a range of autonomic and vegetative disorders for several days until she told her nurse that the surgeon "called me a beached whale." The operating room nurse confirmed the insult. (See also ANESTHESIA AND MEMORY.)

feeling of knowing   A subject's ability to predict whether an unrecalled item will be recognized later.

fipexide   A cerebroactive drug that has been shown in some studies to improve short-term memory. The drug appears to mildly enhance the release of DOPAMINE, the neurotransmitter critical to fine motor coordination, motivation, emotions and immune function. (See NEUROTRANSMITTERS AND MEMORY.)

In laboratory mice studies, the drug appears to consolidate new memories and improve recall. Unlike other nootropic drugs, however, fipexide must be given both before learning new material and during the recall period in order to show an improved recall.

In one double-blind study of 40 elderly patients with severe cognitive problems, fipexide improved cognition and performance, short-term memory and attention. Average improvement in cognition was estimated to be 60 percent.

first-letter cueing The use of the first letter of a word as a cue to remembering the word itself. This cueing usually employs acronyms—making a word out of the first letters of the words to be remembered. For example, it's possible to remember the Great Lakes by the acronym "HOMES" (*H*uron, *O*ntario, *M*ichigan, *E*rie, *S*uperior). Another related type of first-letter cueing is the ACROSTIC, in which the first letter in a series of words, lines or verses form a word or phrase. For example, the notes on the lines in the treble clef can be remembered by this acrostic: Every Good Boy Does Fine (EGBDF).

Because the system is so effective, most organizations and governmental bodies make use of first-letter cueing: NATO (North Atlantic Treaty Organization) or AA (Alcoholics Anonymous).

The only problem with acronyms or acrostics lies in the propensity to forget which strategy has been devised. Therefore, it's a good idea to make the association remind you of the information to be remembered. Imagine HOMES floating on the Great Lakes; when you want to think of the names of all the lakes, the image of HOMES will return to you and with it, the first letter of each lake's name.

First-letter cueing also has been used to help brain-injured patients remember names. In one case, researchers used it to teach a patient with KORSAKOFF'S SYNDROME the names of two hospital staffers. Before this try, the patient had not been able to learn one person's name in five years. The patient was told: "This person's name is John Smith. Try to remember the initials JS." The next time they met, John Smith was introduced as "John S.," and the patient was asked to remember the rest of the last name. Subsequently, each time they met the verbal cues were reduced, and the patient learned two names using this method within two weeks. (See also MEMORY FOR NAMES.)

first-letter mnemonic See ACROSTIC.

flashbacks during surgery A phenomenon of spontaneous recall of distant memories during neurosurgery, when a probe touches certain parts of the brain thought to be associated with memory storage.

The phenomenon was discovered by Wilder Penfield during neurosurgery on a conscious patient in 1933; when he electrically stimulated the brain's surface, the flashback occurred.

"The astonishing aspect of this phenomenon," Penfield wrote, "is that suddenly [the patient] is aware of all that was in his mind during an earlier strip of time. It is the stream of a former consciousness flowing again."

The flashbacks—which are profoundly vivid—cease as soon as the probe is removed from the brain, but they may be repeated many times if the electrode is replaced without too long a delay. Apparently the recall is random, since the retrieved memories are usually neither significant nor important. The patient describes the experience as being like a dream, or "seeing things." Interestingly, these "memories" are often of things the patient was not likely to have witnessed; for example, one woman saw herself during birth, feeling as if she were reliving the experience of being born, and another woman saw herself in a place where she had never been.

Of the 520 patients who received electrical stimulation of the temporal lobes (the area of the brain in which Penfield believed these memories were stored), only 40 produced "experiential responses." Later studies showed that these responses can occur only when the limbic structures, which are thought to be responsible for emotion, have been activated. If these limbic structures are not activated, then the experiential phenomena do not occur.

Other psychologists, however, disagreed with Penfield that the patients were recalling true memories, pointing out that the memories could result from reconstruction of fragments of past experience. Emotions link the ambiguous fragments of "memory" into more coherent wholes that can be related to the immediate setting, later scientists realized. The brain contains only patterns of activity, not symbols, and these patterns acquire different meanings in different contexts.

flashbulb memory A memory formed in relation to dramatic or emotionally upsetting events. The memory is sharply etched in the mind because it involves a sudden powerful emotion: shock, anger, disbelief, outrage, fury. Scientists believe that these flashbulb memories are almost certainly encoded in the brain in a different way from regular, every-day memories. Remembering the day President John F. Kennedy was shot stands out in the memory, whereas remembering the day before can be recalled only in bits and pieces, if at all. The more muted the emotion, the less powerful and enduring the memory.

fluid imbalance and memory Too much or too little water will disturb brain function, because water contains electrolytes (potassium, sodium, chloride, CALCIUM and magnesium) crucial to memory. Especially during hot weather, aging patients are particularly at risk for electrolyte-induced memory loss. The careful administration of water can have dramatic improvements on the memory loss in these patients. (See also MAGNESIUM AND MEMORY.)

folic acid and memory Scientific evidence suggests that low levels of folic acid (a B vitamin) are closely tied to psychiatric symptoms in the elderly; one study has found that elderly patients with mental disorders (especially DEMENTIA) were three times more apt to have low folic acid than others their age. Studies also suggest that among healthy aged people, those with low folic acid intake scored lower on memory and abstract thinking ability. Surprisingly, even borderline deficiencies can be harmful to the mental state, according to E.H. Reynolds, M.D., of Kings College School of Medicine in London.

Folic acid is a vitamin essential to the production of red blood cells by the bone marrow and is contained in a wide variety of food, particularly liver and raw vegetables, legumes, nuts, avocados, cereals, spinach and leafy greens. Scientists have also found that low daily doses of folic acid supplements (200 micrograms, found in 3/4 cup of cooked spinach) may lift mood and relieve depression. Normally, a well-balanced diet provides adequate amounts of folic acid. Low-dose supplements (200–500 micrograms) seem safe, experts say, but high doses require medical supervision.

Folic acid is particularly important during pregnancy, since the vitamin plays an important part in fetal growth, especially the development of the

nervous system and the formation of blood cells. Its lack during pregnancy has been linked to neural tube defects; during pregnancy, some women may need folic acid tablets to supplement their diet. Folic acid deficiency also has been linked to megaloblastic anemia, fatigue and pallor.

football and memory loss New research has found that head injuries in professional football players suggests that head trauma from the sport may lead to later neurological problems. More than half of retired players surveyed had experienced concussions; as a group, these players were more likely to have neurological complaints later in life, ranging from memory problems to numbness in their arms or legs.

Concerned that football players may suffer lasting damage from the repeated head blows and occasional concussions unavoidable in the sport, the National Football League Players Association provided the funds that allowed researchers to study 1,090 former pro players. According to the surveys, 60 percent had suffered at least one concussion during their amateur or professional careers, and 26 percent reported three or more concussions. When compared to players who had no concussions, the group with at least one head injury reported significantly more neurological symptoms, including problems with memory and concentration, confusion, speech or hearing difficulties, numbness or tingling in extremities, and headaches.

Some researchers believe loss of consciousness, motor problems and disorientation that can follow the head trauma don't signal any long-term effects on the brain, but the cumulative and long-term neurological effect of repeated blows to the head has become a major medical concern in contact sports. Many neurologists are convinced that concussions, as well as repeated blows to the head, do lasting damage. The most commonly cited anecdotal example is the "punch-drunk" syndrome of speech and movement impairments and other abnormalities seen in some retired boxers.

forensic hypnosis While experts concede that HYPNOSIS has positive uses, accepting hypnosis in the courts as virtually foolproof is dangerous. Research has shown that the brain is not some sort of 24-hour video camera on which anything that is recorded can be recalled automatically under hypnosis. In fact, witnesses can "remember" information that may be totally inaccurate, and—because of a jury's misperception of hypnosis—this testimony can carry great weight with the court. Juries can convict a person on the strength of a memory that could have been influenced by the questioning techniques of the hypnotist or by a mental quirk in the subject.

When a person wants to remember something, the memory is not plucked intact out of a "memory store" but is constructed from stored available bits of information. Gaps in the information are filled in unconsciously by inference, and when these fragments are joined together, they form memory.

But memories are often faulty. The person may not have perceived the information correctly in the first place, or the data could have been lost or disturbed. Even if the information had been perceived and stored correctly, it could be forgotten upon questioning. And the longer the time between the event and its recollection, the less accurate it will be.

It's not just the length of time that is important during this retention interval, but what occurs during that period of time—conversations the subject hears, other information uncovered, and hypnosis itself, which can supply new information or supplant information already stored by the subject.

Witnesses who are not certain about what they saw can, when hypnotized, recall the events as if they were actually there. They may relive the crime as if it were a scene on TV and become convinced that they saw and heard relevant facts—and then testify in court based not on true recollection but on their response to explicit and implicit suggestions during hypnosis.

Hypnotists try not to ask "leading questions"—but whether a question is leading or not is known only if the hypnotist knows the truth, and if the hypnotist did know the truth, hypnotizing the witness would be irrelevant. For instance, it is very easy for a hypnotist to translate the belief that the witness may have seen something into the memories of a responsive hypnotic subject.

Hypnotic intervention might actually alter memory itself, since some experts believe a memory must be evoked before it can be changed. Since the hypnotic process causes activation of memory, this process may make these memories especially subject to change.

Once a memory has been altered, there may be no practical means of distinguishing between the portions that are derived from the witness's sensory experiences and the parts that come from somewhere else.

Hypnotic intervention may help in those situations where original memories remain intact, but for memories that undergo transformation due to postevent suggestion, no technique results in successful retrieval.

In a legal context, hypnosis may interfere with the constitutional right of confrontation by making a previously uncertain witness certain, according to hypnosis expert Martin Orne. After being hypnotized, witnesses are no longer the same witnesses as they were before, especially since they now may be profoundly resistant to cross-examination. (See also MEMORY FOR EVENTS.)

forebrain   One of three major subdivisions of the brain, including both the cerebral hemispheres and the thalamus and hypothalamus.

forgetting   When the memory for a past event has not been called up for days or months, the memory itself begins to fade. Some researchers suggest that passing time actually alters the physiological basis of memory, gradually clouding and eroding the neural engram (the memory trace in the brain). Currently, no neurochemical basis of memory has been found to account for this chemical description of forgetting.

Behavioral theories suggest that forgetting may be based on the phenomena of interference: RETROACTIVE INHIBITION would mean that new learning interferes with the old memories; in PROACTIVE INHIBITION, memories interfere with the retention of information. There are many different explanations for why information may be "forgotten." Forgetting is part of the memory mechanism, because it allows concentration on one subject at a time. At some point the brain must sift, choose and eliminate some memories or else it would face a daunting overabundance of memories. This sifting, whether conscious or not, often occurs amid the tapestry of emotion. "We forget," said the poet Matthew Arnold, "because we must, not because we will."

In one study that looked at people who tended to have problems with forgetting, it was discovered that both children and adults shared common problems that explained their reduced memory performance. They tended to have shorter attention spans and a lack of awareness, they weren't spontaneously organized and they had difficulty focusing and selecting the most important elements of any information. They were passive, did not visualize well and did not set goals.

At least five main reasons can explain why we forget something: DECAY, REPRESSION, distortion, interference and cue dependency. No single explanation can account for all instances of forgetting.

Decay   Decay is one of many theories of forgetting that suggests memories leave a physical trace in the brain that gradually fades away with time after a period of non-use. Decay is believed to affect short-term memory almost exclusively.

Repression   Forgetting occurs because unpleasant memories are intentionally forgotten, or repressed.

Memory Distortions   Memory can be affected by a person's interests or values so that an experience is remembered the way a person wants to remember it. In other words, memories can be changed, or distorted, to fit what we want them to be or how we think they ought to be.

Interference Theory   The interference theory (also called retroactive inhibition) holds that forgetting may be affected more by what happens after something is learned—such as interference by other learning—than by how much time passes. It does not imply, however, that there is a limited memory capacity that pushes old information out when new data are learned. Rather, what we learn, not how much we learn, determines forgetting by interference.

Cue Dependency   Memories are cue dependent when they do not fade away or are displaced by other information; instead, the right cue must be used to retrieve the memories.

Research suggests that most forgetting occurs because we haven't used the right cue and that much other forgetting is caused by interference. In addition, studies suggest that most forgetting occurs right after the information has been learned; as time passes, the rate of forgetting slows and levels off. But material that has been learned thoroughly, or that is very important to an individual, can be remembered throughout a lifetime.

Researchers also discovered that "slow" learners don't forget any quicker than fast learners. If a slow learner is given enough time to learn something, the rate of forgetting is about the same as for a fast learner, because when it comes to forgetting, how well a person learns something is more important than how fast the information was learned. And while young people generally learn faster than the elderly, once the information has been learned, forgetting rates are about the same for both age groups.

This fact holds important implications for students. If both a fast and a slow learner are given only one hour to study a subject, the fast learner will likely perform better on a subsequent test of the material. But if the slow learner is given an extra hour or two to master the subject, that student can do just as well on the test.

It's possible to cut down on forgetting by practicing active recall during learning, by periodic reviews of the material and by overlearning the material beyond the point of bare mastery. A mechanical technique devised to improve memory is called MNEMONICS, involving the use of associations and various devices to remember particular facts. (See also CUE-DEPENDENT FORGETTING; DISTORTIONS, MEMORY; INTERFERENCE THEORY.)

forgetting curve   A graph of forgetting rates drawn by Hermann Ebbinghaus in 1885 showing that we forget very rapidly immediately after an event, but forgetting becomes more and more gradual as time passes. Ebbinghaus's classic experiment is the most often cited study that reveals the loss of retention with an elapse of time.

In his study, Ebbinghaus tested how well he could remember a list of nonsense syllables after a lapse of time and then how well he could relearn them. He plotted his results on his forgetting curve.

(See also EBBINGHAUS, HERMANN E.; EYEWITNESS TESTIMONY; MEMORY FOR EVENTS.)

fornix One of four areas of the brain associated with memory, the fornix is the bridge between the temporal lobes and the diencephalon. Some researchers believe that AMNESIA is a result of a disconnection between the fornix and MAMMILLARY BODIES. (See also LOCALIZATION OF MEMORY.)

Freeman, Walter (1895–1972) The inventor of the LOBOTOMY and a prominent neurologist, Freeman was a scion of a well-known Philadelphia medical family who had worked for many years at St. Elizabeth's Hospital in Washington, D.C. At a conference in London in 1935, Freeman met Portuguese neurologist Antonio Egas Moniz, who had been conducting psychosurgical experiments with animals and who soon began operating on humans with a procedure called LEUCOTOMY.

After studying Moniz's book on the procedure, Freeman and his partner, James Watts, performed the first American leucotomy on a depressed patient in 1936. Impatient with the procedure and convinced he could perform it faster with a minimum of preparation, Freeman adapted the technique that he began calling lobotomy. Instead of opening the skull, he inserted an ice pick through the eye socket directly into the frontal lobe. This allowed him to operate more quickly on far more patients, on an outpatient basis. By 1946 Freeman started performing the lobotomies "assembly-line style," operating on ten patients a day in his office.

Based on 80 lobotomies, Freeman and Watts published their textbook *Psychosurgery* in 1942. Before the procedure eventually faded into disrepute as dangerous and inhumane, more than 40,000 lobotomies had been performed in the United States through the 1950s.

As public sentiment turned against lobotomies and the development of psychoactive drugs made them unnecessary, Freeman left Washington in 1954 and abandoned his assembly-line lobotomies. He performed his last lobotomy at the age of 72 in Berkeley.

free recall The production of material from memory without the aid of specific cues.

freezing effect A high degree of persistence of a memory. Early comments are frozen into place in the memory and later reappear often when the witness recalls the experience. For example, when a person is asked to recall some prelearned information, statements that appear in an early recollection tend to reappear later. Therefore, when a witness reports that a bank robber carried a gun, this detail would probably appear in later recollections regardless of whether it was true or not.

The freezing effect may occur because after an event takes place but before a witness recalls that event (called the retention interval), details about the event aren't just lying in memory waiting to be recalled. Instead, the details are prone to influences, such as personal thoughts or external information. (See also AGE AND EYEWITNESS ABILITY; CROSS-RACIAL WITNESS IDENTIFICATION; EVENT FACTORS; EYEWITNESS TESTIMONY; GENDER AND EYEWITNESS ABILITY.)

Freud, Sigmund (1856–1939) A Viennese specialist in nerve and brain diseases who is best known for the creation of psychoanalysis and his theories on sexuality. Freud also was fascinated with the idea of memory, including the baffling questions of how—and why—we forget. It was Freud who compared memory to a magic slate: the clear celluloid receives the imprint of short-term memories, soon to be wiped clean, and the waxy cardboard underneath becomes etched with the lasting impressions.

Freud accepted the belief popularized by his contemporary, psychologist Hermann Ebbinghaus, that the brain files away all memories, but his angle of approach was wildly different. Freud studied memory not from the position of what we remember or how we remember, but on how little we remember—and why. He believed that any failure of recall had a specific cause, and since people forget things every day, he had plenty of material with which to work. For example, Freud found it implausible that childhood, filled with the richness of new experience, pleasure and pain, should be so totally forgotten.

He argued that recalled experiences and ideas were related to other symbolically and emotionally important thoughts and feelings and that much of what a person forgets is simply repression. He believed that the lack of memories of early childhood (usually before age four in most people) was caused by repression of infantile sexuality, which peaks in the third and fourth years of life. This repression is caused by the "psychic forces of loathing, shame, and moral and aesthetic ideal demands," he said. His basic theory describes both the unconscious and conscious mind, noting that the unconscious mind can have a great effect on a person's conscious actions. We remember something, he postulated, because it is meaningful to us and significant, although that significance may be hidden.

Freud believed it was conflict, followed by repression, that made the problem of deciphering early memories so difficult. Because he thought there is nothing accidental or arbitrary about the things we forget, he believed that everyday absent-mindedness could be divided into "forgetfulness" and "false recollection" (also called a "Freudian slip," or substituting one word for another). The process that should have produced the actual memory was interrupted and the memory was "displaced" by another.

And displacement isn't simply a quirk, he argued—it followed a routine as logical as summoning up the actual memory. For example, he analyzed a number of his own "Freudian slips" in his book *The Psychopathology of Everyday Life*. When he couldn't remember the name of Rosenheim, a major railway station (translation: Rose's home), he decided that the name was lost in his memory because he had just come from visiting the home of his sister, Rose, and the name was taken away by his "family complex." He concluded that forgotten names were associated—sometimes very indirectly—with painful and unpleasant memories. In other words, we eliminate from the conscious mind everything that makes us anxious, which, he believed, explained the loss of memories during the first four years of life.

frontal lobe The area just forward of the central fissure of the brain. One of the functions of the frontal lobe is concerned with intellectual functioning, including thought processes, behavior and memory.

frontal lobe lesions and memory The frontal lobe of the brain deals with intellectual functioning, including thought processes, behavior and memory. Abnormalities, or lesions, in this area of the brain can cause a wide variety of memory problems, especially if the damage is bilateral (affecting both lobes).

Some patients with frontal lobe lesions experience a problem in learning complex material. Some researchers have reported that patients with lesions of the lateral frontal zones can't form stable intentions to memorize new material and therefore can learn new information only in a passive way. For example, such subjects could pick up four or five words on a list but could not learn the rest. In addition, other researchers note that similarly affected patients can't learn weakly associated word pairs very well (such as horse–tree).

It is also believed that frontal lobe lesions may disrupt recall more than recognition, although this view is not universally accepted. Patients with lesions of the frontal lobe usually can recognize recently presented material, even though their recall may be severely disrupted. Even though some patients with these lesions do badly in both recall and recognition, there is evidence that they are likely to do worse on recall.

Third, patients with bilateral frontal lobe lesions (but not unilateral) show a disturbance in metamemory—the knowledge of one's own memory and memory strategies. This supports other researchers' idea that frontal lobe lesions impair patients' ability to monitor their own effectiveness. This inability to monitor the effectiveness of plans and actions may also underlie another group of retrieval disorders that may be caused in part by frontal lobe lesions. The best known of these is CONFABULATION, the recall of incorrect information in response to standard questions, usually to cover up a memory deficit. Researchers have discovered that the degree of confabulation is not related to the extent of memory disturbance but is related to the inability to self-correct.

Frontal lobe lesions also have been linked to reduplicative paramnesia, in which a patient insists that two places (such as his home) exist with identical properties when only one such place exists. Reduplicative paramnesia is linked to CAPGRAS SYNDROME, in which the reduplication concerns close relatives, so that a wife may insist her husband is a "double" and not her true spouse. While the precise cause of the reduplicative disorders is not known, they have been linked to massive frontal lobe lesions. Another group of frontal lobe lesion effects relates to a patient's sensitivity to high levels of interference during learning. (See also AGNOSIA.)

fugue   A period during which a person forgets his or her identity and often wanders away from home or office for several hours, days or even weeks. The belief that psychogenic disorders may be a way of avoiding depression or suicide is expressed in the term *fugue*, which is derived from the Latin *fugere* (to "run away" or "flee"). Causes include DISSOCIATIVE DISORDERS, depression, HEAD INJURY and DEMENTIA. In addition, psychomotor or temporal lobe epileptics who suffer from complex, partial seizures may experience long periods of aimless wandering, or poriomania.

Other cases of fugue are clearly psychogenic in nature. Some researchers believe that the tendency to wander away from home while experiencing an attack of AMNESIA often occurs together with other symptoms, including a history of a broken home, periodic depression and predisposition to states of altered consciousness. On the other hand, psychoanalysts see the fugue state as a symbolic escape from severe emotional conflict.

In fugues of long duration, behavior may appear normal but certain symptoms, such as hallucinations, feeling unreal or unstable moods, may coexist.

One of the most celebrated cases of fugue involved a patient of psychologist William James, the Reverend Ansell Bourne, who wandered away from home for two months. During this time, the patient acquired a new identity and—once he returned home—claimed no memory of the entire two months he had been away. His memory for this time period finally surfaced after he underwent HYPNOSIS. (See also FREUD, SIGMUND; HYSTERICAL AMNESIA.)

functional amnesia   See PSYCHOGENIC AMNESIA.

fuzzy trace theory   The idea that human cognition is primarily a system in which inferences are drawn by processing vague, gistlike representations (fuzzy traces) and that stored information is recalled by reconstructively processing these representations.

The theory, developed by psychologist C. J. Brainerd of the University of Arizona, is an experimental concept of intuition. The term *fuzzy trace* was borrowed from mathematics, where it also emphasizes creativity and imagination. This theory is an alternative to the two most comprehensive theoretical approaches in the field: Swiss psychologist Jean Piaget's belief that a child's mind evolves through a series of set stages to adulthood and the theory of information processing. See also PIAGET, JEAN.

Ganser's syndrome   A rare "factitious disorder" that occurs as a response to severe stress in which a person tries (consciously or unconsciously) to mislead others regarding his or her mental state. Its symptoms also include AMNESIA and clouded consciousness.

Also called prison psychosis, it was found almost always among prisoners and was first described by German psychiatrist Sigbert J. M. Ganser (1853–1931). However, most cases have been found among those who are not confined.

The hallmark of Ganser's syndrome is that the sufferer often displays symptoms that simulate psychosis (episodes of intense agitation or stupor) and often gives approximate answers—that is, 4 + 2 = 7. The choice of an answer near the correct one suggests that the person does know the correct answer. Other symptoms reveal that patients with Ganser's syndrome also experience a clouded consciousness, hallucinations, delusions and periods of amnesia for the intervals when the symptoms were present.

In his 1897 lecture on this hysterical state, Ganser noted the "inability" of the prisoners to answer the simplest question correctly even though it was obvious by their answers that they understood the question. Further, their answers showed that they lacked a great deal of knowledge that they once clearly had—or still have. He believed these patients were not malingerers; rather, their answers were a true symptom of mental disorder of a hysterical origin. Ganser's syndrome is most often considered either a true psychotic disorder or simple malingering, but it is classified among the nonspecific dissociative disorders under that category in the *Diagnostic and Statistical Manual of Mental Disorders*, 3rd ed., revised (DSM-III-R).

While this syndrome is sometimes referred to by the German word *Vorbeirden* ("to talk past the point"), Ganser never used this term himself.

gender and eyewitness ability   While men and women in general are about equally reliable as witnesses, both men and women pay more attention to items that catch their interest and therefore store more or better information in memory about those items.

In a study of 50 subjects who were tested after looking at 24 slides of a wallet-snatching incident, women were only slightly more accurate overall. But women were far more accurate than men on questions dealing with women's clothing or actions, and men were far more accurate on questions concerning the thief's appearance and the surroundings.

In another study of 200 men and women who saw slides of a man and a woman who witness a fight, women were more accurate and less suggestible on the female-oriented questions and less accurate and more suggestible on the male-oriented items. Men were more accurate and less suggestible on the male-oriented questions and less accurate and more suggestible on the female-oriented questions. According to researchers, this indicates that men and women tend to be accurate on different types of items, perhaps because they differ in their interest in particular items and differ in the amount of attention they pay to those items.

Other researchers note that people are more readily influenced to the extent that they lack information about a topic or think of it as trivial or unimportant. (See also AGE AND EYEWITNESS ABILITY; CROSS-RACIAL WITNESS IDENTIFICATION; EYEWITNESS ABILITY.)

generalized amnesia   A type of PSYCHOGENIC AMNESIA in which a patient cannot recall anything of his or her entire life. (See also HYSTERICAL AMNESIA.)

generation-recognition theory   The theory that retrieval of information involves an initial search stage in which possible "targets" are generated; each of these possible targets is then subjected to a recognition process to determine whether it is the information needed.

Both stages must be implemented for recall to take place, whereas for recognition only the second stage is required. Recall is therefore less reliable, because there are two stages at which problems can occur.

ginkgo biloba   The oldest known species of tree, also known as the maidenhair tree, this allegedly memory-enhancing tree dates back 300 million years and is the only living representative of the order Ginkgoales. Called a living fossil because it does not exist in the wild, it has been planted since ancient times in China and Japanese temple gardens and is now used throughout the world as an ornamental tree.

Used for millennia in China as a valuable medicine, today it is used throughout Europe for the same purpose. Leaves from the ginkgo tree are said to improve short-term memory loss and may be of some benefit to ALZHEIMER'S DISEASE patients.

The leaves work by boosting blood flow throughout the body and the brain, increasing the production of adenosine triphosphate (ATP) and streamlining the brain's ability to metabolize GLUCOSE. They also prevent platelet clumping in arteries, improving nerve signal transmission and serving as a powerful antioxidant.

Ginkgo is thought to have both antioxidant and anti-inflammatory properties, to protect cell membranes, and to regulate neurotransmitter function. In a study published in the October 22, 1997 issue of the *Journal of the American Medical Association* (October 22/29, 1997), researchers found ginkgo biloba had a positive effect in individuals with Alzheimer's disease. This 52-week study initially involved 309 patients suffering from mild to moderately severe dementia, caused by either Alzheimer's disease or multi-infarct dementia.

Participants were tested for improvement in cognition, daily living and social behavior, and positive changes in overall impairment. Researchers found those who took ginko had modest improvements in cognition, activities of daily living (such as eating and dressing), and social behavior, but no measurable difference in overall impairment. Results from this study show that ginkgo may help some individuals with Alzheimer's disease slightly, but further research is needed in order to determine the exact mechanisms by which ginkgo works in the body. (Results from this study are considered preliminary because of the low number of participants involved and methodological issues associated with the research).

Few side effects are associated with the use of ginkgo as a dietary supplement, although it does reduce the ability of blood to clot, potentially leading to more serious conditions such as hemorrhaging. This possibility of hemorrhaging may increase if ginkgo biloba is taken in combination with other anticoagulants, such as aspirin.

ginseng   This herb and its root of the family Araliaceae (*Panax quinquefolium* and *Panax schinseng*) have been used for centuries by Chinese healers as a way to increase resistance to stress. The herb is said to improve memory, brain function, concentration and learning.

Ginseng is an important component of Chinese medicine that has numerous beneficial properties. Indeed, the generic name *panax* is derived from the same Greek word as *panacea*, an indication of the many uses the Chinese have found for this herb. The action of ginseng is said to be linked to its saponins, a group of chemicals that influence the metabolism of neurotransmitters such as serotonin and ACETYLCHOLINE, which are important for memory function. Ginseng also appears to interfere with the activation of the adrenal cortex, the seat of stress. In addition, saponins increase the activity of lymphocytes, which would enhance immune function.

Panax quinquefolium is the North American ginseng, which is found in woodlands from Quebec to the Gulf coast. The plant also is cultivated for its root in the United States.

Chinese medical experts caution that people with high blood pressure should not use ginseng. Also, it should be used only as an occasional "tonic," not on a daily basis. Most health food stores carry several varieties of ginseng; the amount of active ingredients found in different preparations varies greatly.

global aphasia A total or near-total inability to speak, write or understand spoken or written words. Global aphasia usually is caused by widespread damage to the dominant cerebral hemisphere.

glucose A simple sugar carbohydrate, the body's chief source of energy, which also seems to play an important role in declarative memory (memory for events and things). In studies at the University of Virginia, scientists found that increasing the level of glucose circulating in the blood improved a person's ability to store memories while not affecting other cognitive functions.

Despite wide variations in carbohydrate intake, the concentration of glucose in the blood (the blood sugar level) is usually kept within narrow limits through the action of hormones including insulin, glucagon, epinephrine, corticosteroids and growth hormone.

Animal studies suggest that raising blood glucose levels helps some brain cells transmit ACETYL-CHOLINE, a chemical messenger involved in memory. It is believed that acetylcholine becomes less available to the brain as people age.

In one study, researchers found that after drinking glucose-sweetened lemonade, elderly subjects performed better on certain memory tests by 30 to 40 percent. The glucose reversed most of the age-related deficits, according to psychologist Paul Gold and colleagues. Subjects performed better on tests of declarative memory (memory for events and things), the type of memory most often impaired in the elderly. Gold also discovered that those subjects whose bodies did not process glucose well performed less well on the declarative memory tests.

Results suggest that glucose seems to enhance memory storage for at least 24 hours. Glucose also improves sleep—another problem the elderly face. In related research, scientists found that in animal studies, those who have memory deficits also have sleep problems. Perhaps the same neural system is influencing memory storage and sleep.

Other scientists at McGill University have noted that glucose levels are monitored by the liver, which sends signals to the brain by the autonomic nervous system. When nerves from the celiac ganglion (the structure through which most of the nerves connect the liver to the brain) were cut, memory improvement following glucose did not occur.

In the late 1980s memory researchers found that epinephrine and glucose are partly responsible for signaling the brain that "here's something important to remember." The first step in storing a memory is the release of epinephrine, which then triggers the release of glucose into the blood, which may act on the central nervous system and enhance memory storage. Older people may begin to have memory problems because the neuroendocrine responses responsible for the demand to "store this memory" are wearing out.

Recent findings also suggest that glucose increases the effects of the memory-enhancing cholinergic agonists (drugs that increase the function of acetylcholine systems). Studies also show that glucose interferes with the effects of cholinergic antagonists (drugs that impair memory storage).

Glucose may regulate a system in the brain that handles the inhibition of cholinergic functions. Scientists do not know yet what parts of the brain are affected by the glucose.

Despite its possible memory benefits, frequent glucose consumption may not be a healthy way to boost memory for elderly patients, however, since high glucose levels increase the risk of developing health problems such as diabetes.

glutamate A common nerve cell stimulator found in every cell in the body, this amino acid also plays a central role in the workings of the brain and memory. Glutamate is important in the proper function of the hippocampus, among other brain areas, and an imbalance will cause epileptic seizures, memory disorders or both.

Glutamate is the best known of a group of excitatory amino acids that plays an important part in initiating and transmitting signals in the brain. Almost half of the brain's neurons use glutamate as a primary transmitter.

Normally glutamate is bound tightly in the cells, and only tiny amounts are allowed into the spaces between brain cells at any one time. But new research suggests that abnormal glutamate activity also may be responsible for brain damage following lack of oxygen from injury, stroke or seizure. When the brain is deprived of oxygen and some of the cells that store glutamate shut down, glutamate comes flooding out; in such high levels, it kills brain cells. Just five minutes of excess glutamate is enough to kill cells.

habituation A decrease in the intensity of a behavioral response because a stimulus has been presented so often that it is no longer consciously noticed. Perhaps the most common form of learning, habituation enables humans and other animals to ignore unimportant stimuli and focus on those that are rewarding or important for survival.

Memory experts believe that habituation is the very first learning process found in infants, who learn, for example, to ignore harmless household noises. (See also POTENTIATION.)

head injury Even the mildest bump on the head can damage the brain by causing a subdural hematoma, especially in those who are taking corticosteroids or who have rheumatoid arthritis or osteoporosis. In fact, research suggests that 60 percent of patients who sustain a mild brain injury are still having symptoms after three months. These patients often develop bizarre symptoms (called postconcussion syndrome) including memory loss following even the slightest bang on the head.

The fact that head injury can have effects throughout the body has been known for at least 3,000 years; the Edwin Smith Surgical Papyrus, written between 2,500 and 3,000 years ago, contains information about eight cases of head injuries affecting other parts of the body. In reports in the 1800s, physicians also knew that memory impairment often followed closed head injuries.

Mild head injury symptoms can result in a puzzling interplay of behavioral cognitive and emotional complaints that make the problems difficult to diagnose.

Symptoms following head injury may be caused by direct physical damage to the brain as well as secondary factors (lack of oxygen, swelling and

vascular disturbance). A penetrating injury also may cause a brain infection. The type of accident determines the kind of injury the brain receives in a closed head injury; injuries vary depending on whether the head was unrestrained upon impact and the direction, force and velocity of the blow. If the head was restrained upon impact, the maximum damage will be found at the impact site; a moving head will cause a "contrecoup" injury where damage will be on the side opposite the point of impact.

Both kinds of injuries cause swirling movements throughout the brain, tearing nerve fibers and causing widespread vascular damage. There may be bleeding in the cerebrum or subarachnoid space leading to hematomas, or brain swelling may raise intracranial pressure, blocking oxygen to the brain.

Both direct and diffuse effects may cause memory deficits after a head injury; the temporal lobes are particularly vulnerable to this type of trauma. In most cases, however, permanent severe memory loss with intact functioning in other areas does not occur. Severe diffuse damage may lead to posttraumatic dementia with general intellectual impairment.

After a head injury, patients suffer from a period of impaired consciousness followed by a period of confusion and impaired memory known as posttraumatic amnesia (PTA), with confusion, disorientation, RETROGRADE AMNESIA and impairment in the ability to store and retrieve new information. For some reason, the physical and emotional shock of the accident interrupts the transfer of all information that happened to be in the short-term memory just before the accident; this is why some people can remember information several days before and after the accident, but not information right before it occurred. The length of both the unconsciousness and PTA have been linked with how well a person recovers after head injury.

Temporary retrograde amnesia following head injury often begins with a memory loss for a period of weeks, months or years prior to the injury, but it will diminish as recovery proceeds. Permanent retrograde amnesia, however, may extend for just a few seconds or minutes before the accident; in very severe head injuries, however, the permanent retrograde amnesia may also cover weeks or months before the accident.

Until recently, diagnostic tools were not sensitive enough to detect the subtle structural changes that can occur and sometimes persist after mild head injury. Many patients are plagued by symptoms, including headache, dizziness, confusion and memory loss, which may continue for months. Typically, computerized tomography (CT) scans of this group of patients reveal no damage. But studies involving magnetic resonance imaging (MRI) and brain electrophysiology indicate that contusions and diffuse axonal injuries associated with mild head injury are likely to affect those parts of the brain that relate to functions such as memory, concentration, information processing and problem solving.

In fact, a 1981 study of 424 patients diagnosed with mild head injury showed that many had recurrent problems with deviant behavior, headaches, dizziness and cognitive problems; only 17 percent were symptom-free three months after the accident. A third study in 1989 reached the same conclusions.

Only 12 percent of patients with mild head injury are hospitalized overnight, and instructions they receive upon leaving the emergency room usually do not address behavioral, cognitive and emotional symptoms that can occur after such an injury.

Diagnostic Tests

CT Scans   While CT scans are widely available in emergency rooms to help in the diagnosis of neural hematomas, many experts believe these scans may not pick up the subtle damage following a mild head injury.

MRI   Many researchers believe MRI is more sensitive in diagnosing many brain lesions beyond a basic hematoma. For example, MRI is more sensitive in detecting the diffuse axonal or shearing injury and contusions often seen in mild head injury.

Quantitative EEG (qEEG)   In many patients, neither CT scans nor MRI can detect the microscopic damage to white matter that occurs when fibers are stretched in a mild, diffuse axonal injury. In this type of mild injury, the axons lose some of their covering and become less efficient, but MRI detects only more severe injury and actual axonal degeneration. Mild injury to the white matter reduces the quality of communication between different parts of the cerebral cortex. A quantitative EEG is different from a regular electroencephalogram in that the signals from the brain are played into a computer, digitized and stored. EEGs can measure the time delay between two regions of the cortex and the amount of time it takes for information to be transmitted from one region to another.

Evoked Potentials   The electrophysical technique of measuring evoked potentials (EPs) generally is not useful in patients with less serious mild head injury. EPs are not sensitive enough to document any physiologic abnormalities, although a patient may be having symptoms. If testing is done within a day or two of injury, an EP may pick up some abnormalities in brain stem auditory evoked potentials.

Neuropsychological Testing   Neuropsychological tests may show positive results when imaging tests and neurologic exams are negative. In some patients with persistent symptoms following mild head injury, neuropsychological tests are part of a comprehensive assessment. The tests also can provide information when litigation is an issue.

Future Tests   PET (positron emission tomography), which evaluates cerebral blood flow and brain metabolism, may provide useful information on functional pathology. Single-photon emission computerized tomography (SPECT) is less expensive than PET and might provide data on cerebral blood flow after mild head injury.

Patients who do experience symptoms are advised to seek out the care of a specialist in mild head injury. Experts caution that there is a great chance that patient complaints will be ignored by most family physicians. Patients with continuing symptoms after a mild head injury are advised to call a local head injury foundation, which can refer them to the most suitable nearby practitioner. (See also CONTRECOUP EFFECTS.)

Hebb, Donald (1904–1985)   A Canadian neuroscientist who revived the idea that memories are stored as patterns of newly connected neurons. In his book *The Organization of Behavior* (1949), Hebb speculated that the new circuits might be made during a learning situation, when one neuron tends to fire another, strengthening the synapse between them.

Two neurons that tend to be active at the same time will form a new connection automatically; if they are already weakly connected, the synapse between them will be stronger, and if not, an entirely new synapse will be made. This has come to be called the HEBB SYNAPSE.

Hebb's theory also includes ideas about long-term potentiation (LTP), which explains how when an axon of one cell excites its neighbor cell repeatedly or consistently, some growth process or metabolic change takes place in both cells. This increased synaptic efficacy may last for weeks.

While today the idea does not seem unusual, in the early 1940s when Hebb came up with the notion, there was no evidence to believe that experience caused any kind of physiological change in the brain.

Hebb's rule   If two neurons fire at the same time, they increase the strength of the connection between them. The rule is named for Canadian neuroscientist Donald Hebb, who explored the idea of long-term potentiation in his book *The Organization of Behavior* (1949). (See also HEBB, DONALD.)

Hebb synapse   The name given to a synapse strengthened by a link formed when two connected neurons fire together. It also refers to a new synapse formed if there is no connection between firing cells.

The idea, formulated in 1949 by Canadian neuroscientist Donald Hebb, is part of his learning theory that explains how neurons are connected to form neural assemblies that are integrated into still larger structures called phase sequences. (See also HEBB, DONALD.)

hedonic selectivity   The idea that unpleasant memories are harder to remember than pleasant ones. (See also FREUD, SIGMUND; REPRESSION.)

herpes simplex encephalitis   A highly contagious and frequently fatal disease that leaves patients with extensive brain damage in the MEDIAL TEMPORAL LOBE, where it affects the HIPPOCAMPUS, AMYGDALA and uncus, causing a pronounced AMNESIC SYNDROME. In extreme cases, it causes the KLÜVER-BUCY SYNDROME, including AMNESIA, visual AGNOSIA and altered sexual behavior. (See also ENCEPHALITIS AND MEMORY.)

high blood pressure and memory   High blood pressure might make it more difficult to remember details, and lead to problems in thinking, learning and remembering. In one study, 21 percent of those with untreated high blood pressure experienced severe decline in thinking and remembering skills, compared to just 7 percent of those with normal blood pressure. Less than 8 percent of those people with high blood pressure who were taking medication showed a similar decline.

hippocampus   Called the gatekeeper of memory, the hippocampus is a ridge along a fissure of the brain that is crucial to learning and memory. Part of the LIMBIC SYSTEM, the hippocampus is one the most ancient parts of the brain and is named for its curving shape, which reminded early neuroscientists of a seahorse. A paired organ found on each side of the brain, it directly links nerve fibers involved in sense (touch, vision, sound and smell) as well as the limbic system. Most researchers consider the hippocampus to be involved in learning and memory, but they don't agree on exactly how it is involved or on the extent of its involvement. In fact, there are countless debates as to exactly how this task is carried out.

Most scientists believe that the hippocampus and interconnected neural structures register and temporarily hold new information, binding together the elements of environment, odors, sounds and people that constitute a remembered episode. When people remember a lover or the first day of school, they are aware of what they remember. But memory also involves nonconscious skills, like riding a bicycle or knowing how to jump rope.

New research suggests that the hippocampus, long believed to help form only conscious memories, also creates certain memories that we aren't aware of. The finding bolsters an emerging theory that the role of the hippocampus in memory is to relate different elements of experience—especially since it receives information from many other brain regions.

In the past, scientists tended to think that *all* memory was centered in the hippocampus. Currently, many scientists agree that the hippocampus seems to be part of a larger learning system, working in parallel with other forebrain learning systems. The prevailing current view is that the hippocampus serves primarily to boost the capabilities of the underlying neocortical memory system. The hippocampus has access to the highest-level information that is being processed by the neocortext at any given moment. It may then combine and store spatial and sensory cues into trace memory (ENGRAMS) that are stored immediately.

These engrams can be retrieved by several kinds of cues. During sleep and also during quiet waking periods this information is written back onto the neocortex by creating very high-level associations between the components of the episodic memory (which already reside within the cortex).

Associative memory is the kind that makes you think of your childhood breakfast 30 years ago when you smell oatmeal. This kind of memory, it turns out, is not exclusive to humans. It seems likely that as well as being involved in spatial memory, the hippocampus plays a broad role in other kinds of memory in rats and other mammals, including humans. (See also PET.)

Many researchers believe that the hippocampus links the separate parts of a memory as it is formed, enabling all to be evoked when the memory is recalled. The hippocampus, whose role in memory storage may be time-limited, receives nerve cell input from the cortex and appears to consolidate information for storage as permanent memory in another brain region (probably also the cortex). It

seems to be particularly important in learning and remembering spatial information.

In order to store a memory, the nerve messages reaching the hippocampus from a perception must be passed back through the medial temporal lobe and out onto the relevant regions of the neocortex; the specific memory then can be recalled from its various storage sites through the links made by the hippocampus.

The hippocampus can recall a memory by using a single moment or sensation to trip off the recall of others. Repeated recall gradually strengthens the connections between the various elements of each perception, boosting their strength each time the memory is called upon. Only after months or years of recall is a memory laid down permanently in storage, where one detail may call up the others without the help of the hippocampus.

The hippocampus is intimately related to memory because of its response to repetitive stimulation; its synapses change according to previous experience, which may form the structural basis of memory itself. But because research shows that a person with a damaged hippocampus can still retain long-term memory, it is not likely that the hippocampus is the primary storehouse for this type of memory.

Scientists suggest that the actual memories involved in integrating stimuli may be in the neocortex all along, and the hippocampus—together with the AMYGDALA—may simply play a role in their storage and retrieval. Scientists theorize that memory gateposts such as the nucleus basalis keep the brain free of inconsequential bits of information by allowing only certain impressions into the cortex.

In addition, while the hippocampus does not play a vital role in storing older memories, it is profoundly important in the short-term memory of contextual information (such as the series of clues a person would recall when trying to find a parked car in a crowded lot, for example). It is also important in converting new sensory information into a form that can be preserved elsewhere in the brain.

In studies at the University of California at Los Angeles, researchers discovered that the hippocampus is involved in learning that requires integrating various stimuli (such as the look, feel and smell of

and seafood. It's also found in a range of products, including milk of magnesia (magnesium hydroxide), magnesium oxide powder and magnesium carbonate. Exactly which form of magnesium is most easily absorbed is unclear.

magnetic resonance imaging (MRI)   Also known as nuclear magnetic resonance (NMR), this is a brain scanning technique that constructs cross-sectional images of the living human brain (among other structures and organs) by detecting molecular changes in neurons exposed to a strong magnetic field.

During the imaging process, the patient lies inside a hollow cylindrical magnet that emits short bursts of a powerful magnetic field. Because patients must lie very still during this procedure, children are sometimes given a general anesthetic. A scan usually takes about 30 minutes and can be done on an outpatient basis.

While the nuclei of the body's hydrogen atoms normally point in different directions, in a magnetic field they line up in parallel rows. If they are then knocked out of alignment by a strong pulse of radio waves, they produce a radio signal as they fall back into alignment.

Magnetic coils in the machine pick up these signals, which are then transformed by computer into an image according to the strength of the signal produced by different types of tissue. Tissue (such as fat) with a great deal of hydrogen produce a bright image, whereas tissue with little hydrogen (such as bone) look black.

MRI is particularly helpful in studying the brain and spinal cord, revealing tumors very clearly. MRI images are very similar to those produced by CT scan; however, MRI allows for far greater contrast between normal and abnormal tissue.

There are no risks or side effects associated with this technique, and because it does not use radiation the test can safely be repeated as often as necessary. However, a pacemaker, hearing aid or other electrical apparatus may be affected by the electrical field.

malnutrition   Lack of adequate diet can lead to dementing brain disease if the deficiency includes lack of the B-complex vitamins (especially NIACIN, thiamine and B_{12}). This is one reason for the memory problems of serious alcohol abusers, who typically lack thiamine because they don't eat properly. In addition, a serious lack of dietary niacin can lead to pellagra, a symptom of which is memory loss. (Niacin is found in meats, poultry, fish and brewer's yeast.)

Vegetarians who don't get enough vitamin B_{12} (which is found in liver, kidney, meats, fish, eggs and dairy products) may experience symptoms of memory loss; recent research suggests that those with low-normal levels of B_{12} in their blood tend to experience depression and memory problems; a more serious lack of this vitamin can lead to spinal cord degeneration and associated brain diseases, including memory loss. (See also CHEMICALS AND MEMORY LOSS; KORSAKOFF'S SYNDROME; PYROGLUTAMATE.)

mammillary bodies   Part of the DIENCEPHALON, which is the uppermost portion of the brain stem; the top surface of the diencephalon forms the floor on which the mammillary bodies lie.

The mammillary bodies seem to be profoundly important to memory function and are the most commonly reported structures involved in the memory problems common in KORSAKOFF'S SYNDROME. In addition, those with surgical lesions or tumors in the mammillary body area also often have memory disorders.

While not the only brain structure involved in memory (memory loss can occur even in patients with intact mammillary bodies), the mammillary bodies do appear to be crucial to memory.

marijuana   The Indian hemp plant *Cannabis sativa* whose dried leaves and flowering tops have been implicated in a variety of memory problems—especially long-term memory loss—among habitual users.

Marijuana contains the active ingredient THC (tetrahydrocannabinol), which is also found in hashish (*Cannabis resin*). The leaves usually are smoked, although they can be eaten in food, and they produce feelings of well-being and calmness lasting for about an hour. Large doses may result in panicky states, fear of death and illusions, although true psychosis rarely occurs. There is evidence that regular users can become physically dependent on the drug.

Marijuana's negative effects on memory have been recorded for some time; in 1845 French psychiatrist Jacques Joseph Moreau de Tours noted that hashish could gradually weaken the power to direct thoughts at will. More recent studies suggest that the most obvious problem with memory occurs within three hours of smoking, with a direct effect on the HIPPOCAMPUS, the memory center of the brain.

Some researchers suggest marijuana may affect the way a person processes and remembers different kinds of information. It appears to reduce the amount of ACETYLCHOLINE necessary for cell communication, resulting in problems in retrieving words and making it difficult to recall numbers; the ability to store new memories also seems to be affected. Some scientists believe the chronic use of marijuana may cause the same kinds of memory effects as those experienced in patients suffering from brain infections, KORSAKOFF'S SYNDROME and ALZHEIMER'S DISEASE.

Other studies suggest marijuana may interfere with memory because it increases the number of intrusive thoughts (ideas that pass through the mind while the subject is trying to concentrate on something else).

meaningfulness effect The more meaningful the data, the easier they are to learn; if information doesn't make sense, it will be hard for a person to memorize it. The opposite of meaningful learning is ROTE LEARNING, in which information is remembered by repeating over and over without making any of the details meaningful.

Since information should be meaningful to be remembered, it follows that nonsense syllables are not remembered as easily as words, that abstract terms are not as easy to remember as concrete words and that words in random order are harder to recall than words grouped in a meaningful way.

In one study of meaningfulness, subjects memorized 200 words of poetry, 200 nonsense syllables and a 200-word prose passage. The poetry took ten minutes to learn, the prose less than 30

minutes, and the nonsense syllables took $1^1/_2$ hours. Therefore to memorize information, the more meaningful the material is, or can be made by organization into meaningful units or into a pattern, the better.

medial temporal amnesia A type of amnesia caused by a bilateral lesion in the HIPPOCAMPUS, either alone or in combination with AMYGDALA damage. When only one side of the hippocampus is damaged, the most common outcome is a specific memory deficit: damage to the left hemisphere impairs the retention of verbal information, whereas right-hemisphere damage affects nonverbal memory. (See also HM; MEDIAL TEMPORAL LOBE.)

medial temporal lobe An area of the brain important in memory formation. Direct evidence of the importance of this area of the brain comes in the wake of neurosurgery to remove parts of the temporal lobe as a treatment for epilepsy.

In a series of operations during the mid-1950s, surgeons removed the medial temporal lobe in ten epileptic patients in order to lessen seizures. While the operations were successful, eight of the ten suffered pronounced memory deficits. The most famous of these was known as HM, whose AMNESIC SYNDROME is considered to be among the purest ever studied. After the operation, HM was unable to remember anything other than moment-by-moment events since the time of his operation and has been described as living in the "eternal present," HM's case provided valuable information about the primary importance of the HIPPOCAMPUS in memory; amnesia was present only in those who had lost both the hippocampus and the AMYGDALA, and removal of the amygdala alone did not produce amnesia.

memorist A person skilled in ARTIFICIAL MEMORY or trained in one of a wide variety of memory strategies. (See also LOCI, METHOD OF; MNEMONIC STRATEGIES.)

memory Traditionally understood as the process of storing and retrieving information in the brain, which is central to learning, thinking and remembering, memory is really not so much a retrieval as an active construction. While people often talk about their memory as if it were a "thing," such as a bad heart or a good head of hair, in fact memory doesn't exist in the way an object exists. Instead, it is an abstraction that refers to a process—remembering. If we say we know something, we are speaking metaphorically—we are assuming that we can construct the answer. A person's memories don't spring fully formed from little file folders in the brain, but instead represent an incredibly complex constructive power that each person possesses.

Memory provides a sense of self and of familiarity with people and surroundings, a past and present and a frame for the future. But even as psychologists and brain researchers have learned to appreciate memory's central role in our mental lives, they have come to realize that memory is not a single phenomenon.

Instead, memory functions at the level of synapses scattered in a weblike pattern throughout the brain. There is not one memory system, but a group of memory systems, each playing a different role. When the brain is processing information normally, these different systems work together perfectly. If a person is driving a car, for example, the memory of how to drive the car comes from one set of neurons; the memory of how to get from here to the bank comes from another; the memory of driving rules comes from another, and that nervous feeling as a policeman passes by comes from still another. Yet the driver is never aware that all of these mental experiences are put together from various areas of the brain, because they all work together so well.

In fact, there is no firm distinction between how we remember and how we think. Scientists don't fully understand completely how a person remembers or what occurs during recall. The search for how the brain organizes memories and where those memories are acquired and stored has been an enduring quest among brain researchers. In order to study memory, traditional researchers have used drugs or surgery on animals to affect parts of the brain, and then used behavioral tests to measure those effects. Today, imaging methods

such as COMPUTERIZED TOMOGRAPHY (CT) SCANS and MAGNETIC RESONANCE IMAGING (MRI) allow more precise views of these damaged animal brain sections. PET (positron emission tomography) scans have allowed scientists to study the human brain as it functions for clues to the relationship between brain structure and function.

Types of Remembering
Four different types of remembering are ordinarily distinguished by psychologists: recollection, recall, recognition and relearning:

- Recollection: the reconstruction of events or facts on the basis of partial cues, which serve as reminders.
- Recall: the active and unaided remembering of something from the past.
- Recognition: the ability to correctly identify previously encountered stimuli as familiar.
- Relearning: may show evidence of the effects of memory; material that is familiar is often easier to learn a second time than it would be if it were unfamiliar.

Tracing a Memory
Memory is a biological phenomenon with its roots firmly in the senses. The latest research suggests that all memory begins with perception. For example, if a person's earliest memory is of nestling in the arms of one's mother, the visual system identified that this shape is a sweater, this shape is the mothers' face, this is its color, this is its smell, this is its feel—binding them into the experience of being held by the mother. Each of these separate sensations travels to the HIPPOCAMPUS, which rapidly integrates the perceptions as they occur into a single, memorable experience. The hippocampus thus consolidates information for storage as permanent memory in another brain region (probably the cortex).

While memory and perception can't be split into two, it is possible to speak of visual and verbal memory as two separate things. About 60 percent of Americans have primarily a "visual" memory, easily visualizing objects, places, faces and the pages of a newspaper. The rest seem better at remembering sounds or words, and the associations they think of are often rhymes and puns.

While memory may begin with perception, many researchers believe its language is written with electricity and chemicals. Nerve cells (called NEURONS) connect with other cells at junctures called SYNAPSES. All the action in the brain occurs at these synapses, where electrical pulses that carry messages leap across gaps between cells. This electrical firing across the junction between cells triggers the release of neurotransmitters (such as acetylcholine) that diffuse across the spaces between cells, attaching themselves to receptors on the neighboring nerve cell. Each neuron can form thousands of links, giving a typical brain about 100 trillion synapses.

The parts of the brain cells that receive the electric impulses are the dendrites, the wisps at the tip of brain cells that connect to the next one. It is suspected that when an electrical impulse reaches the brain cell, the impulse may compress the dendrite. When the dendrite springs back into its original shape, the electrical pulse disappears—along with the memory. This, then, could be the description of a short-term memory. Memory occurs as a result of functional changes in these synapses or dendrites caused by the effects of outside stimuli prompted by training or education.

As a person learns, behaves and experiences the world and stores memories, changes occur at the synapses, and more and more connections in the brain are created. The brain organizes and reorganizes itself in response to experience and sensory stimulation, and these changes are reinforced with use. As a person learns and practices new information, intricate circuits of knowledge and memory are laid down. Play a bar of music over and over, for example, and the repeated firing of certain cells in a certain order makes it easier to repeat the firing pattern later on.

The interconnections between neurons are not fixed, but change all the time. Researchers at Rockefeller University have discovered that neurons don't act alone, but work together in a network, organizing themselves into groups and specializing in different kinds of information processing. For example, if one neuron sends many signals to another neuron, the synapse between the two gets stronger. The more active the two neurons are, the stronger the connection between them grows. Thus, with every new experience, your brain slightly rewires its physical structure. In fact, how a person uses his or her brain helps determine how the brain is organized. It is this flexibility, this "plasticity," that helps the brain rewire itself once it has been damaged, helping a person recover lost or damaged functions in the wake of stroke, for example.

As people learn, the synapses are reinforced, creating a complex network of associations. But as people age, the synapses begin to falter, which affects the ability to retrieve memories effectively. What's happening when the brain forms memories (and what fails with aging, injury and disease) involves a phenomenon known as "plasticity." It's obvious that something in the brain changes as we learn and remember new things, but it's equally obvious that the organ doesn't change its overall structure or grow new nerve cells wholesale. Instead, it's the connections between new cells—and particularly the strength of these connections—that are altered by experience. Hear a word over and over, and the repeated firing of certain cells in a certain order makes it easier to repeat the firing pattern later on. It is the pattern that represents each specific memory.

Something in the brain changes as a person learns and remembers new things, but the brain doesn't change its overall structure or grow new nerve cells with each memory. Instead, it's the connections between new cells, and especially how strong they are, that are changed by experience.

Memory Stages
Once a memory is created, it must be stored, however briefly. Most experts believe that there are three stages of memory storage: sensory storage, short-term storage and long-term storage.

Sensory Storage Sensory storage retains a sensory image for a brief moment, just long enough to develop a perception. The formation of a memory begins with registration of the information during perception in this brief "sensory storage." It is then filed in a short-term memory system.

Short-Term Memory Short-term memory seems to be very limited in the amount of material it can store at one time. Unless it's constantly repeated, it lasts for just minutes before being replaced with other material. If the information is rehearsed, short-term memory will last as long as the rehearsal continues.

The capacity of short-term memory isn't infinite; it's limited by the number of items it can hold (the capacity is about seven items). However, it's possible to increase this limit by various memory strategies, such as "chunking" (remember a 10-digit number, such as a phone number by dividing 8005551212 into chunks—800-555-1212).

Originally, short-term memory was perceived as a simple rehearsal buffer, but in fact it is much more complicated. It's possible to think of short-term memory as the ability to store a limited amount of information temporarily while it is being processed (a sort of working memory).

Next, important information must be transferred to long-term memory, called "retaining." Here the process of storage involves associations with words or meanings, with the visual imagery evoked by it or with other experiences, such as smells or sounds. People tend to store material on subjects they already know something about, because the information has more meaning. This is why a person with a normal memory may be able to remember in depth more information about one particular subject. For example, people remember words that are related to something they already know because there is already a file in their memory related to that information.

Long-Term Memory   While most people think of long-term memory when they say "memory," in fact most researchers believe that information must first pass through sensory and short-term memory systems before it can be stored as long-term memory.

Some experts believe that long-term memory is made up of different types of remembering. Others believe that long-term memory is actually permanent—that nothing is forgotten, but the means of retrieving information is lost. Proponents point to the existence of "flashbulb memories" as evidence that nothing is lost. (A flashbulb memory is a vivid recollection of important events, such as when a person first heard about the death of John F. Kennedy). Other experts believe that memories are

not as accurate as once thought, which would mean that long-term memory is not permanent.

Recall

When a person remembers, he or she retrieves the information stored on the unconscious level, bringing it up into the conscious mind at will. How reliable this material is, researchers believe, depends on how well it was encoded. While most people speak of having a "bad memory" or a "good memory," in fact most people are good at remembering some things and not so good at remembering others. When a person has trouble remembering something, it's usually not the fault of the entire memory system—just an inefficient component of that memory system.

For example, if a person wanted to remember where he had put his keys, first he must become aware of where he put them when he walked in the door. He registers what he has done by paying attention to the action of putting his keys down on the hall table. This information is retained, ready to be retrieved at a later date. If the system is working properly, he can remember exactly where he left his keys. If he has forgotten where the keys are, one of several things could have happened:

- He may not have registered clearly to start with.
- He may not have retained what he registered.
- He may not be able to retrieve the memory accurately.

Research indicates that older people have trouble with all three stages, but are especially troubled with registering and retrieving information. If people want to improve their memory, they must work on improving all three stages of that process.

Many factors go into how well a memory is formed, including how familiar the information is and how much attention has been paid. Good health also plays a major part in how well a person performs intentional memory tasks. When mental and physical conditions aren't at their best, the entire memory system functions at a slower pace. Attention (key to memory performance) is lessened and long-term memory weakens, and ideas and images aren't likely to be registered as strongly, and memory traces become fainter, making them harder to retrieve or file into long-term memory.

Where Is Memory?

Little is known about the physiology of memory storage in the brain. Some researchers suggest that memories are stored at specific sites, and others say that memories involve widespread brain regions working together; both processes may in fact be involved. Theorists also propose that different storage mechanisms exist for short-term and long-term memories, and that if memories aren't transferred from one to the other, they will be lost.

Several brain structures are involved in the process of memory, including the hippocampus, hypothalamus, THALAMUS, and TEMPORAL LOBES. Damage to any one of them can cause memory problems.

The hippocampus plays a vital role in transforming short-term memories into permanent ones, which makes this part of the brain crucial to learning. It was in the hippocampal area that the best-documented link to memory was discovered with the patient HM, an epileptic whose temporal lobes were destroyed to alleviate seizures. After surgery, HM was unable to learn any new information and showed symptoms of a classic amnesic syndrome. From these data, scientists realized that an intact hippocampus was essential for normal memory function. Further research has shown that removing the left temporal lobe causes verbal memory deficits and removing the right lobe impairs nonverbal memory (such as remembering mazes, patterns or faces).

However, memory problems following damage to the hippocampal structures do not occur only after surgery; injury following a stroke also can cause a profound short-term memory problem.

The thalamus is one of the main parts of the DIENCEPHALON, and is involved in many cases of memory disorder in WERNICKE-KORSAKOFF patients. One of the best-known cases of thalamic damage and memory problems is NA, a man who was stabbed in the thalamic region at age 22 and suffered extensive memory problems as a result. Other cases of thalamic tumors have been reported, which can lead to a rapidly developing dementia.

But permanent memories are also stored elsewhere in the brain. Another region, an almond-size bit of tissue known as the AMYGDALA, seems to be crucial in forming and triggering the recall of a special type of memory tied to strong emotion, especially fear. The hippocampus allows a person to remember having been afraid; the amygdala evidently calls up the feelings that go along with each such memory.

Animal studies indicate that structures in the brain's limbic system have different memory functions. For example, one circuit through the hippocampus and thalamus may be involved in spatial memories, whereas another, through the amygdala and thalamus, may be involved in emotional memories. Research also suggests that "skill" memories are stored differently from intellectual memories.

In general, memories are less clear and detailed than perceptions, but occasionally a remembered image is complete in every detail. This phenomenon, known as eidetic imagery, is usually found in children, who sometimes project the image so completely that they can spell out an entire page of writing in an unfamiliar language that they have seen for a short time.

Types of Memory

Scientists believe there are two types of memory, implicit and explicit memory. Implicit memory is another name for spontaneous or unintentional memory. The effortless and automatic recall of a person's name is an example of implicit memory. Struggling to recall a person's name uses explicit memory.

The two terms were formulated in 1985 by psychologists Peter Graf and Daniel Schacter of the University of Arizona, although five years before that researchers recognized that two memory systems existed. Traditionally, memory experts have tested only explicit memory by giving subjects lists of items to recall intentionally during a study period before a test. A test of implicit memory would require subjects to respond to questions that don't require any sort of intentional recall, but only respond to whatever comes to mind.

Within the category of implicit (or nondeclarative) memory lie the subcategories of associative memory—the phenomenon that led Pavlov's dogs to salivate at the sound of a bell, which they had learned to associate with food—and of habituation, in which we unconsciously file away unchanging features of the environment so we can pay closer attention to what's new and different upon encountering a new experience.

Explicit (or declarative) memory is just another name for intentional recollection. With explicit memory, there are specific subsystems that handle shapes, textures, sounds, faces, names—even distinct systems to remember nouns vs. verbs.

Researchers believe there may be two separate biological systems for implicit and explicit memory, and that the implicit memory system develops first. The explicit memory system is then built onto the implicit system and, being more vulnerable, suffers from life stresses. Moreover, techniques that improve explicit memory don't improve implicit memory, and vice versa. Studies also show that people with memory loss who have serious problems with explicit memory don't show problems with implicit memory.

memory, associative   See ASSOCIATION.

memory, disorders of   There is a wide range of specific impairments to memory that can occur from more than 100 types of disorders and other causes, ranging from organic (brain dysfunction) to psychogenic (psychological) problems.

The most common memory problems are specific memory dysfunctions involving language. While APHASIA is a general term for loss of language ability, experts classify the many different forms of aphasia. For example, a patient suffering with BROCA'S APHASIA has a very disturbed speech and some problems in comprehension; patients with WERNICKE'S (RECEPTIVE) APHASIA have fluent speech with a meaningless content.

ALEXIA refers to the loss of the ability to read, and AGRAPHIA is the loss of the ability to write; when these abilities are only partially dysfunctional, they are referred to as dyslexia and dysgraphia respectively. ACALCULIA is a problem in dealing with arithmetical concepts, and AMUSIA sufferers have lost the ability to understand music.

AGNOSIA refers to a patient's inability to recognize something despite no sign of sensory dysfunc-

tion; in visual agnosia, patients can't identify visual information although they can indicate recognition by other means (such as gestures). Agnosia is often limited to certain types of stimuli, such as objects or colors. Auditory agnosia (deficit in sound recognition) may take the form of pure word deafness (the inability to recognize spoken words even though the patient can read, write and speak) or cortical deafness (in which the patient can't discriminate sounds). In somatosensory agnosia, the patient can't recognize objects by shape or size.

PROSOPAGNOSIA is a selective impairment in recognizing faces and sometimes other classes of objects, such as species of dogs or makes of cars. In reduplicative paramnesia, patients can't recognize people and places they know well, but claim that doubles have replaced them. While some scientists believe the disorder is psychogenic, recent research suggests that sometimes there is an organic cause.

Disorders of memory can be caused by a problem at any of the three stages of memory: registration, long-term memory and recall. Most problems involve an inability to recall past events because of a failure at the retention or recall state. (See AMNESIA.) A person who can't store new memories suffers from ANTEROGRADE AMNESIA, while a pronounced loss of old memories is RETROGRADE AMNESIA. These two forms of amnesia may appear together or alone.

Sometimes, however, the problem occurs at the registration stage—for example, depressed people can't remember because their preoccupation with personal thoughts and feelings gets in the way.

A problem with memory is one of the most common symptoms of impaired brain function; memory defects may be transitory (such as those after an epileptic seizure) or long term, such as after a severe HEAD INJURY.

In addition, memory problems may be the result of an organic problem in the brain. These could include ALZHEIMER'S DISEASE and the dementias, in which cognitive functions are progressively lost. In the early stages of Alzheimer's disease, there is usually a selective amnesia caused by degenerative processes in the parietemporal-occipital association neocortex, the cholinergic basal forebrain and the limbic system structures, such as the HIPPOCAMPUS and AMYGDALA.

Organic amnesia (or global amnesia) is a memory disorder featuring very poor recall and recognition of recent information (anterograde amnesia) and very poor recall and recognition of information acquired before brain damage occurred (retrograde amnesia). It is caused by lesions in various brain regions, including the hippocampus and amygdala, by bursting aneurysms, and other problems.

HUNTINGTON'S DISEASE, an inherited disorder causing involuntary movements, also causes cognitive problems and memory deficits. Huntington's disease is caused by the increasing atrophy of the caudate nucleus in the basal ganglia and the frontal association neocortex.

KORSAKOFF'S SYNDROME causes a form of organic amnesia resulting from chronic alcoholism, probably related to thiamine deficiency and poor diet. PARKINSON'S DISEASE is a progressive motor disorder that also may include cognitive problems and poor memory arising from dysfunction of the frontal association neocortex.

Postencephalitic amnesia is caused by a viral infection of the temporal lobes of the brain; while the term covers various viruses, the herpes simplex virus is most commonly the cause. The amnesia in these cases is probably caused by destruction of the hippocampus and amygdala; the destruction of the temporal association neocortex probably causes retrograde amnesia.

Schizophrenia, the most common form of psychosis, affecting 1 percent of the population, also has been linked to memory disorders. However, it is unclear to what extent the memory problems depend on subtype of schizophrenia and to what extent they are the result of the effects of an inability to pay attention to external events.

BRAIN TUMORS are abnormal growths that destroy brain tissue and put pressure on nearby brain structures. Tumors that cause particular memory problems similar to Korsakoff's syndrome are often found on the floor of the third ventricle near the DIENCEPHALON. But memory deficits are likely to show up in a wide variety of brain tumors.

memory and brain development   While scientists have long believed that basic language skills are a prerequisite for memory development, new research at Rutgers University suggests that infants as young as six months may be able to store information about their surroundings in a systematic way. Even more surprising, researchers at Johns Hopkins University discovered that even before birth there are signs that a fetus develops the rudimentary ability to remember. For example, a fetus—after an initial reaction of alarm—eventually stops responding to a repeated loud noise. It displays the same kind of primitive learning (known as habituation) in response to its mother's voice.

But the fetus has shown itself capable of far more. Researchers discovered that within hours of birth, a baby already prefers its mother's voice to a stranger's, suggesting it must have learned and remembered the voice (although perhaps not consciously) during the final months before birth. In addition, scientists discovered that a newborn prefers a story read to it repeatedly in the womb over a new story introduced soon after birth.

In addition, newborns can not only distinguish their mother from a stranger speaking, but would rather hear her voice (especially the way it sounds filtered through amniotic fluid), and prefer her native language than to hear her or someone else speaking in a foreign tongue.

By monitoring changes in fetal heart rate, French psychologists have found that fetuses can tell strangers' voices apart and seem to like certain stories more than others. It's probable that the fetus is responding to the cadence of voices and stories, not their actual words, but the conclusion remains: The fetus can listen, learn and remember at some level, and, as with most babies, likes the comfort and reassurance of the familiar.

Researchers found that six-month-olds rely on specific aspects of their surroundings (such as the color or design of a crib liner) to retrieve memories of a simple learned task. This so-called place information seems to be the first level of retrieval for memories among infants and adults, according to researchers. Scientists tested how infants learned to move a mobile by kicking it, how long they remembered it and what changes in their environment affected their memories.

Six-month-olds remember how to move the mobile up to two weeks after training sessions, but only if the background design of their crib liner remains the same. Even three-month-olds learn that kicking sets the mobile in motion, and they retain this knowledge for up to five days. But a three-month-old who trains in the bedroom and gets tested in the kitchen, or who goes from crib training to testing in a lower portable crib, stares blankly at the previously encountered mobile. Apparently, researchers say, young infants learn what happens in what place long before they are able to move from one place to another or learn the spatial relations between those places.

Scientists theorize that the context information serves as an "attention gate"; the context during learning matches context at recall, and recognition of basic perceptual cues (such as color or form) permits attention to focus on memories for a learned task. This fact suggests that sensory receptors and the brain break information down into elementary perceptual units and then put them back together to form a coherent perception.

memory curve   See FORGETTING CURVE.

memory exercises   Therapists sometimes use games such as Pelmanism, Mrs. Brown-went-to-town and Kim's game to reduce memory impairment. While research suggests that stimulation does not improve memory of severe global amnesiacs, it is not known whether this is true for those with less severe impairment. Some scientists believe that mental exercises may have some benefit for this group. Patients and relatives usually believe the exercises may help. Other research has suggested that neural regeneration may be enhanced by mental exercise.

memory for colors   Both strategy and instinct are useful in the recording of sensory information such as color. The best way to remember colors is to analyze them by studying a color chart to understand the scale of tones and values within each primary or secondary color. (For example, a red may have tinges of red or orange.) The more a color is analyzed, the better it will be recalled. It's also a good

idea to associate colors with familiar objects such as "the green in my favorite dress" or with points of reference—"sky blue, salmon pink."

Intensely visualizing color will help develop visual memory so that colors can be recognized more accurately.

memory for crime   See AMNESIA AND CRIME.

memory for events   Failure of reality monitoring shows that people sometimes can't distinguish in memory between what they have really perceived and what they have only heard about or imagined. Memory for events tends to be incomplete; in everyday life situations, if an event is not very unusual, people probably won't pay much attention to it or may simply fail to see what is going on. However, if the event is dramatic, observers are more likely to pay attention—but if the event is at all frightening or emotional, stress can make their subsequent recall less reliable.

It is possible actually to alter a person's memory of a witnessed event, either through leading questions or subsequent misleading information. Once an alteration has occurred in a person's memory, resurrecting the original memory as it was first experienced is almost impossible.

The VACANT SLOT HYPOTHESIS holds that the original information was never stored, so that false information after the event was simply popped into a "vacant slot" in the memory representation. However, many leading experts in the field, including witness expert Elizabeth Loftus, reject this hypothesis on the grounds that 90 percent of subjects who are tested immediately after witnessing an event and aren't exposed to postevent information can correctly recall the event.

Those who believe the COEXISTENCE HYPOTHESIS state that both the original memory and the false postevent memory coexist, as two competing alternatives. When asked about the event, witnesses usually respond with the false version because it is the more recent memory and is therefore more accessible. This hypothesis suggests that even if a person produces a false memory, the original is recoverable.

The DEMAND CHARACTERISTICS HYPOTHESIS is similar to the coexistence hypothesis in that it also holds that both memories exist—but this theory argues that the memories are equally accessible. People produce the false memory because that is the one they think is what is demanded of them, not because it is more or less accessible. When Loftus tested this theory by asking subjects after witnessing an event to recall both the original and false memory versions, however, very few subjects could comply.

The SUBSTITUTION HYPOTHESIS explains that false information after an event replaces or transforms the original memory, which then is irretrievably lost. This theory, which is supported by Loftus's research, assumes a destructive updating mechanism in the brain; it assumes that subjects would have remembered the correct information if their knowledge hadn't been interfered with by false postevent information.

Finally, the RESPONSE BIAS hypothesis claims that misleading information after the event biases the response but has no effect on the original memory. This theory argues that in most experiments, people have forgotten the original information by the time it is tested, and when they respond with false data they are not remembering incorrectly but are simply choosing the wrong answer.

memory for faces   The memory of a face activates a region in the right part of the brain that specializes in spatial configurations. But recent research has found that the brain systems that learn and remember faces are found in a completely different place from those that learn and recall manmade objects. While the face memory is stored in the part of the brain responsible for spatial configurations, the memory of a blender, for example, activates areas that govern movement and touch.

Scientists believe the difference in remembering types of information lies in how the brain acquires knowledge. The theory says that memories are stored in the very same systems that are engaged with the interactions—in the case of the blender, the memory is found in the same part of the cortex that originally processed how the blender felt and how the hands operated it.

Other studies have shown that it's often easier to recognize someone's face than to remember the name that belongs to that face. This is because recognition requires a person to choose among a limited number of alternatives, but remembering requires a far more complex mental process; therefore, it is usually easier to recognize a person than remember the person's name. The following quiz will illustrate the difference.

Recall

Who was president of the United States during the Civil War?

Recognition

Who was president of the United States during the Civil War?
(a) Robert E. Lee
(b) Abraham Lincoln
(c) Ulysses S. Grant

memory for languages   In order to maintain memory for language, a person must experience the language in written or verbal form; otherwise, active vocabulary will shrink, although passive understanding will be maintained. Recognition and recall of a language both depend on proficiency, exposure and practice.

The best way to do this is to listen to the radio or tapes, read books or newspapers and read at least once a week in the language to be maintained.

Although it is harder to learn a foreign language later in life, the more previous knowledge of the language, the more references there will be to facilitate new learning.

Vocabulary can be actively increased by putting the words in context and reviewing them often for several weeks.

memory for music   Even as a young child, Mozart could memorize and reproduce a piece of music after having heard it only once. Since he learned to read music and started composing at almost the same time, it is believed that he visualized the sounds on the musical staff as well as on the keyboard and mentally re-created the notes of the melody. He could play a piece immediately after hearing it, which crystallized the memory when the trace was freshest.

While few musicians can perform to the level of Mozart, they can mentally hear whole pieces of music, enabling them to rehearse anywhere—even far from their instruments.

Certain strategies can boost one's memory for sounds and music. One should concentrate on the sounds, analyze them and dwell on them. When hearing a piece of music, one should study in particular the transitions between movements, because they act as cues for what will follow. By rehearsing the links, the associations between musical elements will be strengthened.

memory for names In everyday memory, remembering other people's names seems particularly problematic. In fact, poor memory for names appears to be quite common. While most people seldom forget the names of objects, names of individuals are often forgotten; it appears that memory for proper names appears to be different from memory for common nouns. Memory for names is a particularly difficult and embarrassing everyday problem for those who have suffered brain damage.

In fact, one study found that when subjects were given a brief history of a named individual and then asked to repeat this information, recall of first names and surnames was poorer than the recall of information about place names, occupations and hobbies. Furthermore, research suggests that last names tend to be harder to remember than other names, probably because they are less common. Recent studies have found that 13 percent of people age 18 to 44 have trouble sometimes or frequently remembering names, compared with 35 percent for ages 45 to 54, 48 percent for ages 55 to 64 and 51 percent at ages 75 and above.

Experts say that people forget a name because they haven't paid enough attention or rehearsed the name enough to register it, or they were tense, preoccupied or distracted as they heard the name. It is not clear, however, why proper names are organized differently from object names, or why they are particularly susceptible to age and stress. While it is true that names of new people we meet are hard to remember because we often aren't paying enough attention during the introduction, even well-known names elude us from time to time. Scientists suggest that our memory systems treat proper names more like the vocabulary of a foreign language than the words of our mother language.

Fortunately, research also has discovered several methods to help people with this problem, including external aids such as wearing name tags or keeping a notebook with photos and names of certain people likely to be encountered during the day. External aids have strengths and weaknesses, and there are several other options.

Rote learning is sometimes used to treat amnesia patients. In rote learning success and reinforcement is combined with a slowly increasing distribution of practice: The new name is presented followed by testing after a short time and then gradually increasing the interval of repeating the name and testing as learning proceeds. However, this method is rarely effective for severe amnesics.

There are two main groups of internal strategies, or "mnemonics"—verbal techniques (such as alphabetical searching and FIRST-LETTER CUEING) or the VISUAL IMAGERY METHOD.

Among the various memory strategies included in visual imagery, the FACE-NAME ASSOCIATION METHOD was designed specifically for learning names. Research has indicated that amnesic patients can learn some paired associations if they are based on a logical association (that is, if they rhyme or are phonetically similar). In research with Korsakoff's patients, subjects who were taught the face-name method (select a distinctive feature, transform the person's name into a noun, and then link the feature with the noun) were able to learn names.

A simpler type of visual imagery is simply to turn the name to be remembered into a picture, which is then drawn on a card. For example, Bill Smith could be drawn as a blacksmith with a long, rounded nose like a duck's bill. This type of system does not require mental imagery, and a person doesn't need to have any distinctive features.

However, research suggests that imagery is probably of limited value in a patient's day-to-day life. It works best when only the names of those who are regularly contacted are taught.

memory for numbers To remember a number, a person's eyes first register the individual numbers; once this visual sensory input enters the brain, the information is retained just long enough to be remembered briefly. Selected bits of information may enter long-term memory if the numbers are rehearsed or repeated over and over, or if there is a strong sensory or emotional component to the number.

Remembering numbers is probably one of the hardest memory chores—but it can be solved by using any of several memory strategies. For example, the number 8005552943 might be difficult to memorize, but by grouping the numbers, the task is much easier. Instead of the long series of 8005552943, by writing it as a telephone number, suddenly it becomes (800) 555–2943, a fairly simple number to maintain in short-term memory.

Other, more complicated techniques have been developed to memorize long strings of numbers, such as employing a simple phonetic alphabet with just ten pairs of digits and sounds to represent the numbers to be remembered.

Some researchers believe that short-term memory for numbers also can be improved through aerobic exercise. While researchers aren't sure why, they suspect it may be linked to the increase in oxygen efficiency or a rise in GLUCOSE metabolism. Good examples of aerobic activities include walking, cycling, swimming, jogging and racquet sports done three times weekly for 30 minutes at a time.

memory for objects   In everyday life, memory for objects involves both object identification and object location. Humans identify and classify objects by relying on memory representations—to recognize what the objects are and to what category they belong. We must remember where objects are in our vicinity, not just what they are.

However, forgetting or misplacing objects happens every day. We may forget an object's location because we are feeling absentminded—it was put in an out-of-the-way place and we can't remember where that place is. Its loss might be attributed to being put in several different places lately, and we can't remember which place we put the object last (updating errors). Or the object may be lost because of a detection failure—it was put in its proper place, but hasn't been detected there.

memory for odors   Of all the senses, smell is most directly linked to memory because scent perceptions are recorded in the limbic system, which is considered to be the seat of emotions. In addition, smells are encoded exactly as they are without needing to be processed verbally in order to be retrieved.

Research has found that those born between 1900 and 1929 associate their childhood with fragrances of nature, including pine, hay, horses, sea air and meadows. Those born between 1930 and 1979 remember the smell of plastic, scented markers, airplane fuel, VapoRub, Sweet Tarts and Play-Doh.

Other research suggests that the happiness of a person's childhood influences which smell triggers childhood memories. The one in 12 subjects studied who reported having unhappy childhoods were most likely to remember somewhat unpleasant odors in connection with their youth, including mothballs, body odor, dog waste, sewer gas and bus fumes.

memory for places   Information about location, orientation and direction is encoded in spatial memory, which is used to remember places and how to find our way, and to locate objects and remember to find things. In each case, the problem is to locate some thing (either oneself or an object) within a spatial layout.

In looking at individual differences in memory for places, such as the ability to read a map or find one's way in a strange environment, scientists testing students have discovered that those with "a good sense of direction" are those who can benefit from experience and acquire an accurate cognitive map. In addition, subjects with a good sense of direction also rated themselves as better at giving and following directions, remembering routes as a passenger, liking to read maps and finding new routes.

It is not clear whether a sense of direction is a particular ability that affects performance on a variety of spatial tasks, or whether a good sense of direction is a grouping of different abilities (such as good visualization, visuospatial memory, spatial reasoning, and so on) that reinforce each other.

In a study of the ability to use maps, researchers discovered large individual differences based on different acquisition strategies. Good learners allocated their attention, used visuospatial imagery to encode patterns and spatial relations, tested their own memory to find out how they were doing and focused on areas they hadn't learned. Poor learners tried to learn the whole map at once, used no imagery, relied on verbal rehearsal of named elements and did not evaluate their own memory. According to some researchers, maps are stored mentally in the form of a network of propositions instead of a visual image.

There are two kinds of spatial information—stored and computable. Stored spatial information is already stored in memory as a proposition (that is, Paris is in France). The knowledge that Paris is north of Marseilles is not stored directly but can be deduced logically from a set of propositions. New information also can be figured out by analysis of existing knowledge, such as finding a new route to a destination.

To remember places one visits, one must look at the scene with interest, identifying anything that is peculiar, and dwell on strong images, flashing back to them occasionally for the job of mentally traveling back there. The more one involves the senses, the stronger the memory trace will be.

memory for rote movements   New studies suggest that the cerebellum may house the memory of rote movements, such as touch typing or violin fingering. Interestingly, this is the same part of the brain that controls balance and coordination.

memory for stories   It appears that there is a general rule allowing the meaning of stories (the most important, most relevant facts) to be preserved in memory, along with a few specific details that also are stored for a fairly short period of time. (The exception to this is material that has been deliberately memorized; in this case, verbatim memory can persist as long as a person lives, although it may take many repetitions to acquire this lifetime memory.)

In one study of students who had years ago memorized certain famous writings (the 23rd Psalm, the Preamble to the Constitution, and Hamlet's soliloquy), the students revealed similar characteristics in what they remembered using very long-term verbatim memory.

There were very few constructive errors—either recall was perfect or it completely failed. For Hamlet's speech and the Preamble, most people showed a marked PRIMACY EFFECT; they could recall about the first 20 words and then memory completely broke down. Recall of the psalm did not show such a strong primacy effect, probably because its rhythmic structure made recalling the entire thing easier.

Researchers conclude that recall is organized in terms of surface structure, since the breakdown of memory occurred at syntactic boundaries. The surface units are remembered as associative chains, and if a part of the chain is broken, the rest is usually lost.

memory for taste   While all of the senses of a human being can evoke memory, taste is one of the most powerful aids to remembering, partly because the olfactory fibers make an immediate connection with memory structures in the brain—they interact directly with the HIPPOCAMPUS and AMYGDALA, whereas vision requires several intermediate cell connections. (See also PROUST, MARCEL.)

memory for voices   While it is not unusual to be able to identify the voice of a friend not heard for many years over the telephone, identification of once-heard voices is not nearly as good. In one study, subjects were 98 percent correct in identifying the familiar voices of coworkers, but much less for strangers. And the memory for the unfamiliar voices decreases rapidly as time passes.

In addition, accuracy of voice recognition is reduced if the voice is whispering. Even the determination to remember an unfamiliar voice does not help recall after two or three days.

memory games   See MEMORY EXERCISES.

memory in infancy   For many years, researchers were convinced that infants had no memory because they had no language, but recent research has discovered otherwise. In fact, scientists have found that babies have very specific memories and can slowly retrieve seemingly forgotten information when given a retrieval cue. Infants' memories of events in which they have actively participated are quite enduring and they become even more so after repeated retrievals, including repeated encounters with reminders.

Researchers at Johns Hopkins University discovered that even before birth there are signs that a fetus develops the rudimentary ability to remember. For example, a fetus—after an initial reaction of alarm—eventually stops responding to a repeated loud noise. It displays the same kind of primitive learning (known as habituation) in response to its mother's voice.

But the fetus has shown itself capable of far more. Researchers discovered that within hours of birth, a baby already prefers its mother's voice to a stranger's, suggesting it must have learned and remembered the voice (although perhaps not consciously) during the final months before birth. In addition, scientists discovered that a newborn prefers a story read to it repeatedly in the womb over a new story introduced soon after birth.

In addition, newborns can not only distinguish their mother from a stranger speaking, but would rather hear her voice (especially the way it sounds filtered through amniotic fluid), and prefer her native language than to hear her or someone else speaking in a foreign tongue.

By monitoring changes in fetal heart rate, French psychologists have found that fetuses can tell strangers' voices apart and seem to like certain stories more than others. It's probable that the fetus is responding to the cadence of voices and stories, not their actual words, but the conclusion remains: The fetus can listen, learn and remember at some level, and, as with most babies, likes the comfort and reassurance of the familiar.

In fact, infants' memories are highly detailed and include information about the incidental context in which events occur. Infants are so sensitive to their learning environment that when anything about it changes, they aren't able to remember what they had previously learned, according to research at Rutgers University.

Not long ago, most scientists believed that early memories are short-lived, highly generalized and diffuse, without any place information for most of the first year of life. For many years, experts did not believe that infants who had no language could remember over the long term. This belief is rooted in the phenomenon of infantile amnesia (adults' inability to remember events before age three or four) and the belief that the brain mechanisms necessary for long-term memory are functionally immature in infancy.

At various times, memory experts believed infants were capable only of automatic memory for motor skills or procedures, unable to recognize stimuli or remember specific events. Infants were likened to aging amnesics, KORSAKOFF SYNDROME patients or monkeys with brain lesions. In fact, however, more and more evidence suggests that even before infants possess language skills, they can remember for days, weeks or months the events in which they actively participate. Researchers also have discovered that older infants remember longer and retrieve memories more quickly than younger infants.

While scientists used to believe basic language skills were a prerequisite for memory development, in fact even very young infants can store information about their surroundings in a systematic way. Scientists tied a ribbon from a baby's ankle to a mobile hanging over the crib. Within a few minutes the babies learn that kicking the foot moves the mobile. The researchers then measure how often the babies will kick when the mobile is not attached to the child's foot. The tests are performed in the child's home and so far have included more than 1,500 infants. Regardless of socioeconomic background, race or gender, babies of similar ages tend to perform about the same on the basic test.

Researchers found that infants rely on specific aspects of their surroundings (such as the color or design of a crib liner) to retrieve memories of a simple learned task. This so-called place information seems to be the first level of retrieval for memories among infants and adults. Scientists tested how infants learned to move a mobile by kicking it, how long they remembered it and what changes in their environment affected their memories.

While the six-month-olds remember how to move the mobile up to two weeks after training sessions, they remember only if the background design of their crib liner remains the same. Even three-month-olds learn that kicking sets the mobile in motion, and they retain this knowledge for up to five days. But a three-month-old who trains in the bedroom and gets tested in the kitchen, or who goes from crib training to testing in a lower portable crib, stares blankly at the previously encountered mobile. Apparently, researchers say, young infants learn what happens in what place long before they are able to move from one place to another or learn the spatial relations between those places.

Scientists theorize that the context information serves as an "attention gate"; the context during learning matches context at recall, and recognition of basic perceptual cues (such as color or form) permits attention to focus on memories for a learned task. This theory suggests that sensory receptors and the brain break information down into elementary perceptual units and then put them back together to form a coherent perception.

As language develops, the child practices his or her descriptive skills. Spontaneous strategies to recall information (active intervention) don't develop until about age 9 or 10. By then the child has learned, for example, that she can boost her memory by placing her clarinet next to her school bag to remember to take it to band practice. The adolescent years are the most important for the development of learning strategies, and memory development peaks with cognitive development.

memory in myth Myths involving memory and forgetting are found throughout history in all parts of the world and play a role in many cultural traditions.

In cultures where the idea of reincarnation and rebirth are strong, the mythology of memory is very important. For example, some North American medicine men claim to remember a prenatal existence, a memory they believe is lost to "common" people. Many practicing Buddhists claim to remember many lives, and a few—including Buddha himself—remember their very first existence.

In Indian myth, the veil of *maya* (illusion) prevents a person from remembering his or her true origin. The ancient Gnostics also warned of a similar forgetfulness, which they believed should be resisted. The ancient Greek goddess of memory, MNEMOSYNE, was believed to know the past, present and future and formed the basis of all life and creativity.

Forgetting this true origin of things was believed to be tantamount to death, as illustrated by the Greek's idea of the river of death (Lethe), which destroyed memory.

In the Christian religion, the anamnesis (commemoration or recollection) is one of the crucial aspects of the celebration of the Communion, through which the passion and death of the Lord is "applied" to the congregation.

memory palace One of the most ancient mnemonic strategies known, in which items are mentally placed in a huge architectural edifice; to recall the item, a person recalls the location where the object or words are placed. The use of memory palaces (part of the method of loci) was the most popular artificial memory system until the middle of the 1600s, when other strategies were introduced. (See LOCI, METHOD OF.)

To make use of a memory palace, a person begins (preferably) with an architectural edifice that is already well known. The person visualizes a series of locations within the palace in a consistent order, beginning at the front door, and then continues logically from room to room. The person visualizes all of the contents in each room and holds these locations clearly in the mind's eye, making sure that a set of locations has been established that will always be seen in the same order.

To remember an object, a person simply associates the object in the order it must be remembered with a location in the palace. It is important to associate each object in as colorful, brash and dramatic a way as possible. To remember a shopping list, one could imagine a large Bermuda *onion* reclining on the front porch of the palace wearing sunglasses; upon entering the hall, one could picture a loaf of *bread* loafing on the umbrella stand; upon entering the living room, one could see a carton of *milk* toasting *marshmallows* over the fireplace, and so on.

To remember words (such as a speech), the person should begin again in the memory palace, but instead of objects associate words that sound the same or chunks of words that will serve as a memory cue to the next words that are to be remembered.

With a memory palace, the individual can be certain of remembering the correct thing at the correct time since the order is fixed by the sequence of places in the building.

memory practice   Practicing memorization can help improve memory, but what a person does during that practice is more important than how much time is spent in practice. There is no substantial evidence that practicing alone makes a significant difference in the function of memory. One study found that three hours of general memory practice did not improve long-term memory, but three hours of practicing using certain techniques did do so.

The idea that the mind can be strengthened through exercise in much the way that the body's muscles can be improved was an idea popular in educational circles in the early 1900s. This belief of the memory as muscle was behind the impetus to teach Greek and Latin in the schools, on the theory that studying these subjects exercised and disciplined the mind. But follow-up studies on thousands of high school students found that the reason why students who took Greek did better in school than those who did not was because brighter students took Greek in the first place. The study of Greek did not make them more intelligent.

In the late 1800s psychologist William James tried to test whether he could improve his memory through mental exercise. He memorized some works by Victor Hugo and then went on to memorize Milton for 38 days. After this, he memorized more from Hugo, and discovered that he was actually memorizing more slowly than he had before the memory practice. Several other subjects James tested reported similar results.

We remember a wide variety of different kinds of things: events, such as our 40th birthday party; facts, such as the capital of France; and procedures, such as how to bake a cake. While there is no substantial evidence that practice, by itself, significantly improves memory, it is possible to help improve memory by the *way* a person tries to remember something.

Improving overall memory involves three basic principles: concentration, visualization and association.

Concentration   It's impossible to remember much of anything while juggling four or five activities at once. The best way to remember a fact, an event or a face is to focus on the information during learning. Writing is one of the best ways to do this, but repeating information out loud or leaving a visual reminder (such as a string tied around a finger) is also effective.

Visualization   The more absurd or silly an image, the better it will be remembered.

Association   Linking what must be remembered with something else provides a memory "hook" that may help retrieve it from storage.

Absentmindedness is another form of forgetting that really is tied to a failure to pay attention in the first place.

If a person is struggling with the TIP-OF-THE-TONGUE PHENOMENON, the best approach is to relax and try filling in the details of the context so it can be visualized clearly. The harder a person tries to remember in this instance, the more anxiety will be generated, and the word will not be retrieved.

People who forget what they came for when they arrive in a room or a store should repeat out loud whatever it is that is needed as they head to the location where it is found. Repeating "I'm going to the store to get some milk" as they drive toward the store will help.

Study Aids   Several shorter study sessions rather than one marathon session are more useful to those who are trying to master new material. The methods used to learn should be varied—notes may be taken one day, an outline made the next, the material spoken out loud the next, then discussed with another person.

memory prodigies   Individuals with exceptional memories. Very few have been studied very intensively. One such person was the Russian mnemonist known only as "S," who was studied and treated by the psychologist Aleksandr Luria. S's exceptional mnemonic ability depended on an outstandingly vivid, detailed visual memory with an unusual degree of SYNESTHESIA (stimulation in one sense activates other senses). Although S had a highly developed concrete visualization that allowed him to perform astounding feats of memorization, his abstract thinking was weak and he was only marginally successful in life.

Exceptional memory capacity sometimes also is found among mathematicians and others with talent for fast calculation. Some composers and musicians have an exceptional auditory memory, capable of remembering incredibly complex scores of music. AUTISTIC SAVANTS often are capable of prodigious feats of calculation or memory despite being developmentally disabled in every other facet of life. (See also LURIA, ALEKSANDR R.)

memory questionnaires There are two types of memory questionnaires: *Memory questionnaires* ask subjects about world knowledge or events and assess a person's memory performance; *metamemory questionnaires* ask about a person's memory functioning and assess beliefs about his or her memory performance.

Traditionally, clinical assessments of memory problems are carried out with a standardized laboratory memory test, such as the WECHSLER MEMORY SCALE, which consists of a series of tests in several intentional verbal learning paradigms. Memory questionnaires and laboratory memory tests may draw on different memory skills and are not regarded as equivalent measures of a single memory aptitude.

Memory questionnaires test two types of memories—semantic and episodic. Within each type of memory questionnaire, different questions address either a different body of knowledge (such as historical facts) or personal experiences (high school performance, hospitalizations).

Metamemory questionnaires, on the other hand, can be used to investigate the relationship between a person's self-knowledge and performance. These tests ask questions about a person's memory performance as a way of eliciting a subject's beliefs about his or her own memory. These questionnaires use self-reports to assess one or more aspects of people's memory performance—how often they forget, how well they remember, how memory changes, how easily they learn, what memory strategies they use and how they feel about personal memory performance.

While both these questionnaires may not be reliable enough to assess how well a person remembers, they can indicate how people process information in memory tasks, since beliefs affect performance. A person's beliefs about personal memory may affect whether he or she chooses to do something or how he or she performs a memory task. Research has shown that those who believe their memory is poor are more likely to have cognitive problems when stressed.

memory quotient (MQ) An assessment of memory that is measured like IQ on a scale in which 100 indicates average performance. The WECHSLER MEMORY SCALE is the most widely used clinical memory test.

memory span The amount of information that can be held in our short-term memory storage, also called the span of awareness. Memory span is measured by the DIGIT SPAN technique, which measures the number of randomly arranged digits that a person can repeat in the correct order immediately after hearing or seeing them. Normal subjects can recall about seven digits (plus or minus two). (See also MULTISTORE MODEL.)

memory stages The three stages of remembering material—acquisition (also called encoding), retention (or storage) and retrieval (or recall). Encoding is the act of learning the material; storage is keeping that information "on file" in the brain until it is needed; retrieval is finding the information and getting it back when it is needed.

If a person can't remember something, it may be because the information was never recorded in the first place (a failure of encoding); it could be that the information was never stored; or it might be that the information was not stored in a way that makes it easy to find. Most problems in remembering occur in the retrieval stage, not the storage or encoding level. While there is not much to be done to improve retrieval directly, it is possible to improve it indirectly by polishing the methods of recording and retaining. Such polishing usually involves some type of mnemonic method that stores information in a way designed to improve its retrieval.

memory trace See ENGRAM.

meningitis An acute infection and inflammation of the meninges (the membranes that cover the brain and spinal cord) that can cause symptoms of DEMENTIA.

Cause

Meningitis is usually caused by infection from a variety of microorganisms; while viral meningitis is fairly mild, untreated bacterial meningitis can cause brain damage and dementia; it also can be fatal.

Organisms that go on to infect the brain usually travel through the bloodstream from an infection somewhere else in the body. The most common form of bacterial meningitis is meningococcal meningitis, which sometimes occurs in small epidemics and affects primarily youngsters under age five.

Symptoms

Symptoms include fever, severe headache or vomiting, confusion or drowsiness and stiff neck—and sometimes seizures. All of these symptoms may not develop early.

Diagnosis

To diagnose the disease, a physician will examine the head, ears and skin (especially along the spine) for sources of infection, together with samples of pus from the middle ear or sinuses, take X rays of chest, skull and sinuses (or a COMPUTERIZED TOMOGRAPHY SCAN to detect abscess or deep swelling). The definitive diagnosis is made by analyzing spinal fluid extracted by lumbar puncture for low glucose level and increased white blood cell count.

Treatment

Meningitis is considered to be a medical emergency and is treated with large doses of antibiotics. In some cases, treatment for brain swelling, shock, convulsions or dehydration may be necessary.

mental status examination A relatively quick psychological assessment, often administered to determine a person's general level of psychological functioning. In emergency and hospital settings, the mental status exam may be used to quickly separate those who need a more comprehensive psychological or psychiatric examination from those who don't.

The typical mental status exam begins with a quick series of observations of the examinee's appearance, behavior and activity. Additional assessments, determined by talking with and questioning the examinee, include:

- mood (long-range emotional state)
- affect (outward emotional state and expression during interview)
- thought disturbances
- thought processes (as determined through various tasks, such as the MINI-MENTAL STATE EXAMINATION.)

Mesmer, Franz Anton (1734–1815) An Austrian physician who first practiced a form of hypnotism called "mesmerism" in the 18th century.

While still a student at the University of Vienna in 1766, Mesmer began studying the works of the Renaissance mystic physician Paracelsus, developing theories based on what he thought were the astrological influences on human health as the result of planetary forces transmitted through an invisible fluid. Nine years later, he revised his theories, asserting that some occult force—which he called "animal magnetism"—flowed through the hypnotist into the patient.

He designed therapeutic interventions based on these theories loosely resembling a seance in which patients sat around a vat of dilute sulfuric acid while holding hands or grasping iron bars sticking out of the vat.

Unfortunately, it was a treatment method his fellow physicians felt was uncomfortably close to black magic, and Mesmer was forced to leave Vienna in disgrace. He settled in Paris, where he built up an extensive practice until once again his medical colleagues turned against him. So controversial were his methods that in 1784 King Louis XVI of France appointed a scientific commission (including statesman and inventor Benjamin

Franklin, guillotine inventor J.I. Guillotin and French chemist Antoine Lavoisier) to investigate Mesmer's theories.

Although the committee concluded that Mesmer's methods were worthless, his practice was destroyed not by ridicule but by politics: The French Revolution forced him to flee the country and resettle yet again, this time in London.

Despite his unhappy experience with the animal magnetism method, his theories continued to interest other physicians. In his absence from France, his disciples continued to practice mesmerism. Among his former students was the Marquis de Puysegur of Buzancy, who treated a young peasant who went into a state that would today be described as a hypnotic trance. Because the peasant's condition was similar to sleep but more like sleepwalking, Puysegur called the state *artificial somnambulism;* the term later became associated with a highly hypnotizable person. Despite the peasant's alertness during the trance, when he awoke he had no recollection of what had happened—the first case of posthypnotic amnesia.

After Mesmer died in 1815, his followers became known as mesmerists and their technique was known as mesmerism. The practice was renamed *hypnotism* after Hypnos, the Greek god of sleep, but it was not fully understood until the mid-19th century.

mesmerism   Also known as animal magnetism, this 18th-century system of treatment was the forerunner of modern-day HYPNOSIS. Mesmerism was named for its creator, Austrian physician Franz Anton Mesmer, who developed the practice while trying to uncover a link between astrology and health.

Mesmerism was based on the theory that there were astrological influences on human health as the result of planetary forces transmitted through an invisible fluid.

Therapeutic interventions based on these theories loosely resembled a seance in which patients sat around a vat of dilute sulfuric acid while holding hands or grasping iron bars sticking out of the vat. Mesmerists believed that a person may transmit universal occult forces to others in the form of "animal magnetism" during these sessions. (See also MESMER, FRANZ ANTON.)

metamemory   The overall knowledge and understanding of our own memory processes—that which allows us to know that we know something.

metamemory questionnaires   See MEMORY QUESTIONNAIRES.

Metrodorus of Scepsis   Counselor of kings and world famous in his time, this Greek rhetoric expert devised a secret mental writing system that was used to jog the memory. Called "almost divine" by the Roman orator Cicero, Metrodorus used not only architecture but the 360 degrees of the zodiac to place memory images. By placing images on a circle, he opened up new ways to make associations in the memory systems of his day.

Astrologers divided the zodiac not only into 12 signs but also into 36 decans, each covering 10 degrees. It is believed that Metrodorus grouped 10 artificial loci under each decan figure; he would thus have a series of loci numbered one to 360 in which to place information. Since all were arranged in numerical order, he could ensure against missing a locus.

It is believed that Metrodorus wrote several books on mnemonics that were subsequently lost; it is also conjectured that these lost works were part of the Greek memory system the unknown author of *AD HERENNIUM* consulted. (See also LOCI, METHOD OF.)

milacemide (2-n-pentylaminoacetamide)   A drug shown in some studies to improve human selective attention, word retrieval, numeric memory and vigilance. Milacemide crosses the blood-brain barrier, where it is converted in the brain to glycinamide and then glycine, and interacts with brain receptors associated with long-term potentiation of memory.

In one study, milacemide enhanced the speed and accuracy of word retrieval in healthy humans, although the effect was selective. Source memory (memory of the context in which a fact was learned) improved significantly, but item memory (memory of the fact itself) did not.

However, the drug appears to enhance memory only in normal subjects; according to studies, it was not effective in the treatment of ALZHEIMER'S DISEASE patients. It is not currently approved by the Food and Drug Administration for use in the treatment of age-associated memory impairment.

mild cognitive impairment   A type of memory loss more serious than that associated with normal aging, but less severe than the memory loss of ALZHEIMER'S DISEASE. People with MCI perform worse on memory tests than healthy people, but they are just as healthy in other cognitive areas— they aren't disoriented, generally confused or unable to perform activities of daily living that are characteristic of Alzheimer's disease.

Over time, the mental and functional abilities of people with MCI declined more quickly than did healthy people, but less rapidly than with those diagnosed with mild Alzheimer's disease.

Research also suggests that people with MCI appeared to be at increased risk of developing Alzheimer's disease at a rate of 10 percent to 15 percent per year. In one study at the Mayo Clinic, about half the patients with MCI developed Alzheimer's disease within four years. In the control group, only 1 to 2 percent progressed to Alzheimer's.

Diagnosis

MCI can't be diagnosed by one test; instead, a doctor must assess both physical and neurological assessments to reveal memory problems that are abnormal for age and education—together with normal ability to carry out everyday activities, normal cognitive function and the absence of dementia.

Treatment

Scientists hope that with the ability to identify those with MCI, research can focus on finding a treatment that will slow the subsequent development of Alzheimer's disease.

Unfortunately, there is still quite a bit of uncertainty about mild cognitive impairment and how it will progress in any one patient. Some critics object to the idea of MCI as a separate condition instead of simply a very early form of Alzheimer's disease.

While there is currently no approved treatment for MCI, the National Institute on Aging is conducting studies at medical research institutions in the United States and Canada to assess the effectiveness of large doses of vitamin E or DONEPEZIL (Aricept) in slowing the progression from mild cognitive impairment to Alzheimer's disease.

mini-mental state examination (MMSE)   A standard brief mental status exam routinely used as a quick way to measure a person's basic cognitive skills, such as short-term memory, long-term memory, orientation, writing and language. It is often used to screen for dementia or monitor its progression, and provides a brief but relatively thorough measure of cognition.

It doesn't measure mood, perception and the form and content of thought, and therefore isn't a substitute for a full mental status examination. It is also not a substitute for neuropsychological evaluation, but may well indicate when and what kind of such evaluation is appropriate. It's most suitable for detecting the cognitive deficits seen in syndromes of dementia and delirium and for measuring these cognitive changes over time.

Questions might include today's date, "where are you?," the ability to name three objects slowly and clearly, the ability to count backward from 100 by 7, the ability to spell a common word backward, and the ability to follow a command such as "take this piece of paper with your left hand, fold it in thirds and put it on the table." (See also ASSESSMENT OF MEMORY DISORDERS; WECHSLER MEMORY SCALE; RIVERMEAD BEHAVIORAL MEMORY TEST.)

mirror drawing   A motor task used in AMNESIA assessment in which subjects must trace between the two lines of a star while looking at their hands in the mirror.

misidentification syndromes   A group of syndromes characterized by the delusion that objects or individuals are something other than what they appear to be. Familiar people may be considered to be imposters (as in CAPGRAS SYNDROME), strangers are believed to be persecuting the patient (as in

Fregoli's syndrome) or individuals in the patient's vicinity can be misconstrued as other individuals (a nurse is believed to be a first-grade teacher). All of the misidentification syndromes are usually part of one of the psychotic disorders and are not diagnostic categories themselves.

mixed amnesia   The complex intermingling of a true organic memory defect with psychogenic factors that prolong or reinforce the memory loss. It is quite common for a brain-damaged patient to experience a hysterical reaction as well. For example, one patient who developed a severe amnesia that impaired the formation of new memories after carbon monoxide poisoning went on to develop a hysterical amnesia that continued to sustain the memory loss. (See also PSYCHOGENIC AMNESIA.)

mnemonics   The art of improving short-term recall that depends on strong visual images and meaningful associations—sort of a cross-index for memory storage.

The term was derived from the Greek MNEMOSYNE, the goddess of memory, and its techniques have been practiced since 500 B.C. Mnemonics can be verbal or visual; verbal mnemonics make word associations, and visual mnemonics use visual imagery to associate the information.

Mnemonic techniques work because they seize the attention and demand concentration. Some of the more common techniques include:

Loci (Latin for "place")   One of the oldest methods (devised by Roman orators) that relate facts to various rooms or places a person knows well. For example, to remember points in a speech, the subject would match each fact to a specific site that can be visualized—a living room, bedroom or street. When giving the speech, the person would move mentally around the living room, picking up the "facts" where they had been "placed." (See also MEMORY PALACE.)

Rhymes   Nobody likes grammar, but a rhyme makes it easy: "I before E, except after C."

Mental Pictures   This is particularly helpful in trying to remember names: When meeting Art Black, for example, one might picture a large black painting.

Repeat Facts   Another easy way to remember names is simply to repeat a person's name when introduced. For example, when someone is introduced to the new vice president, Bob Green, at a business meeting, he or she would say: "Hello, Bob," and a few seconds later repeat the name silently: "That's Bob Green." A minute or two later, the person should use Bob's name again out loud.

Chunking   While it's hard to remember a number of ten digits, everyone can remember a telephone number because it's grouped in three parts: (800) 555–2222.

Acronyms   An easy way to remember a string of words is to use acronyms. To remember the six New England states, one might try: Maybe Nobody Visits Mary's Red Car (Maine, New Hampshire, Vermont, Massachusetts, Rhode Island, Connecticut).

Lists   While it's helpful to write a list and refer to it, many people find that the act of writing something down fixes it in the memory.

Structure   If a person always places eyeglasses into a glass by the door, that's a mnemonic—by structuring activities so they don't have to be thought about, the person is better able to remember.

mnemonic strategies   Techniques (usually verbal) to aid memory, such as "Thirty days hath September . . ." Most mnemonic strategies do not have any inherent connection with the material to be learned, but they impose meaning on material that is otherwise disorganized. In general, these strategies usually involve adding something to the material to be learned to make it easier to remember and are referred to as "elaboration" by memory experts.

mnemonist   A person who has achieved spectacular mastery of mnemonic encoding strategies.

Mnemosyne   The Greek goddess of memory (and origin of the word MNEMONICS), she is the Memory that is the basis of all life and creativity and is said to know everything: past, present and future. In Greek mythology, Mnemosyne was a Titan, daughter of Uranus (heaven) and Gaea (Earth) and the mother (with Zeus) of the nine Muses. Tradition holds that after the Olympians defeated the Titans, they asked Zeus to create divinities who were capable of celebrating their victory. Zeus then went to Pieria and stayed with Mnemosyne nine consecutive nights, after which she gave birth to the Muses. Some experts argue that Mnemosyne is memory personified and as a pure abstraction could not have been a Titan.

Still, her art was of profound importance to the ancient Greek culture, and every one of the educated class practiced mnemonics. The memory palaces built by these early memory experts allowed them to perform outstanding feats of memory. Many believed memory was the path to immortality itself. (See also LETHE; MEMORY IN MYTH.)

mnemotechnics   Invented by the Greeks, this is the art of memorization by using a technique of impressing places and images on memory. Such techniques were critically important in an age before printing.

mnestic syndromes   A mixed group of disorders in which memory disturbances are the dominant clinical problem. The disturbances may be of different kinds (AMNESIA, dysmnesia or HYPERMNESIA) due to organic damage that is specific rather than generalized and usually involves lesions in the HIPPOCAMPUS or the MAMMILLARY BODIES. People with a variety of mnestic syndromes show intellectual impairment as well; there may be clouding consciousness, loss of abstract reasoning or mental confusion. The best known of the mnestic syndromes is KORSAKOFF'S SYNDROME. (See also AGNOSIA; AGRAPHIA; ALEXIA; ALZHEIMER'S DISEASE; ANOSOGNOSIA; APHASIA; APRAXIA; BROCA'S APHASIA; CRYPTOMNESIA; DIENCEPHALIC AMNESIA; DISSOCIATIVE DISORDERS; DYSMNESIA/DYSMNESIC SYNDROME; DYSPHASIA; HYSTERICAL AMNESIA; ISCHEMIC AMNESIA; MIXED AMNESIA; ORGANIC AMNESIA; RETROGRADE AMNESIA; SELECTIVE AMNESIA; TRANSIENT GLOBAL AMNESIA.)

Moniz, Antonio Egas (1874–1955)   A Portuguese neurologist who performed the first LEUCOTOMY (the severing of nerve tracts connecting the frontal association cortex with deeper structures in the brain). Moniz was deeply interested in the practice of psychosurgery (another term he invented), and he won the 1949 Nobel Prize in Physiology and Medicine for his leucotomy work.

The term *leucotomy* is derived from two Greek words meaning "white" and "to cut." In leucotomy, the skull of a person is opened and the white fibers connecting the frontal lobe to the rest of the brain are cut. Moniz developed the idea after hearing of experimental lobectomies performed on chimpanzees. His work inspired American neurologists Walter Freeman and James Watts to perform the first American leucotomies in 1936.

Moniz described his procedure in the 1936 textbook on psychosurgery, *Tentatives Opératoires dans le Traitement de Certaines Psychoses (Experimental Surgery in the Treatment of Certain Psychoses)*. In 1955, he was beaten to death in his office by one of his patients. (See also FREEMAN, WALTER.)

motor association   The type of memory responsible for the fact that once a human learns certain motor skills—say, to ride a bicycle—the motor memory of the experience is never forgotten. It is the oldest form of memory in the biological world.

Birds and mammals can remember both sensory and motor associations, but animals farther down the evolutionary ladder (such as fruit flies, cockroaches and flatworms) can form only motor associations.

Research with cabbage butterflies in 1986 revealed that motor associations enhance survival; while individual butterflies visit flowers of one species, the motor memories of experienced butterflies enable them to work more quickly and obtain more nectar from flowers. Because a different method is required to obtain nectar from different types of flowers, cabbage butterflies that can select one single species are more productive. Scientists know that recognition depends on memory and not on instinct because different cabbage butterflies favor different species; experiments have shown that if necessary, cabbage butterflies will change to a new species and become faithful to those flowers.

MQ   See MEMORY QUOTIENT (MQ).

MRI   See MAGNETIC RESONANCE IMAGING (MRI).

multi-infarct dementia   One of the two most common incurable forms of mental impairment in old age, caused by a series of small strokes that result in widespread death of brain tissue. Multi-infarct dementia causes a step-by-step degeneration in mental ability, with each step occurring after a stroke; memory (especially of recent events) is affected first.

It accounts for about 20 percent of the irreversible cases of mental impairment. In the early stages before severe damage has been done, the person usually is aware of impaired ability, which can lead to frustration and depression. Multi-infarct dementia (and the strokes that cause it) are usually the result of an underlying medical condition, such as high blood pressure and artery damage.

Multi-infarct dementia usually develops more quickly than ALZHEIMER'S DISEASE, and is usually linked to stroke-related physical problems such as paralysis or slurred speech, which aren't symptoms of Alzheimer's disease. Nonetheless, it may be hard to tell the difference between the two dementing conditions. It's also possible for someone to have both Alzheimer's disease and multi-infarct dementia. About one in five of those with senile dementia show signs of both conditions.

Cause

Multi-infarct dementia occurs when brain tissue dies (*infarct* means "tissue death"). The tissue dies as a result of cumulative damage to the brain after a series of mini-strokes known as TRANSIENT ISCHEMIC ATTACKS (TIAs)—strokes that are so mild they may not be noticed. TIAs occur when a blood clot temporarily blocks an already narrow artery in the brain, briefly cutting blood flow to the brain. These mini-strokes occur suddenly, and may lead to numbness, fainting, dizziness, clumsiness or loss of speech or vision. Other mini-strokes are ignored or unnoticed. Although most people seem to recover from TIAs completely, each episode kills some brain tissue. Those who experience several TIAs ("multi-infarcts") may eventually have enough brain damage to develop multi-infarct dementia.

Symptoms

Symptoms include confusion, problems with recent memory, wandering or getting lost in familiar places, loss of bladder or bowel control, laughing or crying inappropriately, problems following instructions or handling money. At first the symptoms may be slight, but as more small vessels are blocked, mental ability and memory gradually decline. Multi-infarct dementia usually begins between ages 60 and 75, affecting more men than women.

Diagnosis

Those who are suspected to have multi-infarct dementia should have thorough physical, neurological and psychiatric evaluations, including a complete medical exam and tests of mental state together with a brain scan. The brain scan can rule out curable diseases and also may show signs of normal age-related changes in the brain, such as shrinkage.

Treatment

Prevention is really the only effective treatment for multi-infarct dementia; patients with high blood pressure, transient ischemic attacks or earlier strokes should continue treatment for these diseases to minimize the chance of developing dementia. It is possible to prevent and (to some extent) treat the condition with low-dose aspirin. While the dose isn't strong enough to cure a headache, it can help prevent internal blood clots that cause TIAs. A 1989 study at the Cerebral Blood Flow Laboratory at the Veterans Administration Medical Center in Houston showed that aspirin can slow the progression of multi-infarct dementia and in some cases, reverse it.

While there is no cure, careful use of drugs can lessen agitation, anxiety and depression, and improve sleep. Proper nutrition is especially important, and patients should be encouraged to maintain normal daily routines, physical activities and contact with friends. Information about time of day, place of residence and what is going on in the home and the world can help prevent brain activity from failing at a faster rate. Memory aids, such as a visible calendar, lists of daily activities, safety guidelines and directions to commonly used items, also may help people in their day-to-day activities.

multiple personality disorder   A disorder in which a person has two or more distinct personalities, each of which dominates at a different time. The personalities are almost always very different from each other and are often total opposites. While the personalities may have no awareness of each other, each is aware of lost periods of time. Multiple personality is often the mind's response to trauma in childhood, often including severe sexual or physical abuse.

An expanded diagnosis of multiple personality disorder is now known as dissociative identity disorder.

Before 1910 it had been widely recognized, but between 1910 and 1975 its description disappeared from psychiatric literature. Some experts suggest this was because most people with multiple personality disorder were misdiagnosed as schizophrenics. In fact, a 1988 study found that 41 percent of 236 people with this disorder had previously been diagnosed with schizophrenia. Since the 1980s it has been diagnosed much more often; some experts believe inappropriately so.

Because the nature of the condition is so dramatic, multiple personalities have been the subject of books and movies for some time, including *The Three Faces of Eve* (1957), a book later made into a movie.

Evidence of multiple personality also has been used as a criminal defense, such as in the case of the Hillside Strangler in Los Angeles. When Kenneth Bianchi strongly denied his guilt of rape and murder of several women, under hypnosis another personality called "Steve" emerged. This Steve was very different from Ken, and he claimed responsibility for the murders; even after returning to consciousness, Ken remembered nothing of the conversations between "Steve" and the hypnotist.

The presence of another personality inside Ken involved a moral dilemma for the court, which had to decide on the criminal responsibility of Ken, although it apparently was "Steve" who committed the crimes. In this case, the court refused to accept that Bianchi was a genuine multiple personality, because the second personality emerged only during hypnotic sessions after the examiner had already informed him that he would reveal another part of himself. (See also AMNESIA AND CRIME.)

multiple sclerosis   A degenerative disease of the central nervous system believed to involve the immune system, which attacks the myelin (protective covering of nerve fibers), disrupting function and causing paralysis and, in some patients, memory loss. It is believed that this memory loss is a result of dysfunctioning frontal and temporal lobes. The severity of the disease varies considerably among patients.

Cause

The cause of multiple sclerosis (MS) is unknown, but it is thought to be an autoimmune disease in which the body's own defense system treats myelin as an invader, gradually destroying it. There seems to be a genetic factor, since relatives of affected people are eight times more likely than others to contract the disease, although the environment also may play a part. (MS is five times more common in temperate zones, including the United States and Europe.) Some researchers believe it may involve a slow virus, picked up during a susceptible time of early life. The disease occurs in one in every 1,000 people in temperate zones.

Symptoms

The disease usually appears in early adult life, with brief periods of remission; symptoms vary depending on the part of the brain that is affected. Memory loss often does not appear immediately, but may occur years later.

Diagnosis

Confirmation of the disease usually comes only after other diseases have been ruled out; a neurologist may perform tests to help confirm the diagnosis, including lumbar puncture (removal of a fluid from the spinal canal for lab analysis) or testing electrical activity in the brain.

Treatment

At present, there is no cure. Corticosteroid drugs may alleviate some acute symptoms, and other drugs may help incontinence and depression.

multistore model   The theory that memory is a series of "stores," each representing a different stage in the processing of information.

New information first enters a "sensory store" via the nervous system and one or more of the senses. Researchers have found that the pattern of stimulation set up remains for a short period after the stimulus itself ceases. For visual information, for example, this type of sensory storage is called ICONIC MEMORY: When subjects are shown three rows of letters (such as PDT, ZRT, SNR) for 50 milliseconds, afterward they could name only four or five sets of them. But when subjects were shown the letters and immediately afterward were given a signal indicating which of the three rows should be reported, they named all three letters correctly most of the time. Since subjects weren't warned ahead of time as to which row they would have to name, they must have had the whole sequence available when the signal was given, even though the stimulus itself was no longer visible.

During sensory storage, information is identified before it passes into short-term store (or "primary memory"), the basis of conscious mental activity. Short-term store determines what information is attended to and how information is processed; it also is responsible for retrieving existing memory. Short-term store can hold only so much information—called the "span of awareness," or memory span.

This short-term type of memory storage is necessary in order to perform many tasks; for example, when reading a book, the beginning of the sentence must be kept in mind while reading the last part of the sentence in order for the whole phrase to make sense. However, research suggests that the information in short-term storage is highly vulnerable to distraction or negative interference (for example, when a person loses the train of thought during a conversation after being interrupted).

Once placed in short-term storage, information can be either transferred into long-term store (or "secondary memory") or forgotten. If data are to be transferred into long-term store, a permanent memory trace is formed that provides the basis for restoring the information to consciousness.

However, these early memory processes are extremely complex and require word identification and object recognition. By the time information has reached short-term store, a great deal of processing has already occurred of which we are not consciously aware. What passes into consciousness and short-term store is simply the result of those unconscious processes. Researchers suggest that only information that has been consciously perceived is transferred from short- to long-term store. (See also ENGRAM.)

Nakane's mnemonics   Extensive mnemonic programs based on stories, rhymes and songs, developed by Japanese educator Masachika Nakane for learning mathematics, science, spelling and grammar and the English language.

This system has been used for children as young as kindergarten age for solving algebraic problems, performing calculus, generating formulas for chemical compounds and learning English.

In the United States, Nakane's system has been used for more basic learning. One group of third graders using his mnemonic devices learned all of the mathematical operations with fractions in three hours—just as well as sixth-grade students had learned the same calculations in three years. Extensive mnemonic programs have also been developed in the United States for reading, spelling, grammar and basic math skills.

narrative chaining   A type of mnemonic strategy in which items to be remembered are incorporated into a story.

neocortex   The part of the brain that lets us store logic, language, mathematics and speculation about the future and enables us to change the behavior patterns that are set in motion by the more primitive parts of our brains.

nerve growth factors   Also called neurotrophic factors, this is a naturally occurring hormone that stimulates the growth of neurites (tiny projections growing from each neuron that carry information between cells). Nerve growth factor is one of the human growth factors currently being studied for its potential to restore function in the aging. Human growth hormone, another growth factor, also is being investigated for its potential to strengthen the memory in the elderly.

Nerve growth factors (at least eight different varieties currently are being studied) each have a different target cell in the body, and each has a possible role in protecting the body's nerve cells against damage from diseases such as Alzheimer's, Parkinson's and amyotrophic lateral sclerosis (Lou Gehrig's disease).

POTENTIAL USES FOR
NERVE GROWTH FACTOR HORMONE

Nerve Growth Factor	Used for
Nerve growth factor	Alzheimer's disease
Basic fibroblast growth factor	Wound healing and Parkinson's disease, stroke
Brain-derived neurotrophic factor	Parkinson's disease
Neurotrophin-3	Nerve damage following trauma, chemotherapy or diabetes, and in the treatment of Alzheimer's disease
Neurotrophin-4/5	Alzheimer's and Parkinson's diseases
Ciliary neurotrophic factor	Lou Gehrig's disease
Glial growth factor	Peripheral neuropathy
Glial maturation factor	Nerve injuries

Scientists at the University of California at San Diego found that in a variety of learning and memory tests, infusions of nerve growth factor into the brain could improve learning capacity and increased the size of brain cells that had previously shrunk. In Sweden, a human Alzheimer's patient is reportedly being treated with a similar approach.

Some scientists are now developing a new class of drugs called K252 compounds, which are designed to boost the body's production of nerve growth factor. Other studies are investigating a possible treatment for Parkinson's disease, Lou Gehrig's disease and stroke patients. (See chart, page 163.)

The problem with using the different nerve growth factors is that most of the molecules are large and difficult to handle, and must be pumped directly into the brain because they will not cross the blood-brain barrier. Researchers hope that new kinds of drug delivery systems, such as patches and nasal sprays, may simplify research and treatment with these growth factors.

neurofibrillary tangles   Abnormal accumulations of fibrous filamentary material within the brain's neurons are one of the hallmarks of ALZHEIMER'S DISEASE. The tangles were first described by German neuropathologist Alois Alzheimer in 1906, who realized that the tangles differentiated Alzheimer's disease from other problems. Although scientists knew of the existence of neurofibrillary tangles in 1906, it was not until the 1980s that scientists discovered the tangles were associated with the internal structure of the neuron and a protein called TAU. In a healthy neuron, the internal structure (called a microtubule) exists in a parallel shape, much like a set of train tracks. The structure is held together by crosspieces made up of tau protein. The microtubules are responsible for carrying nutrients from the body of the cell down to the ends of axons.

In patients with Alzheimer's disease, the tau forming the crosspieces begins to twist and tangle, which leads to the collapse of the microtubule. (See also ALZHEIMER, ALOIS.)

neuron   Another name for nerve cell, the neuron is the basic functional unit of the nervous system.

Neurons carry on information processing in the brain. Each consists of a relatively compact cell body containing the nucleus, several long branched extensions (dendrites) and a single long fiber (the axon) with twiglike branches along its length and at its end.

Dendrites lie adjacent to one another in a gigantic web; to send a signal, one neuron squirts out a chemical (called a neurotransmitter) that crosses the gap (synapse) between adjacent dendrites. The receiving dendrite has receptors that recognize the chemical transmitter and speed the signal through the neuron. In a series of complicated steps, the receptor changes shape and opens a channel. Information in the form of electrically charged molecules passes through the channel and into the neuron. There the information can be either stored or passed along. At the same time, the first neuron emits substances that terminate the transmission and reabsorb any excess transmitter chemicals left in the synapse.

The average human brain contains many billions of brain cells, each with up to 60,000 synapses, but the average number of neurons varies dramatically and seems to have nothing to do with intelligence. (Some animals have more neurons than humans do.) Apparently, quantity is less important than the quality of the connections between them.

It also appears that memories are encoded in the brain's neurons, which convert chemical signals to electrical signals and then back to chemical signals again.

A single neuron can receive signals from thousands of other neurons, and its axon can branch repeatedly, sending signals to thousands more. While researchers have long understood the mechanism of neurons, only recently have they begun to understand how these cells might be able to store memories.

Most scientists agree that when a person experiences a new event, a unique pattern of neurons is activated in some way and, within the entire configuration of brain cells, certain cells "light up." In order to store a new memory, there must be a way to save the memory—to forge connections between neurons to create a new circuit that acts as a symbol of something in the outside world. By reactivating the circuit, the brain can retrieve the memory—a replica of the original perception. The memory can be evoked again when the person encounters something that brings up a neural pattern similar to the one that was already stored in the brain.

Unlike the wiring in a home, however, the brain's circuits are not permanent; as knowledge is acquired, circuits break apart and reform, constantly rewiring themselves and influencing our representations in the world.

Any one memory can be found not in one particular neuron in one particular place, but along a neuronal circuit within the vast, weblike structure of neurons sprawling throughout the brain.

neuropeptides   Building blocks of proteins that are made of amino acids. Normally they are produced by the pituitary gland and function as neurotransmitters. They include adrenocorticotropic hormone (ACTH), melanocyte-stimulating hormone (MSH) and vasopressin. Some researchers believe ACTH improves sustained attention and diminishes depression in dementia patients. Vasopressin is being studied as a possible memory enhancement drug.

neuropsychological assessment   Tests that can evaluate the extent of brain damage and memory deficits, including assessment of language, memory, perception, reasoning, emotion, self-control and planning. (See chart below.) This kind of test-

ing was first used as a way to distinguish between those whose abnormal behavior was caused by brain dysfunction and those whose problems were caused by psychological factors. Disorders caused by brain dysfunction are called organic; psychological disorders are referred to as functional or psychogenic.

Early tests were based on the assumption that there were common characteristics in all organic impairments. These tests gave a general assessment of "organicity" instead of details about the status of different mental functions.

Although the idea of "brain damage" as a single concept persists, in fact there is no one simple test that can uncover the often-diffuse problems experienced by those who have brain problems. Because brain damage may be caused by lesions of different sizes and shapes in different parts of the brain, uncovering the exact source of brain damage requires a more sophisticated, comprehensive assessment. In order to rehabilitate patients with brain deficits properly, it is imperative to have a clear picture of their cognitive strengths and weaknesses, to help choose the treatment technique and to measure response to treatment. (See also ASSESSMENT OF MEMORY DISORDERS.)

neurosis and memory   Neurosis is a term often used to describe a range of relatively mild psychiatric disorders in which the patient remains in touch with reality; memory problems are primary symptoms in several neurotic disorders.

FREQUENTLY USED NEUROPSYCHOLOGICAL TESTS

General Intelligence
Wechsler Adult Intelligence Scale
  Revised (WAIS-R)

Reading, Writing, Arithmetic Skills
Wide Range Achievement Test Revised
Woodcok-Johnson Revised Test of Academic
  Achievement

Memory
Wechsler Memory Scale Revised
Buschke Selective Reminding Test

Visual Perception Processes
Hooper Visual Organization Test
Judgment of Line Orientation Test

Visual Form Discrimination Test
Visual Scanning and Speed
Halstead-Reitan Trailmaking Test

Abstraction and Problem-Solving
Wisconsin Card Sorting Test
Receptive Listening/Vocabulary
Peabody Picture Vocabulary Test Revised

The major neurotic disorders include mild forms of depression, anxiety disorders (including phobias and obsessive-compulsive disorder), somatization disorder and DISSOCIATIVE DISORDERS and psychosexual disorders. Of these, both depression and dissociative disorders feature memory loss as a primary symptom.

Repression—an explanation of forgetting that suggests unpleasant memories may be forgotten intentionally—was the underlying theme of the theories of Sigmund Freud; he considered repression the keystone to his entire theory of neurosis. According to Freud, to enable people to survive mentally, unacceptable, traumatic or unpleasant memories are forgotten intentionally by being pushed into the unconscious on purpose. Repression is a form of coping and often occurs, Freud believed, during childhood. He also believed that childhood amnesia is caused by the repression of infantile sexuality; many modern memory researchers now say it is due to the lack of early development of various mental abilities (such as language) used to cue memory.

neurotransmitters and memory Specialized chemical messengers synthesized and secreted by neurons that affect most connections between the nerve cells. A neurotransmitter is released into the synapse (space between neurons), moves across the space and attaches to a receptor in the outer wall of a neighboring neuron. Some neurotransmitters stimulate the release of neurotransmitters from other neurons, while others inhibit the release of other neurotransmitters.

Many different neurotransmitters appear to be involved in the memory process, including ACETYLCHOLINE, CALPAIN, NOREPINEPHRINE, DOPAMINE, ACTH, endorphins and the opioid peptides.

New Adult Reading Test A list of 50 increasingly difficult words that can indicate premorbid intelligence in those of high-average or superior intelligence. Psychologists who are trying to test for brain damage face a problem in quantifying loss in the absence of evidence of how well the person performed before deterioration began. For example, a person with an IQ of 140 could lose 20 or 30 points and still test as "average," but if the person's previous intellectual ability had been known the comparison would reveal a significant loss of intellectual ability.

Studies have found that, in fact, language skills seem to deteriorate more slowly than other memory aspects; a group of patients with dementia retained their ability to pronounce unusually spelled words despite gradual deterioration in other intellectual areas.

The New Adult Reading Test (NART) was developed to take advantage of this persistence of language skills; scores on this test are considered to be a good predictor of intelligence before deterioration took place in those with high-average or superior intelligence.

next-in-line effect A phenomenon related to attention in which self-concern erases memory for events immediately preceding a person's own performance. In one experiment, scientists assembled groups of subjects to read word lists. The group of subjects who knew the order of performance showed a marked next-in-line effect; that is, they could recall the performances of those who came before the person immediately preceding them but retained no memory of the person who read the word list immediately before their own performance. When told that subjects would have to report on the list read immediately before their own, the next-in-line effect was abolished simply because subjects had a reason to pay attention.

niacin Also called vitamin B$_3$, this vitamin has shown in some studies to be a memory enhancer. In one double-blind study, normal healthy subjects improved their memory between 10 and 40 percent after taking 141 milligrams of niacin daily.

Niacin should never be taken without a physician's approval by those with diabetes, high blood pressure, ulcers or porphyria. Some patients experience skin flushing or dizziness shortly after taking niacin; flushing is more likely to occur when taken on an empty stomach.

The principal dietary sources of niacin include liver, lean meat, poultry, fish, whole grains, nuts and dried beans. (See also MALNUTRITION; XANTHINOL NICOTINATE.)

nicotine and memory While smoking may give the impression of sharpening concentration, in fact studies have shown that smokers puffing on a regular nicotine cigarette fared 24 percent worse than subjects smoking nonnicotine cigarettes on a memory test of item recall. Similarly, a British study paired 37 smokers and 37 nonsmokers in another study and asked them to remember a list of a dozen names. Ten minutes later the nonsmokers could recall significantly more names than the smokers.

In fact, smoking cigarettes can impair memory performance about as much as several alcoholic drinks. Nonsmokers are able to remember lists of numbers more quickly than smokers, and they also score higher on the standard Wechsler Memory Scale.

In addition, research indicates that smokers who want to remember something should put off lighting up right before a memory task—but putting off smoking too long beforehand can make a person so jittery that it distracts from the task.

Scientists suspect that the nicotine may interfere with the blood supply carrying oxygen to the brain, resulting in poorer memory efficiency.

nimodipine (Nimotop) A possible "memory drug" that has been used successfully to treat stroke victims and is being studied for the treatment of ALZHEIMER'S DISEASE and age-associated memory impairment. The drug can minimize brain damage after a stroke by helping to keep brain arteries open, maintaining blood flow to the brain. Nimodipine also seems to increase ACETYLCHOLINE levels.

It was approved by the Food and Drug Administration in 1989 to treat hemorrhagic stroke, as it improves blood flow in the brain and lessens oxygen deprivation.

However, a recent review of existing studies can find no convincing evidence that nimodipine is a useful treatment for the symptoms of dementia, whether caused by Alzheimer's disease or stroke. On the other hand, scientists concluded that larger and more complete studies are needed to independently evaluate this drug.

NMDA A molecule whose full name is N-methyl D-aspartate, this substance is found at the ends of dendrites, the branchlike projections that protrude from nerve and brain cells, waiting to respond to incoming signals. Like other receptor molecules, NMDA reacts to a chemical cue (when it comes to learning and memory formation, it's glutamate) sent by the axon from a neighboring cell. But unlike other receptors, NMDA must also receive an electrical discharge from its own cell. Only when both cells are communicating at the same time does the NMDA receptor turn on.

It then triggers calcium ions to flow into the host cell, which somehow makes the cell easier to excite the next time. This phenomenon, known as long-term potentiation, is believed to underlie one type of memory formation.

Scientists have solid evidence of the importance of the role of NMDA in learning and memory. For years, researchers have known that blocking NMDA receptors with drugs interferes with learning in animals. Some even appear to lose their memory completely. Administering drugs that stimulate the receptor, on the other hand, seems to improve their memory.

nominal aphasia Difficulty in naming objects or finding words, although the person may be able to choose the correct name from several offers. Nominal aphasia may be caused by generalized cerebral dysfunction or damage to specific language areas. While some recovery is usual after a stroke or injury, the more severe the type of aphasia, the less the chance of recovery. (See also APHASIA; BROCA'S APHASIA; GLOBAL APHASIA; OPTICAL APHASIA; WERNICKE'S [RECEPTIVE] APHASIA.)

nootropic drugs A class of drugs designed to improve learning, memory consolidation and memory retrieval without other central nervous system effects. The name "nootropic" was taken from the Greek words *noos* (mind) and *tropein* (toward). The search for a "magic pill" to improve memory continues to this day, and the success of the search remains controversial.

Many neuroscientists argue that the complexity of the brain suggests that cognition is the result of the coordination of many processes, so that it seems unlikely that a single chemical could improve memory.

Still, some studies suggest that indeed there are drugs that improve memory. As early as 1917, researchers discovered that caffeine and strychnine speeded up a rat's ability to learn, and many other studies show that different drugs can improve the learning or recall process in rats, monkeys and humans.

The mechanism by which these drugs seem to improve memory is not completely understood, but many studies suggest they work by affecting the cholinergic system (the part of the nervous system that uses ACETYLCHOLINE as a neurotransmitter). In addition, there may be some involvement with adrenal steroid production in the adrenal cortex. The nootropics can be divided into several different categories:

Cholinergic Agonists: Strychnine and picrotoxin, nicotine and related substances act by influencing the release of acetylcholine in the HIPPOCAMPUS; it is known that this neurotransmitter plays an important role in the ability of the synapses to change.

Hormones such as vasopressin, EPINEPHRINE, NOREPINEPHRINE and ACTH act by activating the cholinergic signals in the hippocampus.

Stimulants such as caffeine and amphetamine likely act by increasing alertness and attention, which in turn improves memory consolidation.

The piracetam family of compounds (piracetam, aniracetam, oxiracetam and others) may act by influencing growth of the synapses.

Ampakines might act by enhancing the signal activity just before memory encoding in the hippocampus and elsewhere.

Other substances such as ginkgo biloba extract, choline and acetyl-L-carnitine don't seem to enhance memory, but may support increased attention or make neurons healthier.

Many of these chemicals act on very basic processes in the brain where simple adjustments can affect higher-level processes such as memory encoding. Most studies to date have assessed these drugs on animals; most human studies focus on treating dementia or aging.

There are, however, drugs that improve reaction time and attention; the most well known are nicotine and caffeine, and ACETYL-L-CARNITINE.

In any case, it appears that the effect of these chemicals is highly individual; many of the nootropics may react differently among different patients, and even differently in one patient at different times. For example, caffeine appears to improve recognition and recall differently, depending on how much a person is paying attention, or the time of day the person takes the caffeine.

Indeed, some researchers believe that timing very much affects how well a drug works to improve memory. In many cases the drug has no effect if given before or during the learning experience. Other drugs work only when given before the experience.

Some memory drugs may even improve subsequent memory if given before birth. For example, researchers found that if the diet of pregnant rats is supplemented with choline, offspring will show improved spatial memory. This appears to be due to changes in the density of receptors in the brain; whether it would work in humans is not known.

Unfortunately, while some nootropics may improve some aspects of memory, this improvement may come at a price. Caffeine, for example, improves attention, but impairs the ability to deal with contradictory or uncertain stimuli. This means that a person might learn very well, but might remember details at the expense of general knowledge or abstraction ability. Finally, many of the nootropics, such as strychnine or amphetamines, have serious drawbacks and can be highly toxic.

norepinephrine A chemical messenger in the brain (also called noradrenalin) involved in alertness, concentration, aggression and motivation, among other behaviors, which also seems to be associated with memory. Norepinephrine is produced in the brain by the amino acids L-phenylanine and L-tyrosine. It controls the release of endocrine hormones that control metabolism.

Some scientists believe that this chemical triggers long-term memory; when we have an experience that strongly affects us, norepinephrine may tell the brain to save the memory. In studies at the

University of California at Irvine, researchers gave rats a shock when they stepped on a shelf. When the rats were placed in the cage weeks later, they remembered not to step on the shelf; when their production of norepinephrine was blocked, however, the rats forgot what they had learned about the shelf and endured repeated shocks.

Alterations in this neurotransmitter also have been implicated in several mental disorders. (See NEUROTRANSMITTERS AND MEMORY.) Neurons in the locus coerulus (the source of the forebrain norepinephrine system) appear to alert the forebrain to incoming stimuli such as lights, tones and skin contact; norepinephrine, therefore, could be expected to influence learning and memory.

normal-pressure hydrocephalus (NPH)   Also known as water on the brain this uncommon disorder involves an obstruction in the normal flow of cerebrospinal fluid, causing it to build up in the brain. It is called "normal pressure" hydrocephalus because the pressure in the spinal fluid is normal, unlike most cases of water on the brain.

Symptoms

A person with NPH may show all of the symptoms of classic ALZHEIMER'S DISEASE, especially the dementia. However, a COMPUTERIZED TOMOGRAPHY (CT) SCAN will show that the ventricles of the brain are enlarged from an excessive amount of fluid. Other symptoms include urinary incontinence and difficulty in walking. Presently, the most useful diagnostic tools include imaging techniques.

Cause

While the exact cause is unknown, NPH may be associated with the interference of circulating fluid in the brain as a result of meningitis, encephalitis, brain surgery, head injuries, or brain hemorrhage.

Diagnosis

A spinal tap shows normal pressure of cerebrospinal fluid in the spine, while a CT or MRI scan of the head shows changes that indicate NPH.

Treatment

In addition to treating the underlying cause, the condition may be corrected by a neurosurgical procedure called a shunt, which will divert excess fluid from the brain. About 50 percent of cases are cured with this treatment. Patients whose NPH is caused by a brain hemorrhage or inflammation do not usually benefit from shunting.

nuclear magnetic resonance (NMR)   See MAGNETIC RESONANCE IMAGING (MRI).

ondansetron A new drug that increases the release of ACETYLCHOLINE, a neurotransmitter in the brain linked to improved learning and memory. Acetylcholine deficits often are found in most forms of memory impairment. By selectively blocking serotonin, a brain substance that inhibits the release of acetylcholine, ondansetron increases acetylcholine release and enhances memory and performance, according to some research.

According to Glaxo, the British drug company that manufactures ondansetron, the drug increases acetylcholine only in parts of the brain concerned with memory; this fact might eliminate the side effects associated with acetylcholine release in other parts of the body.

It has been shown to increase learning and memory in animals. Initial research suggests that drugs like ondansetron may improve memory in some healthy older adults with age-associated memory impairment. In one study, memory improvement still occurred after three months of ondansetron administration on tests of immediate and delayed name-face recall. In studies of 250 subjects with age-associated memory impairment sponsored by Glaxo, 12 weeks treatment significantly improved the patients memories as compared to a placebo. The extent of the improvement in memory function was about equivalent to the amount of memory that is lost every six years with aging.

Other studies have found that ondansetron improves memory and learning ability in marmosets, rats, mice and primates. In some studies, scientists first injected SCOPOLAMINE to induce memory impairment and then employed ondansetron to reverse the cognitive deficits. Still other studies are investigating another serotonin antagonist, ZATOSETRON, available in tablet form in England and suspected to improve cognition in older adults with age-associated memory impairment.

The drug (trade name: Zofran) is approved by the Food and Drug Administration for use only as an antivomiting/nausea medication following chemotherapy.

optical aphasia The inability to name the object that one sees. A person with optical aphasia who sees a bowl of soup can recognize the soup but cannot name the object. If a person with optical aphasia can taste or smell the soup, the person can name it; it is only the visual recognition that is lacking. (See also APHASIA, BROCA'S APHASIA, GLOBAL APHASIA, OPTICAL APHASIA, WERNICKE'S [RECEPTIVE] APHASIA.)

oral traditions The memory feats of storytellers and singers in nonliterate societies are impressive; these memory experts do not recite verbatim, letter-perfect tales, but they provide reconstructions according to formulaic rules. The storyteller introduces new ingredients to suit the current audience while adhering to a traditional structure. In oral traditions long stories usually are told in verse instead of prose because the rhythm makes verse easier to remember. Storytellers also make use of group chanting to aid retrieval.

organic amnesia Amnesia due to brain dysfunction. Organic memory disorders can be either global or specific; that is, they can affect either a large part of memory (global) or only particular memory bits (specific).

organic brain syndrome A disturbance of consciousness, intellect or mental functioning of physical (organic) as opposed to psychiatric origin. Possible causes include degenerative diseases such as ALZHEIMER'S DISEASE, metabolic imbalances, infections, drugs, toxins, vitamin deficiencies or the effects of brain trauma, stroke or tumor.

In the acute phase of the condition, symptoms can range from a slight confusion to stupor or coma and may include disorientation, memory impairment, hallucinations and delusions. The chronic form of the syndrome causes a progressive decline in intellect, memory and behavior.

Treatment is more likely to be successful with the acute form of organic brain syndrome if the underlying cause can be identified; in chronic cases irreversible brain damage may already have occurred. (See also BRAIN TUMOR.)

organic mental disorders   Conditions that affect the brain and cause problems with memory, thinking, behavior and mental health. These disorders represent a broad grouping of diseases, including ALZHEIMER'S DISEASE. Organic mental disorders that can cause clinical problems like those of Alzheimer's disease, but which might be reversible or controlled with proper diagnosis and treatment, include:

- **circulatory disorders:** Heart problems or strokes.
- **drug side effects:** Unusual reactions, too much or too little of prescribed medications, or toxic combinations of medications
- **infections:** Viral or fungal infections of the brain, such as MENINGITIS or ENCEPHALITIS
- **metabolic disorders:** Thyroid problems, nutritional deficiencies, or anemias
- **neurological disorders:** NORMAL PRESSURE HYDROCEPHALUS or MULTIPLE SCLEROSIS
- **substance abuse:** Abuse of legal and/or illegal drugs or alcohol
- **toxicity:** Carbon monoxide, methyl alcohol, etc.
- **trauma:** Head injury
- **tumors:** Any type within the skull, whether originating there or spreading from elsewhere.

organic mental syndromes   A cluster of psychological or behavioral signs and symptoms with unknown cause, but associated with brain dysfunction.

A person could be diagnosed with an organic mental syndrome upon admission to the hospital with delirium or dementia from an unknown cause. These symptoms could be due to a stroke, substance abuse, poisoning, brain tumor or neurological disease.

Once the source of brain dysfunction is discovered, the problem is rediagnosed as an ORGANIC MENTAL DISORDER.

organization and memory   Organizing material so it is easier to learn and remember is one of the best ways to improve the memory. In fact, this is such an effective strategy that many people spontaneously organize material as they memorize it.

When researchers gave a list of 24 pairs of scrambled words that were actually highly associated (such as "sleep" and "dream" or "cart" and "horse"), despite the scrambling subjects tended to recall the words in associated pairs. But when information has no inherent organization, subjects often will impose their own subjective organization. That is, they will remember a list of words in order, even though there is no logical reason to do so.

In fact, it is easier to learn any facts if there is some link between them, so that remembering one word automatically drags along its link (called "cueing"). In addition, our ability to learn is based on what we already know about the subject.

The importance of organization rises as the information to be learned becomes more detailed and complex. While learning a simple list of words is not too difficult, digesting and understanding the contents of a book chapter is more difficult. One approach, according to memory experts, is to imagine a tree and place the organization of the book chapter on that tree.

orientation reaction   The Russian physiologist Ivan Pavlov was the first to describe the sudden arousal of orientation reaction, in which trained dogs would turn to investigate a new person entering a room instead of behaving properly. This "investigative" behavior (what Pavlov called the what-is-it reaction) has biological significance for survival, he believed.

Arousal usually changes to fear, aggression or indifference—usually indifference, which means that on the level of factual memory, we have decided the stimulus is not worth paying attention to. (See also PAVLOV, IVAN PETROVICH.)

overlearning   An important aid to LONG-TERM MEMORY, overlearning is what occurs when a person remembers something over a long period of time despite the fact that it no longer serves any useful purpose (such as a person's childhood phone number). Overlearning occurs when information has been thoroughly memorized first, and then periodically rehearsed, even though it is already well known. (See also REHEARSAL.)

oxiracetam   One of a class of nootropic drugs and an analog of PIRACETAM. Findings from a variety of studies suggest that oxiracetam enhances vigilance and attention, with some effects on spontaneous memory and improvements in concentration.

In one Italian mice study, researchers assessing the drug's potential for birth defects gave pregnant mice oxiracetam from the beginning of their pregnancies until birth. But instead of toxicity, the drug appeared to benefit the offspring of the treated mothers. These offspring—which had never received oxiracetam directly—showed signs of being more curious at one month of age than the offspring of controls that had received a placebo. At three months, the treated offspring performed significantly better in memory tests than the control offspring.

In a test of 272 humans, demented patients who received oxiracetam showed significant improvements in memory and concentration after three months of therapy.

Oxiracetam currently is being investigated for the treatment of Alzheimer's disease at a number of centers around the country, but it is not currently available in the United States for other than experimental use.

P

paired-associate learning A type of test that assesses the retention of novel information. In the test, a subject is given a list of word pairs to learn. The next day he is shown one word from each pair and told to supply the missing words.

Pappenheim, Bertha See ANNA O.

paramnesia Errors of memory. The term was introduced by German psychiatrist Emil Kraepelin in 1886, who divided paramnesia into three main types: simple memory deceptions (when a patient remembers a hallucination or imagination as real); associative memory deceptions, or reduplicative paramnesia (when a patient fails to recognize well-known people or places, believing that doubles have replaced them); and identifying paramnesia, or DÉJÀ VU (in which a new situation is experienced as duplicating an earlier situation in every detail). (See also AGNOSIA; CAPGRAS SYNDROME.)

parietal lobes The parts of the cerebral brain hemispheres that are covered by parietal bones. The parietal lobes, together with the upper temporal and occipital lobes, seem to serve as a short-term memory bank for auditory, visual and motion perception impulses. (See also TEMPORAL LOBE.)

Parkinson's disease A progressive degenerative brain disease characterized by nerve cell death in a specific part of the brain, causing muscle tremor, stiffness and weakness. Often, it may lead to memory and thinking problems as well. People who suffer from this disease, once thought to be strictly neuromuscular, lose neurons from a part of the brain called the substantia nigra that produces the neurotransmitter DOPAMINE, which helps brain cells communicate with one another. Parkinson's patients also experience a slowing of some cognitive functions and have difficulty with complex tasks.

Studies have suggested that more than half of people with Parkinson's have mild intellectual changes and about 20 percent have more substantial cognitive problems. Typically, memory problems in Parkinson's are not as severe as in Alzheimer's. In Parkinson's disease, the patient may have trouble concentrating, learning new information and recalling names.

The disease affects between 1 to 1.5 million people in the United States, usually after age 50. However, more and more Americans under age 40 are being diagnosed with Parkinson's.

Cause

The primary symptoms are believed to be caused by a low level of dopamine, an important chemical transmitter in certain brain cells governing movement, balance and walking. In addition, scientists have discovered that Parkinson's patients with memory problems also have smaller hippocampal structures than other Parkinson's patients, and that failure of verbal and visual memory may be related to this hippocampal atrophy in Parkinson's disease.

Other scientists suspect that Parkinson's patients may have problems with their memory for time. Body movement involves a timed sequence of motions, and evidence is accumulating that a central problem in Parkinson's is memory for time—a cognitive function in the brain, not a neuromuscular function, according to Columbia University scientists. This internal timing function acts much like an internal stopwatch, telling a person that, for example, the end of a TV commercial is approaching. That sense must be based in an unconscious cellular or molecular mechanism that allows memories of timed intervals to be recorded and later retrieved, the scientists say.

Parkinson's patients have trouble estimating and remembering timed intervals. Scientists suggest that the jerky motions of Parkinson's may result from a patient's inability to time smooth, fluid movement, like a turn of the head, creating instead a series of separate, stop-and-go motions.

Diagnosis

Although there are no specific tests for Parkinson's disease, there are several ways of making a diagnosis. While initial symptoms are so mild they may be easily overlooked, as the disease progresses it becomes so clear-cut that a doctor may be able to diagnose the condition by a simple exam. However, other possible disorders with similar symptoms must be excluded as well.

Most doctors rely on a neurological exam that covers evaluation of the symptoms and their severity. If symptoms are serious enough, a trial test of anti-Parkinson's drugs may be indicated. Also when indicated, brain scans may be made to rule out other diseases whose symptoms resemble Parkinson's disease.

Treatment

There is no cure for Parkinson's disease at this time. If the disease progresses beyond minor symptoms, medication can be helpful. In some patients, surgery is also of benefit.

The most commonly prescribed medication is L-dopa (levodopa), which helps replenish some of the lost dopamine. This drug is effective in treating movement problems, but is less helpful with cognitive ones; it also becomes less effective as the disease progresses.

Other drugs, designed to stimulate the dopamine system or mimic its controlling effect on other nerve cells, include bromocriptine, pergolide, selegiline and trihexyphenidyl. To date, L-dopa is considered to be the most effective drug. Sinemet, a combination of levodopa and carbidopa, is usually the drug most doctors use to treat Parkinson's disease patients. Unfortunately, these drugs carry side effects, including uncontrollable movements called "dyskinesias." In fact, all medications should

be monitored since high doses of some drugs used for Parkinson's can cause hallucinations or confusion. Drug therapy for Parkinson's typically provides relief for about 10 to 15 years or more.

In recent years, three surgical options are available to individuals for whom more conventional drug therapies have not worked. To ensure the best results, surgical candidates must have the specific symptoms treatable by the procedure. They should be otherwise healthy and relatively young (that is, under age 65 or 70). Surgical candidates should always be evaluated by a Parkinson's specialist (a neurologist with special movement disorder training).

Thalamotomy

This low-risk surgery destroys cells in the brain's THALAMUS to correct a disabling tremor in the hands or arms for patients who don't have many other symptoms. Between 80 percent and 90 percent of patients improve right away after surgery; full recuperation generally takes six weeks.

Pallidotomy

This surgical technique (performed while the patient is awake) destroys certain cells in the part of the brain controlling movement, which can help correct problems in slow movement, tremor and imbalance. The most dramatic result is the decrease in dyskinesia.

Fetal Tissue Implants

This experimental technique is used to restore the brain's ability to produce dopamine. Political and ethical controversy over this procedure may lead to the future development of genetically engineered cells for this type of surgery. There are no long-term studies on the success of this technique, but early findings suggest that it can dramatically decrease the need for medication, although this improvement may not begin until six months after the surgery and may not peak for 12 to 24 months.

In the Future . . .

New drugs under development include chemicals known as "agonists," which mimic dopamine in the brain and may delay the progress of Parkinson's. In addition, research in glial derived neurotrophic factors (GDNF) has shown exciting results in recent testing on primates. COMT inhibitors (such as entecapone and tolcapone) look like a good way to enhance the Sinemet response.

Meanwhile, current surgical procedures are being refined. Fetal tissue implant researchers are exploring the addition of "nerve growth factor," a protein from the patient's own body used to enhance cell growth. Alternatively, it may be possible to use pig fetal tissue transplants.

Finally, electronic stimulators, implanted in pallidotomy and thalamotomy target areas on an experimental basis, may enable patients to activate the benefit themselves.

Pavlov, Ivan Petrovich (1849–1936) A Russian physiologist best known for his development of the theory of the conditioned reflex. In his classic experiments, he trained dogs to salivate when they heard a bell previously associated with food. This is his best example of an after-the-fact association (when one thing reminds a person or animal of a second thing and the creature responds as if to the second thing). Pavlov developed a similar concept (emphasizing the importance of conditioning) in his pioneering studies of human behavior and the nervous system.

The eldest son of the village priest, Pavlov attended theological seminaries in his native Russia, then in 1870 abandoned his ideas of entering the priesthood to enter the University of St. Petersburg to study chemistry and physiology. After receiving his medical degree, he began his first independent research into the physiology of the circulatory system. He married a student and friend of the author Fyodor Dostoyevsky, and he later attributed all of his success to his brilliant wife. While studying digestion he began to formulate his ideas about conditioned reflexes, widening his theories by 1930 to explain human psychoses in these terms. He believed that the excessive inhibition characteristic of a psychotic patient served to protect him or her from injurious stimuli that earlier had caused excess stimulation.

Pavlov also believed that sleep reflected a widespread inhibitory process in the brain, and concluded that hypnosis is a similar state.

peg words A type of mnemonic strategy in which items to be remembered are mentally "pegged" to (associated with) certain images in a prearranged order. (See PEG WORD SYSTEM.)

peg word system A type of VISUAL IMAGERY METHOD for improving learning in which a standard set of peg words are learned and items to be remembered are linked to the pegs with visual imagery. The system can be traced to the mid-1600s, when it was developed by Henry Herdson, who linked a digit with any one of several objects that resembled the number (for example, 1 = candle, 3 = trident).

The peg system gets its name from the fact that the peg words act as mental "pegs" or hooks on which a person hangs the information that needs to be remembered. It is probably one of the most famous mnemonic devices, popular with entertainers and students of memory training. The peg words help organize material that must be remembered, and act as reminders to recall that material.

The best known of the peg methods is the "rhyming-peg method" in which numbers from one to ten are associated with rhymes: one-bun, two-shoe, three-tree, four-door, five-hive, etc. The first item to be remembered is linked with a bun, the second with a shoe, the third with a tree, and so on. When the list needs to be remembered, the pegs are called up first and then the mental images that are linked to those pegs are recalled. This system was introduced in England about 1879 by John Sambrook.

The rhyming scheme is easy to learn, and many people already know many of the rhymes from the nursery rhyme "One-two, buckle my shoe." When learning the rhyming method, each peg word noun should be imagined as vividly as possible: The bun should be a sesame seed bun, a hot cross bun, a toasted and buttered bun. The tree should be specific—an oak, a spindly pine tree, a birch.

1. One is a bun
2. Two is a shoe
3. Three is a tree
4. Four is a door
5. Five is a hive

6. Six are sticks
7. Seven is heaven
8. Eight is a gate
9. Nine is a vine
10. Ten is a hen

The object that each word represents should be visualized; then a picture of each word (bun, shoe, etc.) is drawn. The act of drawing helps to fix the words in the mind, creating a strong mental association between the numbers and the words that rhyme with them.

If a person had a list of groceries to remember, the grocery names could simply be attached to the pegs. To remember ten items, such as peas, pork chops, milk, bread, eggs, butter, tomatoes, soap, peanut butter and swiss cheese, a person would visualize the list of rhyming words, making them as vivid and ridiculous as possible.

The first item (*peas*) would be visualized wearing leotards and tap shoes, tap dancing on a bun. To remember (*pork chops*), a person might think of a pig in tennis shoes. The sillier the image, the more easily it will be recalled. The peg words can be used over and over; with each new list, the previous words will be erased. Each peg is a clue to an association with the item, and to recall the item, all that has to be remembered is the peg.

The phonetic-peg system is more flexible than the rhyming system, but also more complex. This system relies on the relationship between numbers and their consonant sounds; "0" is remembered as "Z" (the first sound in "zero"); "1" is remembered as "T" (both 1 and T have one downstroke). In addition, each sound is remembered as a word; 1 ("T") is also remembered as "ties," and 2 ("N") is remembered as "Noah."

While many people consider the phonetic-peg system as too cumbersome and difficult to bother to learn, it has been used successfully with brain-damaged patients. In at least one study, four out of seven patients with severe verbal-memory problems were helped to learn experimental material and practical information with the system, although it took a long time to learn the system. Others believe that the system may be of some help to those with mild head injuries, but would probably not help those with more severe memory impairments.

There are still other peg word systems. Peg words can be selected on the basis of meaning: 1 = me (there is only one me), 3 = pitchfork (three prongs), 5 = hand (five fingers).

The system is limited, however, in that it is hard to find good peg words to represent numbers beyond ten.

Numbers make a good peg system because they are naturally ordered and everyone knows them. For this reason, the alphabet also makes a good peg system. In order to make the letters concrete, each of them either rhymes with the letter of the alphabet it represents or has the letter as the initial sound of the word. An example of an alphabet peg system would be: A-hay, B-bee, C-sea.

The peg system is similar to paired-associate learning except that the learners provide their own peg words. In a variety of research studies, people have been able to use the peg system effectively on lists up to 40 words. It can also be used to help form concepts in tasks requiring high memory demands, remembering ideas, etc.

Peg words are helpful in remembering lists for shopping or errands, in organizing activities and in giving people a sense of being in control. (See also LOCI, METHOD OF; PHONETIC SYSTEM OF MNEMONICS; REHABILITATION OF MEMORY; VISUAL-IMAGERY METHOD; VISUAL-PEG SYSTEM.)

Penfield, Wilder (1891–1976) The Canadian surgeon who discovered during the 1950s that stimulating various areas of the cortex produced a range of responses from patients; however, only stimulation of the temporal lobes elicited meaningful, integrated experiences, including sound, movement and color. Interestingly, some of these memories that popped up during stimulation were not remembered in the normal state. Furthermore, the memories Penfield stimulated appeared to be far more detailed, accurate and specific than normal recall.

Penfield did not set out to study memory; he wanted to reduce seizures in epileptic patients by removing the damaged tissue in the brain that triggered the seizures. Penfield knew that the seizures always were preceded by a "mental aura" (a warning sensation the patient experiences before a seizure). He hoped to open the skull of fully conscious patients, moving a stimulating electrode across the brain to deliver a weak electrical shock to various areas to find the site that produced the mental aura. If he found such a site, he reasoned, he could destroy it and end the seizures.

While his technique was often successful, his discovery of the ability to stimulate memories radically altered ideas popular at the time of how the brain worked. Stimulating one side of the brain brought back a certain song to one patient, the memory of a moment in a garden listening to a mother calling her child. Interestingly, stimulating the same point elicited the same memory every time. It seemed that Penfield had found an engram—the site in the brain where memory was stored.

As a result of his findings, Penfield believed that the brain makes a permanent record of every item to which a person pays conscious attention, although this record may be forgotten during day-to-day life. (See also HOLOGRAM THEORY OF MEMORY.)

personal memory   All the happenings and occurrences that make up a person's own life history—everything from the first day of school to the most important moment of one's life. This type of memory brings together all the sense impressions and emotions that make up a continuous life, recording all the changes and happenings that make up a person's inner and outer worlds.

Because personal memory is recording a constant flow of change, it doesn't retain many details. And with increasing age, memory problems are often those of recent personal memory. (Personal memory from the past is likely to be intact.)

For most people, their general knowledge memory (where the sun sets, who is president of the United States) as well as memory from their early life is well organized and stable because it has been rehearsed over and over for a long period of time. Because it is history, it has remained unchanged. On the other hand, information from the recent personal memory (lunch menu from last Monday) may not be so easy to retrieve, because there has been less opportunity to rehearse it.

PET (positron emission tomography) scan   An imaging technique that creates computerized

images of the distribution of radioactively labeled glucose in the brain in order to show brain activity. The more active a part of the brain is, the more glucose it uses.

PET sensors are located around the head of a patient, who sits behind black felt to eliminate distractions. The scan can pinpoint the source of the radioactivity and any corresponding heightened activity. These data are sent to computers that produce two-dimensional drawings showing the neural "hot spots"—areas of the brain that are working the hardest at that particular time. In addition, PET scans of the brains of subjects who have been injected with labeled drugs that attach to specific receptors can show the distribution and number of those receptors.

While PET scans accurately track brain function and provide the first pictures of a working brain, they also have drawbacks; principally, they can't be used for high-quality visualizations of brain structures, since they can't resolve brain structures less than .5 inches apart. (See also BRAIN SCANS; COMPUTERIZED TOMOGRAPHY (CT) SCAN; MAGNETIC RESONANCE IMAGING; SPECT; SQUID.)

Peter of Ravenna (Petrus Tommai)   The Italian author of *The Phoenix* (1491), the best known of all early memory-training books, which brought the art of memory training into general knowledge. The book was extremely popular, reprinted in many editions and translations, and made Peter of Ravenna's name known throughout all of Europe's educated classes for a century. Many other books on the subject followed during the next two centuries.

In his book, Peter gives practical advice to everyday people, full of details. He is said to have been able to accomplish astonishing feats of memory, including repeating 300 philosophical sayings, 200 speeches of Cicero and 20,000 legal points. (See also LOCI, METHOD OF.)

Petrarch (Francesco Petrarca) (1304–1374)   An Italian scholar and poet and an important authority on ARTIFICIAL MEMORY, who wrote "Things to Be Remembered" *(Rerum memorandarum libri)* in the mid-1300s.

phonetic system of mnemonics A sophisticated, versatile mnemonic system that is more flexible than the rhyming peg system, but also more complex. This system relies on the relationship between numbers and their consonant sounds; "0" is remembered as "Z" (the first sound in "zero"); "1" is remembered as "T" (both 1 and T have one downstroke). In addition, each sound is remembered as a word; 1 ("T") is also remembered as "ties," and 2 ("N") is remembered as "Noah."

The technique is superior to the PEG WORD SYSTEM because it allows construction of more than 10 to 20 peg words, yet it retains the peg system's advantage of direct retrieval.

This system has been referred to by a variety of names, including figure-alphabet, digit-letter, number-alphabet, hook, number-consonant and number-to-sound. It was developed more than 300 years ago when Winckelmann introduced a digit-letter system in which the digits were represented by letters of the alphabet. These letters were used to form words to represent a given number sequence. In the early systems, the digits were represented by both consonants and vowels, but in 1813 Gregor von Feinaigle refined the system so that digits were represented by consonants that were selected on the basis of their similarity to or association with the digits they represented. The system was further refined during the 1800s, and by the end of the nineteenth century it had evolved into its present form—represented not by consonants but by consonant sounds.

While many people consider the phonetic-peg system too cumbersome and difficult to learn, it has been used successfully with brain-damaged patients. In at least one study, four out of seven patients with severe verbal-memory problems were helped to learn experimental material and practical information, although it took them a long time to learn the system. Although some researchers believe that the system may be of some help to those with mild head injuries, the phonetic-peg method probably would not help those with more severe memory impairments.

phosphatidylserine (PS) A type of fat-soluble substance that is an essential component of cell membranes. Found in highest concentrations in brain cells, it may help preserve (or even improve) some aspects of mental functioning in the elderly, according to some reports.

Controlled and double blind studies have shown mild benefits from PS supplementation in patients with mild ALZHEIMER'S DISEASE when 300 mg per day is taken for three to twelve weeks. In one study, the improvement on standardized tests of mental functioning averaged approximately 15 percent. Continued improvement has been reported up to three months beyond the end of the supplementation period. However, this is certainly no cure; while it may reduce symptoms in the short term, at best PS probably slows the rate of deterioration rather than stops the progression of the disease altogether, scientists report. For example, in

DIGIT-SOUND EQUIVALENTS OF THE PHONETIC SYSTEM		
Digit	Consonant Sound	Memory Aid
1	t, th, d	"t" has one downstroke
2	n	two downstrokes
3	m	three downstrokes
4	r	last sound for the word four in several languages
5	l	Roman numeral for 50 is "L"
6	j, sh, ch, soft g	reversed script "j" resembles 6
7	k, q, hard c, hard g	"k" made of two 7s
8	f, v	script "f" resembles 8
9	p, b	"p" is mirror image of 9
10	z, s, soft c	"z" for "zero"

one six-month trial, benefits began to fade after the fourth month.

PS is found in only trace amounts in a typical diet; very small amounts are present in lecithin. In the past, studies used PS that had been extracted from cows' brains, a product that is not looked upon with favor in the wake of MAD COW DISEASE. Currently, commercially available PS is derived from soy, but researchers aren't sure if it is equal to PS derived from cows.

Adults age 50 and older, especially those with age-related declines in mental function such as memory loss, may not synthesize enough PS, and may benefit the most from supplemental PS. Taken orally, PS is rapidly absorbed and readily crosses the blood-brain barrier to reach the brain.

photographic memory   The long-term persistence of mental imagery, technically known as eidetic memory.

physiological causes of memory loss   Because the brain is susceptible to fluctuating levels of fluids, oxygen and nutrients, anything that affects the physiological health of the body may affect memory systems as well.

Fluid Imbalances   Too much or too little water in the body can disturb brain function, because water contains electrolytes (potassium, sodium, chloride, calcium and magnesium) that are crucial to the function of cells that make up the memory system.

Hypoglycemia   Because brain cells require an adequate amount of sugar (glucose) to maintain metabolic activity, a drop in the body's blood sugar level can lead to a host of memory problems.

Malnutrition   Dementing brain disease can be produced by a diet that lacks enough of the B-complex vitamins (especially NIACIN, thiamine and B_{12}). This is one reason behind the memory problems of serious alcohol abusers, who typically lack thiamine because they don't eat properly. Vegetarians who don't get enough vitamin B_{12} also may experience symptoms of memory deficits; recent research suggests that those with low-normal levels of B_{12} in their blood tend to experience depression with memory problems. A more serious lack of this vitamin can lead to spinal cord degeneration and associated brain diseases, including memory loss.

physostigmine   A drug used as eye drops in the treatment of glaucoma (high pressure in the eyeballs) also produces mild improvement in memory loss among ALZHEIMER'S DISEASE patients. The drug increases levels of ACETYLCHOLINE, the neurotransmitter that is deficient in Alzheimer's. A time-released form of physostigmine allows the drug to be taken just once a day and improves cognition in people with Alzheimer's as much as DONEPEZIL (Aricept), one of the two drugs currently approved to treat the disease.

A 12-week double-blind controlled trial of 176 patients with Alzheimer's disease found that 24 or 30 mg. per day of extended-release physostigmine salicylate (Synapton) was effective in treating cognitive defects of Alzheimer's disease compared with placebo. However, the substantial unpleasant side effects (primarily nausea and vomiting) may limit its usefulness. Nausea and vomiting each occurred in 47 percent of the physostigmine-treated patients.

Piaget, Jean (1896–1980)   The Swiss psychologist who was the first to study the acquisition of understanding in children systematically. Best known for his work on the IQ test, Piaget also wrote *Memory and Intelligence* (1973), based on his ideas about memory in children.

He received his doctorate in zoology in 1918 at the University of Neuchâtel (Switzerland) and soon afterward became interested in psychology. He studied psychology under Carl Gustav Jung and Eugen Bleuler, and then began studying at the Sorbonne in Paris in 1919. There he began his work administering reading tests to children. As part of his work in standardizing IQ tests, he noticed that children at certain ages consistently gave the same wrong answer to a particular question. Although most would consider that a wrong answer is simply wrong, Piaget wondered why children gave that particular wrong answer.

As a result, he abandoned IQ research and began studying the qualitative changes in growing children; by the end of his life, he had moved on to the study of memory. As part of his research, he discovered that children's memories for a particular event can improve over time; a child may not remember an event very well after one week but six months later may have a much better memory of the same occurrence.

Piaget taught at the University of Geneva as professor of child psychology until his death; writing more than 50 books and monographs, he continued to develop the theme that the mind of the child evolves through a series of set stages to adulthood.

He believed in the fundamental unity and the common nature of the memory and the intelligence, not only because both pass through the same stages but also because the evolution of the mnemonic code is a direct function of the construction of operational schemata.

Piaget's work shows the interdependence of memory and understanding—the capacity to learn about the present implies a capacity to learn about the past as well. He believed that memory depends on a person's capacity to construct an experience. He did not believe in a storehouse or file cabinet where memories are preserved; instead, he thought that we construct a memory and remember the construction rather than the original event. When a person recalls items grouped together, they are reorganized because the person has constructed the list in his or her own way.

He tested children's recall for a demonstration in which one rolling ball transferred its energy to a second ball, but the second ball couldn't transfer its energy to a third. The age at which children correctly explained this varied, but most could think of some explanation and they remembered something of the experiment that emphasized their own explanation. Piaget believed that memory depends on a capacity to construct an experience. Theories that try to explain memory as retrieval from storage deny that such improvement can happen.

He also studied memory in infancy and believed that mental development begins with sensory and motor associations. His first was the "sensory-motor stage," which lasted for the first two years of life, during which children grow into active toddlers. He believed the child's exploration and remembering was a circular reaction that develops in accordance with the development of emotional memory, beginning with motor associations and progressing to sensory associations.

The best known of the early circular reactions (Piaget called them primary reactions) was thumb sucking, which depended on motor memory; the baby accidentally inserts a thumb, sucks on it and likes the sensation, and therefore repeats it. The repetition of the behavior, Piaget said, occurs because of a remembered motor association (hand motion associated with pleasure).

Secondary circular reactions such as rattle shaking, Piaget believed, depend on sensory memory and appear at about four months of age. The motor activity (shaking) leads to an objective event (rattling), and the sound causes pleasure. Piaget believed that a four-month-old baby's memory already matches or supersedes the memory of most animals.

As children grow older, interpreting their mental state becomes more difficult, and this is where Piaget's theories become more controversial. After the first birthday, children begin to speak single words (a sign of factual memory), and they associate things with sounds. By two years, children's vocabulary reflects more than factual memory—they can form sentences, showing an ability for complex factual association.

Pick's disease   A form of DEMENTIA characterized by a slowly progressive deterioration of social skills and changes in personality leading to impairment of intellect, memory and language. It is almost impossible to distinguish from ALZHEIMER'S DISEASE except on autopsy, although it's much less common. Alzheimer's disease causes 50 percent to 60 percent of dementia cases; Pick's disease accounts for about 5 percent of cognitive deterioration. The disease is characterized by "Pick's bodies" in the brain cells, which consist of miscellaneous collection of parts of the normal cell. Although the parts are recognizable, their normal relationships have been disrupted.

Cause

The cause is unknown. The disorder usually begins in the frontal lobes; the first symptoms usually are not memory problems, as in Alzheimer's but changes in personality and social behavior. Memory problems soon appear. Eventually, patients become mute, incontinent and immobile. The condition is more common in women than in men; patients contract this disease at about 55 years of age, with death following in about seven years. New cases of Pick's disease are infrequent in patients beyond the middle 50s. There have been only three cases of Pick's disease in the United States in patients over age 70.

Pick's disease was first identified in 1892 by Dr. Arnold Pick, who described the progressive mental deterioration in a 71-year-old man. On autopsy, the brain showed an unusually shrunken frontal cortex, the region involved in reasoning and other higher mental functions. This shrinkage is different from the brain changes associated with Alzheimer's disease.

Symptoms

Although the disease affects people differently, there is a common core of symptoms that may be present at different stages of the disease, including

- memory loss
- lack of spontaneity
- difficulty in thinking or concentrating
- speech disturbances
- gradual emotional dullness
- loss of moral judgment
- progressive dementia.

Diagnosis

Pick's disease is diagnosed in a process similar to Alzheimer's. Often a patient is diagnosed with "probable Alzheimer's," and later the diagnosis is changed to Pick's.

Treatment

There is no cure or specific treatment for Pick's disease, and its progress can't be slowed down. However, some of the symptoms of the disease may be treated effectively. The course of Pick's disease is an inevitable progressive deterioration that may take anywhere from less than two years to more than 10 years. Death is usually caused by infection.

piracetam A family of drugs that may improve the learning ability of animals and protect against memory loss in the absence of oxygen (ANOXIA) by improving the transmission of impulses between neurons. In addition, some studies indicate that mixing piracetam with CHOLINE may boost the brain's metabolism and improve memory function.

Some studies of the piracetam family of drugs show some improvement in the condition of Alzheimer's patients. However, other studies have produced contradictory results and show no improvement among these patients. This difference in results may be linked to the fact that the effect of these chemicals is highly individual; some researchers believe the effects may be linked to the amount of steroids in the bloodstream. (See also NOOTROPIC DRUGS.)

plasticity A neuron's ability to change its structure or function. The brain is not a computer that is wired forever at birth. Instead, it remodels itself constantly in response to experience, aging, hormones, illness, injury and learning. It is plastic—that is, it can be molded. It is this plasticity that helps the brain quickly learn new things, such as memorizing a phone number or practicing the piano. In fact, something as simple as remembering a name or address can't be performed until something changes in the brain.

The new understanding of how much the brain is constantly changing is partly due to advances in brain scan techniques that allow scientists to see inside the living, thinking brain. Images from positron emission tomography (PET) and functional MAGNETIC RESONANCE IMAGING (MRI) let scientists track changes in the brain as they happen. Activated areas of the brain "light up" on these scans, revealing increased blood flow and electrical energy.

It all takes place on the level of the connections between individual brain cells. The human brain has up to 100 billion nerve cells; about 10 billion are in the NEOCORTEX, the outer layer of gray matter responsible for conscious experience. All the action in the brain occurs at the cells' connection points, called the SYNAPSES, where electrical pulses that carry messages leap across gaps between cells. Each neuron can form thousands of links, giving a typical brain about 100 trillion synapses.

As a person learns, behaves and experiences the world and stores memories, changes occur at the synapses, and more and more connections in the brain are created. The brain organizes and reorganizes itself in response to experience and sensory stimulation, and these changes are reinforced with use. As a person learns and practices new information, intricate circuits of knowledge and memory are laid down.

The interconnections between neurons are not fixed, but change all the time. Researchers at Rockefeller University have discovered that neurons don't act alone, but work together in a network, organizing themselves into groups and specializing in different kinds of information processing. For example, if one neuron sends many signals to another neuron, the synapse between the two gets stronger. The more active the two neurons are, the stronger the connection between them grows. Thus, with every new experience, your brain slightly rewires its physical structure. In fact, how a person uses his brain helps determine how the brain is organized. It is this flexibility, this "plasticity," that helps the brain rewire itself once it has been damaged, helping a person recover lost or damaged functions in the wake of stroke, for example.

Periods of Plasticity

Periods of rapid change occur in the brain under four main conditions:

- developmental: when the immature brain first begins to process sensory information
- activity-dependent: when changes in the body alter the balance of sensory activity received by the brain
- learning and memory: when we alter our behavior based on new sensory information
- injury-induced: after damage to the brain

Brain Repair

In the past, scientists thought that the nervous system could not repair itself, and that brain cells, once lost, could never be replaced. But today scientists know that the brain can reorganize itself to an astonishing degree. Some very new research with rats even suggests that new brain cells can be created.

Unfortunately, the brain's ability to adapt is not limitless. Normal plasticity can't fully compensate for severe damage from tumors or trauma, for example. It's also possible for the brain to become *too* plastic, and overreact. This is what happens when an amputee feels a "phantom pain" in a missing limb.

At Any Age

This plasticity means the human brain has the capacity to remodel itself at any age. It is experience—both good and bad—that is behind the brain's continual remodeling. Even illness or trauma is a kind of "learning" for the brain. This could mean that one day, the best treatment for a degenerative disease like Parkinson's might be not a drug but an intense relearning process that could help the patient unlearn the illness.

Twenty years ago, experts thought that the structure of the brain develops during childhood and, once organized, it left very little room for changes. Today we know that this isn't true—adult brains remain plastic to some degree. It is true, however, that while humans never stop learning, this remodeling is harder for adults than for children. Studies of children learning to play the violin showed that their brain plasticity, as evidenced by changes in their brains in response to practicing, is greatest in those under age 13. Scientists believe this is because the younger a person is, the more room in the brain's hemisphere for new connections to be made.

Scientists believe a person loses about 1,000 neurons each day after age 40. However, this loss can be offset by regular stimulation. If a neuron is being used, it secretes substances that affect nearby cells responsible for the neuron's nourishment. These cells, in turn, produce a chemical that appears to keep the neuron from being destroyed. If the neuron doesn't get that substance, it dies. So as long as a person is actively using his brain and learning new things, research suggests it's possible to offset the death of neurons.

No matter how plastic the brain, however, it's still true that memory does deteriorate with aging. Yet while there is some physical breakdown and memory loss as adults age, the biggest obstacle to continued learning is the patterns the brain has already learned. Neurons are shaped much like trees, with branches going off in all directions. Each time a nerve cell branches out, it allows for more subtle connections with other neurons far away, not just those close by that do similar things. Scientists believe this means that an adult's mind may lose details but gain more depth and richness, much like seeing the majesty of the forest instead of the details of an individual oak.

In the Future

Once scientists fully understand how the brain makes its new connections, it would be possible to create more effective drugs or physical exercises to enhance the natural plastic processes.

Plato (428/427 B.C.–348/347 B.C.)   An ancient Greek philosopher and developer of a wide-ranging system of ethical philosophy who also believed that a good memory was the "highest of talents." Possessing a prodigious memory, he was interested not in the "superficial" field of MNEMONICS but in the very essence of memory itself.

Plato believed that memory was the mother of all arts that could lead people back to the realization of their own divinity and wholeness. He also thought that humans have an innate memory of the realities beyond this world—a memory of ideal form. The real art, he believed, is to recover this divine memory and fit sensory impressions into this larger framework. His art of memory, therefore, was really an art of enlightenment.

Pliny the Elder (Gaius Plinius Secundus) (A.D. 23–79)   A Roman savant, Pliny was author of the celebrated *Natural History*, used as an authoritative review of scientific matters up to the Middle Ages. Pliny, whose son attended QUINTILIAN's rhetoric school, discussed memory in *Natural History* in the form of an anthology of memory stories.

The art of memory was invented by Simonides Melicus, Pliny wrote, and perfected by Metrodorus of Scepsis, who could "repeat what he had heard in the very same words." Pliny went on to catalog a list of luminaries and their feats of memory: Mithridates of Pontus knew all 22 languages that were spoken in his area; Charmadas knew the contents of all the books in a library; Lucius Scipio knew the names of all the Roman people; Cyrus knew the names of all the men in his army.

Pollyanna hypothesis   The Freudian hypothesis (also called hedonic selectivity) that unpleasant memories are harder to remember than pleasant ones. (See also FREUD, SIGMUND; REPRESSION.)

positron emission tomography   See PET (POSITRON EMISSION TOMOGRAPHY) SCAN.

postencephalitic amnesia   See ENCEPHALITIS AND MEMORY.

posterior cerebral arteries, infarction of   Stroke originating in the posterior cerebral arteries. Patients who have had infarctions of the posterior cerebral arteries (stroke) may experience problems in short-term memory, inability to learn new facts and skills and RETROGRADE AMNESIA. Often memory problems are associated with visual-field defects. (See also CEREBROVASCULAR ACCIDENT [CVA]; SUBARACHNOID HEMORRHAGE.)

posthypnotic amnesia   Memory of a hypnotic trance is often vague, similar to how a person remembers a dream upon awakening. While in the hypnotic state, if a subject is told that he will remember nothing upon awakening, he will experience a much more profound posthypnotic amnesia. However, if the subject is rehypnotized and given a countersuggestion, he will awaken and remember everything; therefore, experts believe this phenomenon is clearly psychogenic.

Memory for experiences during the hypnotic state also may return, even following a suggestion to forget, if the subject is questioned persistently upon awakening. This observation led Sigmund Freud to search for repressed memories in his patients without the use of hypnosis. (See also FREUD, SIGMUND.)

posthypnotic suggestions   Instructions or suggestions given in a trance and intended to be carried out at a later date after awakening from the hypnotic state. The use of posthypnotic suggestions offers extensive opportunities for directing and guiding behavior without depending on immediate guidance or relationships.

The phenomenon can be used to control weight or stop smoking, for example, by giving a hypnotized subject a series of suggestions about behavior and feelings in response to food or cigarettes. (See also HYPNOSIS; SUGGESTIBILITY.)

posttraumatic amnesia   See TRAUMATIC AMNESIA.

posttraumatic stress disorder   A disorder that can occur after any life-threatening traumatic event that threatens a person's existence. Posttraumatic stress disorder (PTSD) can leave long-lasting scars, including anger, guilt, insomnia, loss of appetite, extreme fatigue, recurrent dreams, nightmares, hypersensitivity and—above all—memory loss and concentration problems.

Recent research has found that many patients with PTSD can develop memory problems that are equivalent to the classic signs of ALZHEIMER'S DISEASE. While eventually (over a period of years) the memory problems may improve, symptoms also are greatly relieved with antidepressants and psychotherapy.

In addition, recent research suggests that excessive and prolonged sensitizing stimulation may lead to changes in the synapses and an oversensitivity to certain stimuli. When scientists exposed 18 PTSD sufferers to 30 seconds of combat sounds while under the influence of anesthetic pentobarbital, 14 immediately reexperienced a Vietnam combat experience with intense emotional fear, rage, indignation, sadness and guilt. (See also COMBAT AMNESIA.)

potentiation   An increase in the intensity of a behavioral response that occurs after a stimulus has been repeated many times. Learning that a particular stimulus poses a threat, the subject becomes more aroused each time the stimulus is presented. Potentiation is the opposite of HABITUATION.

PQRST method   One type of memory technique widely used as a study method in trying to remember facts. This acronym stands for "Preview, Question, Read, State and Test."

Preview   Preview (skim through briefly) the material that must be remembered.

Question   Ask important questions about the information. "What are the primary points in the text? How does the action occur? Who is involved?"

Read   Read the material completely.

State   State answers to key questions.

Test   Perform self-test often to ensure the information has been retained.

While the method was developed as a study technique, it also has been reported to be of at least some benefit for memory-impaired patients to acquire new information.

Researchers suggest that this method might work better than simple REHEARSAL because it provides better retrieval cues. It also may employ the idea of ENCODING SPECIFICITY; that is, a person may remember better if the recall situation is similar to the situation during original learning. With the PQRST method, subjects may be able to answer questions about material because the questions themselves were part of the original learning experience.

Researchers also suggest that the method may work because of the LEVELS-OF-PROCESSING; that is, that deeper processing leads to better retention. PQRST appears to involve deeper processing than simple rehearsal because subjects must think about what they are listening to in order to complete each PQRST step. On the other hand, rehearsal doesn't require so much thought. (Subjects just listen and repeat back.)

To use the PQRST method, scientists suggest that ideally subjects should make up their own questions, since this will lead to better retention.

practice and memory   To retain information in the memory, the material must be practiced before it is firmly entrenched. The question that has plagued researchers is whether learning is most effective with practice in short, concentrated bursts or spread over a long period of time.

The effects of "massed" versus "distributed" practice has been studied for many years, and scientists have concluded that distributed practice is more effective in memorizing information.

While repetition improves memorization, spacing repetitions is far more effective than repeating recalled items immediately. Some researchers believe that immediate and spaced repetition produces differently encoded memory traces. Immediately repeating information may cause the subject to perform exactly the same encoding operations when the information is repeated. But when repetition is delayed, the first presentation is less accessible and the second encoding is probably different. This encoding variability hypothesis stresses that the more differently information is encoded, the more easily it will be remembered because there are more ways the information can be accessed during retrieval.

pramiracetam This nootropic drug enhances the functioning of the cholinergic system in much the same way as its relative, PIRACETAM, but it is effective at much lower doses. (See NOOTROPICS.) In one study, subjects with ALZHEIMER'S DISEASE showed enhanced intelligence and memory following administration of pramiracetam. However, the drug is not available in the United States.

preconscious The initial momentary impressions made by sensory stimuli.

pregnancy and memory Many women say they experience memory lapses during pregnancy, probably because of emotional and hormonal conditions—although, because of a lack of studies, scientists don't really know why.

The physical symptoms that occur during pregnancy (such as nausea and fatigue) can be emotionally disruptive and could cause forgetfulness. Also, the powerful hormonal changes that take place during pregnancy alter the brain's chemistry, which could reduce the capacity for remembering.

The situation is not permanent, however; women who experience memory loss during pregnancy usually report that the problem fades away a few weeks after delivery at the latest.

pregnenolone A simple steroid that, in recent research trials, seems to enhance memory in rats and restore normal levels of memory hormones (such as ACETYLCHOLINE) that decline during aging. The steroid also facilitates rats' ability to remember learned tasks, according to scientists at the City of Hope Medical Center in Los Angeles and St. Louis Veterans Administration Medical Center in Missouri.

A 1992 study conducted with laboratory mice concluded that the clinical administration of pregnenolone in the aging animals could significantly improve memory function. What this study found was that low serum levels of pregnenolone in aging mice contribute to memory and behavioral disorders generally associated with geriatric patients. It also pointed out that certain drugs prescribed for cancer and mental disorders frequently block the synthesis of cholesterol, thereby resulting in a deficiency of pregnenolone.

Scientists suggest pregnenolone might enhance memory because it serves as a raw material for the production of all steroid hormones used in storing information in memory. Concentrations of many of these steroids decline with age; by restoring these levels, pregnenolone may bring back memory abilities that had begun to erode.

premorbid period The period of time before injury or damage to the brain.

presenile dementia In the past, this was the other name for ALZHEIMER'S DISEASE, used to differentiate it from the SENILE DEMENTIA that affects elderly people. However, most experts now believe that this division is based on age only and that the two forms of dementia really reflect the same disease.

presenilins Protein products of two genes that are mutated in some inherited forms of ALZHEIMER'S DISEASE and which help to cause cell death. Genes that code for presenilin 1 (on chromosome 14) and presenilin 2 (on chromosome 1) have been linked to early-onset familial Alzheimer's disease; more recently, scientists have also linked presenilin 1 to the more common, noninherited forms of Alzheimer's as well.

The mutated form of PS1 may be responsible for more than 50 percent of the inherited form of the disease; PS2 is associated with a smaller proportion of disease. Anyone with a defect in either gene will probably develop the illness before 65, experts believe.

In Alzheimer's disease, the brain develops deposits that are thought to kill brain cells. These deposits are created when a long, stringlike protein is cut in two specific places. Scientists now believe that a type of chemical scissors that makes one of these cuts might be a substance formerly theorized as gamma secretase but now believed to be presenilin 1.

Since the genes were first discovered in 1995, scientists have discovered that the mutated forms of the genes may cause illness by boosting production of beta-amyloid42, a substance that creates the plaques found in the brains of Alzheimer's patients. Scientists believe that a buildup of beta-amyloid42 damages cells, and that the presenilins also participate in cellular suicide, sending precise chemical messages to cells urging them to die. This mechanism of cell death begins in healthy people at around age 45. People with the mutated form of the presenilin gene are far more sensitive to these enzymes.

primacy effect   The tendency for the first words on a list to be recalled better than any of the others. While the first words on a list are usually recalled best, the last few words are usually recalled almost as easily (RECENCY EFFECT), while the words in the middle are usually forgotten.

It is possible to disrupt the recency effect by requiring the subject to wait a brief time (as little as 15 seconds) without rehearsing before recalling the list. After the interlude, the recency effect has evaporated, while the first words of the list are still remembered. (See also STORAGE VS. RETRIEVAL FAILURE.)

primary memory   See SHORT-TERM MEMORY.

priming   Facilitation of the ability to process a stimulus due to prior presentation of the stimulus. In other words, a person who has seen a word, picture or some other stimulus in the past hour may have no conscious recollection of it, but still will retain that image in memory.

In an experiment illustrating this phenomenon, a person would be presented with 30 words and then be distracted. After several minutes, the subject would be given a list of 10 word beginnings and asked to complete the words, saying the first word that comes to mind. For the word segment "m-o-t" the subject could reply "motive" or "motor," but those who had previously been shown the word "motel" on the list of 30 words would be very likely to recall it, probably without knowing why. This ability to recall a word without realizing it had been stored in memory is evidence of priming.

prions   Malformed protein segments that cause infection that lead to some types of dementing diseases. Prions were first identified by Stanley Prusiner, M.D., a neurologist at the University of California, San Francisco, who won the Nobel Prize in medicine for his discovery.

Harmless forms of prions exist as proteins in the brain. But if a prion folds in a different shape, it becomes a disease-causing infectious agent. When a malformed prion comes in contact with a healthy protein in the brain, it forces it to change shape. This mutant protein then changes additional proteins, which attack still more, in a chain reaction throughout the brain. As the altered proteins accumulate, the brain tissue begins to clump, leaving holes and killing brain cells. These prions are linked to fatal diseases such as bovine spongiform encephalopathy—also known as BSE or MAD COW DISEASE—and CREUTZFELDT-JAKOB DISEASE, its human form.

Prusiner's idea of prions was considered revolutionary when he proposed it in the mid-1970s, and he suffered years of ridicule before his theory was generally accepted; in 1997, he won the Nobel Prize in medicine for his work. Scientists still don't know what causes ordinary proteins to malform and become prions. Scientists have found that a certain peptide (a piece of the amino-acid chain that makes up the prion) can prevent the abnormality from spreading to the normal proteins. It's hoped that this discovery might one day lead to a treatment to stop the brain deterioration.

proactive inhibition   One type of forgetting due to the "interference" phenomenon, in which material already learned interferes with the acquisition of new information. It is "proactive" because the interference is in a forward direction. In other words, if a person studied an anatomy textbook chapter last week and then studied for a physiology test last night, proactive inhibition would be taking place if the anatomy terms kept popping into the person's mind when he or she tried to recall the physiology terms. (See also EBBINGHAUS, HERMANN E.; INTERFERENCE THEORY; RETROACTIVE INHIBITION.)

proactive interference   One of two forms of interference that results in forgetting, in which older memories impair subsequent learning.

Experts agree that all learning involves the formation of associations; as more learning takes place, some of the new associations have elements in common with those already formed. This interference, called proactive interference, will lead to forgetting.

The other form of interference is retroactive interference, where subsequent learning impairs recall of older memories.

procedural memory   Remembering how to do something, such as typing or solving an algebraic equation. This is the type of memory responsible for skills and habits, which may underlie the simple, unconscious learning that extends from lower animals to humans. Scientists believe there are two basic kinds of memory networks—procedural memory and DECLARATIVE (or factual) MEMORY. (See also HM.)

prosopagnosia   A form of AGNOSIA in which patients have special difficulty recognizing human faces. However, this definition may be too narrow, since these patients also may have problems in recognizing certain other classes of objects, such as species of birds.

protein kinase C (PKC)   A molecule found on the surface membrane of all animal nerve cells; it plays a role in growth, blood clotting and the action of hormones. This molecule was first discovered in the early 1970s by a Japanese scientist.

PKC acts by attaching a phosphate group onto specific sites on the other molecules, changing the function of those molecules, increasing or decreasing their level of activity.

Scientists first realized the potential of PKC in 1986, when Princeton University researchers noted that the protein mimicked cellular changes that occur during learning. Scientists already knew that the electrochemical current in neurons changes as an animal learns and that a protein requiring calcium is involved.

When researchers realized that a single molecule was responsible for learning and memory, they reasoned that its appearance should coincide with learning and its disappearance would indicate forgetting. Research suggests that PKC orchestrates neuronal functions necessary for learning and memory.

Researchers also have discovered that chemicals that block PKC prevent short-term (but not long-term) memory in snails, which suggests that other mechanisms might be responsible for memories that last more than a few minutes.

Scientists also are investigating the role of PKC in memory disorders such as ALZHEIMER'S DISEASE. One recent study at the University of California at San Diego found that the brains of 11 Alzheimer's victims contained only half as much PKC as the brains of seven people who had died of natural causes.

Proust, Marcel (1871–1922)   The novels of this French writer proved that memories are much more enduring than many of us believe; as he grew older, his childhood memories remained crystal clear. Proust is considered to be the greatest creative writer to explore memory and the mystery of recall. His masterpiece, *Remembrance of Things Past* (1913–27), analyzes memory and exalts the miracle of its mechanism.

The experiences that helped Proust remember were sensory ones—smell, sound and the feel of a certain piece of pavement or the sight of a room, almost physically transporting him backward in time to his childhood. Once amid these memories, he found other memories came rushing back, leading him to conclude that each person can develop the negatives of such memories and bring into focus dim pictures of the past. In fact, Proust believed that the only way to find meaning in life is to see what all one's past experiences really meant.

His rumination on madeleines and tea in *Remembrance of Things Past* provided one of the first clues about the relationship between sensation and recollection:

> One day in winter on my return home, my mother . . . offered me some tea . . . She sent for one of those squat, plump little cakes called "petites Madeleines," and soon after a dreary day . . . I raised to my lips a spoonful of the tea in which I had soaked a morsel of the cake. No sooner had the warm liquid mixed with the crumbs touched my palate than a shudder ran through me and I stopped, intent upon the extraordinary thing that was happening to me. An exquisite pleasure had invaded my senses, something isolated, detached, with no suggestion of its origin. Whence could it have come to me, this all-powerful joy? I sensed that it was connected with the taste of the tea and the cake . . . The taste was that of a little piece of Madeleine which on Sunday mornings at Combray . . . my Aunt Leonie used to give me, dipping it first in her own cup of tea . . .
>
> —*Remembrance of Things Past*

After this passage, Proust wondered about the origin of this memory and what it meant. He takes the rest of the novel to explore that memory and how it might have been formed. (See also PROUSTIAN MOMENT.)

Proustian moment   The experience of a sudden flash of recall of some memory apparently forgotten long ago, taking a person completely by surprise. The term gets its name from famed French writer Marcel Proust, author of *Remembrance of Things Past*, a paean to the miracle of memory.

pseudodementia   A disorder that mimics DEMENTIA but that includes no evidence of brain dysfunction. Although both dementia and severe depression feature memory loss and intellectual impairment, nearly one out of ten of those thought to be suffering from true dementia in fact have a depressive illness. Unlike dementia, depression is treatable; many people respond well to antidepressant drugs. Not surprisingly, pseudodementia is found most often in elderly patients.

Like HYSTERICAL AMNESIA and FUGUE, pseudodementia is a defense reaction. In the elderly, it is believed to be a way of avoiding depression or asking for help. When it occurs after a minor brain injury, it is often linked to the patient's desire to avoid an unpleasant experience.

Pseudodementia also can be found among those patients who have experienced a minor organic brain injury that produces a degree of impairment in excess of what would be expected after recovery. For example, one young patient experienced pseudodementia after being involved in a car accident shortly before he was due to be transferred to a dangerous military post abroad. Unconscious for just two minutes, he showed no signs of neurological problems, but he seemed to have lost his personal identity and had a dense RETROGRADE AMNESIA. He appeared to be unable to perform simple motor skills or recognize objects, but over the next six months he relearned his former skills and remembered information about his past life. When interviewed under amylbarbitone narcosis, he revealed that his psychological functions, including memory for his accident, were normal.

pseudopresentiment   Related to both DÉJÀ VU and JAMAIS VU, pseudopresentiment occurs when a person witnessing an event feels that he or she has previously foretold it. There is never any indication that there was actually a prophecy before the event, nor does the person usually claim to have done so. Instead, the dreamlike feeling of pseudopresentiment usually occurs at the moment the person watches the event unfold, suggesting to the person that perhaps the presentiment was revealed in a dream.

pseudosenility   A reversible condition caused by a range of factors including DEPRESSION, medication or disease. (See also AGING AND MEMORY; PSEUDODEMENTIA.)

psychoanalysis   A treatment for mental illness developed by Sigmund Freud at the beginning of the 20th century as a result of his experiences with hypnosis in treating "hysterical" patients. Freud believed that recalled experiences and ideas were related to other symbolically and emotionally important thoughts and feelings and that much of what a person forgets is simply repression. We remember something, he wrote, because it is meaningful to us and significant, although that significance may be hidden. He believed we eliminate from the conscious mind everything that makes us anxious, which he thought explained the loss of memories during the first six years of life.

For this reason, a patient undergoing psychoanalysis is encouraged to reenact the first years of childhood and verbalize any problems so that internal strife can be uncovered and resolved. (See also FREUD, SIGMUND.)

psychogenic amnesia   Loss of memory arising not from physical illness or trauma but from psychological causes. Psychogenic amnesia almost always is caused by some traumatic or emotionally painful event; the degree of impairment varies from one patient to the next. Some patients' amnesia may be limited to a specific episode or event, whereas others may experience a total loss of personal identity and a complete RETROGRADE AMNESIA.

Although psychologically based amnesias which include HYSTERICAL AMNESIA, FUGUE, PSEUDODEMENTIA, MULTIPLE PERSONALITY DISORDER and MIXED AMNESIA, are completely reversible, they have never been fully understood or explained.

Most psychogenic memory disorders are defense reactions, in which various devices are used to repress part or all of a person's memory. It appears that episodic memory is most vulnerable, but other aspects of long-term memory (particularly in pseudodementia) also may be affected. While in hysterical amnesia only one part of the memory is inaccessible, in fugue there is a complete loss of memory. Multiple personalities divide up episodic memory, so that different personalities remember different bits of episodic memory.

In psychogenic amnesia, there is no fundamental impairment in the memory process or registration or retention—the problem lies in accessing stored or repressed (usually painful) memories. This inability to recall painful memories is a protec-

tion against bringing into consciousness ideas associated with profound loss or fear, rage or shame. Under traumatic conditions, memories can become detached from personal identity, making recall impossible.

Psychogenic amnesia usually can be treated successfully by procedures such as hypnosis.

Hysterical Amnesia
Hysterical amnesia is a type of psychogenic amnesia that involves disruption of episodic memory. Unlike organic amnesia, this type of forgetfulness is restricted just to specific emotionally laden groups of memories and is usually linked to a patient's needs or conflicts. During a traumatic event, memories can become detached from personal identity, interfering with recall. Sigmund Freud attributed hysterical amnesia to the need to repress information injurious to the ego. This explains why hysterical amnesia appears only after a traumatic event.

Fugue
Frequently caused by psychogenic reasons, fugue is a period during which a person forgets his or her identity and often wanders away from home or office for several hours, days or even weeks. Some researchers believe that the tendency to wander away from home while experiencing an attack of amnesia often occurs together with other symptoms, including a history of a broken home, periodic depression and predisposition to states of altered consciousness. On the other hand, psychoanalysts see the fugue state as a symbolic escape from severe emotional conflict. In a fugue of long duration, behavior may appear normal, but certain symptoms, such as hallucinations, feeling unreal or unstable moods, may accompany it.

Pseudodementia
Pseudodementia mimics DEMENTIA but includes no evidence of brain dysfunction; it is found most often in elderly patients. Like hysterical amnesia and fugue, psychogenic amnesia is a defense reaction. In the elderly, it is believed to be a way of avoiding depression or asking for help.

Pseudodementia also can be found among those patients who have experienced a minor organic brain injury, which after recovery appears to produce a degree of impairment in excess of what would be expected. For example, one young patient experienced pseudodementia after being involved in a car accident shortly before he was due to be transferred to a dangerous military post abroad. Unconscious for just two minutes, he showed no signs of neurological problems, but he lost his personal identity and had a dense retrograde amnesia. He was unable to perform simple motor skills or recognize objects, but over the next six months he relearned his former skills and remembered information about his past life. When interviewed under amylbarbitone narcosis, his psychological functions, including memory for his accident, were normal.

Multiple Personality Disorder

In multiple personality disorder a person has two or more distinct personalities that are almost always very different from each other and are often total opposites. Many experts believe that multiple personality is the mind's response to severe sexual or physical trauma in childhood. Before 1980, multiple personality was believed to be rare; since then, more than 6,000 cases have been diagnosed. The existence of the phenomenon is not universally accepted by mental health experts, however.

Mixed Amnesia

Psychogenic amnesia also may be found in those with organic (physical) brain problems. In this type of mixed amnesia, an accurate diagnosis may be difficult. This complex intermingling of a true organic memory defect with psychogenic factors can prolong or reinforce the memory loss. It is quite common for a brain-damaged patient to experience a hysterical reaction in addition to brain problems.

psychological testing of memory See ASSESSMENT OF MEMORY DISORDERS.

psychosurgery See LEUCOTOMY; LOBOTOMY.

"punch drunk" syndrome The popular term for dementia pugilistica, a problem caused by multiple repeated blows to the head (such as those experienced by boxers or football players) that can result in a short-term memory problem and other abnormal findings on neuropsychological tests.

The condition was first described in 1928, when it was noted that a patient's brain under microscope showed many signs in common with ALZHEIMER'S DISEASE: widespread neurofibrillary tangles and scarring. It is believed that the brain damage and resulting memory loss is caused by rapid movements of the head, causing hemorrhages and damaged brain cells. In particular, the brains of boxers often exhibit nerve degeneration and loss of nerve fibers in the HIPPOCAMPUS to a degree far exceeding the brains of Alzheimer's disease patients. (See also FOOTBALL AND MEMORY LOSS.)

pursuit rotor task A type of memory assessment in which a subject maintains contact with a revolving target by using a handheld stylus. Performance is measured as the percentage of time the subject can stay on the target.

pyroglutamate (2-oxo-pyrrolidone carboxylic acid, or PCA) An amino acid that is an important flavor enhancer found naturally in a wide variety of fruits and vegetables, dairy products and meat, and in large amounts in the brain, cerebrospinal fluid and blood. It also is suspected to enhance cognitive ability.

PCA is able to penetrate the blood-brain barrier, where some researchers believe it stimulates cognitive function, improving memory and learning in rats. At least one study has shown it is effective in improving alcohol-induced memory deficits in humans and in patients suffering from multi-infarct dementia. Administration of this amino acid increased attention and improved short- and long-term retrieval and long-term memory storage.

When compared with a placebo in studies of memory deficits in 40 aged patients, results indicated that PCA improved verbal memory functions in those who were already affected by an age-related memory decline.

pyrrolidone derivatives A class of nootropic drugs including PIRACETAM and its analogs OXIRACETAM, PRAMIRACETAM, ANIRACETAM and PYROGLUTAMATE. While the mechanism behind their memory-enhancing properties is unknown, most research suggests that the drugs affect the cholinergic system and the adrenal cortex in the brain. (See also NOOTROPICS; SMART DRUGS.)

Quintilian (Marcus Fabius Quintilianus) (c. A.D. 35–c. A.D. 96)   This Latin writer and teacher was the author of an important book on rhetoric, *Institutio oratoria*, a major contribution to educational theory and literary criticism that came more than a century after Cicero's *De oratore*. He also provided important developments on memory systems.

Born in northern Spain, he was educated in Rome and trained by the leading orators of the time. He first worked as a lawyer and then as a teacher of rhetoric, eventually educating the two heirs of Emperor Domitian. An excellent scholar and a sensible, moral man, he was considered to be one of the best teachers of rhetoric in Rome during the first century A.D.

His *Institutio oratoria* is really 12 books, which were published shortly before he died. The books begin with general observations on educational principles, continuing on with the usual depart-ments of rhetoric: invention, arrangement, style, memory and delivery. In the book series, he introduces the topic of memory with the story of Simonides at the banquet, and then goes on to discuss the method of loci as a way of impressing details in memory.

Quintilian wanted to replace the art of memory with simpler precepts of memory training. He gives very clear directions about how to establish places for lodging information to be remembered, and gives very rational reasons as to why the places may help memory. It is now known from experience that a place does, in fact, call up associations in memory.

Quintilian said, in part, that people would have never realized how powerful the art of memory was except for the fact that "it is memory which has brought oratory to its present position of glory." (See also HISTORY OF MEMORY; LOCI, METHOD OF.).

Ramus, Peter (1515–1572) A French dialectician who completed the fragmentation of rhetoric theory by splitting the five "sections" of rhetoric into separate studies, jettisoning the art of memory completely. He was quite aware of the art of ARTIFICIAL MEMORY and supported—as did QUINTILIAN—the idea of dividing and composing the material to be memorized rather than linking the material with places and images. For Ramus, the true art of memory lay in his dialectical method for memorizing, and elocution became the center of rhetorical theory almost solely concerned with figures of speech.

reality monitoring The ability to assess objectively the external world and to distinguish it from the internal state. The term, invented by Sigmund Freud in 1911 (*Realitatsprufung*), also involves the ability to discriminate ego boundaries and understand the difference between self and nonself.

recall The patching together of clues from stored memories to reconstruct an item of consciousness. In a free-recall test, a subject might be asked to write down as many words as possible on a list first memorized the day before.

recency effect As common sense tells us, recall is best for the most recent experiences. Most people know that, if given a list of words, it's easiest to recall the last few words on the list. This enables people to think about experiences that have just passed.

What is unusual, however, is that it is almost impossible to disrupt the recency effect. Ordinary verbal recall can be confused if all the words begin with the same letter, if words are repeated or words are very similar to each other. However, no matter what confusions are introduced in the last few words, people almost always can name them all correctly.

Normally, the recency effect works for a maximum of four items; paying attention does not enhance this ability. However, if the subject is required to wait for a brief time (even as short as 15 seconds) before recalling the list, the recency effect completely disappears. (See also PRIMACY EFFECT.)

receptive aphasia See WERNICKE'S (RECEPTIVE) APHASIA.

receptors Brain receptors are bits of protein embedded in the wall of nerve cells that bind neurotransmitters. Each receptor binds a specific neurotransmitter, turning a particular biochemical or cellular mechanism on or off. Receptors are generally found in the dendrites and cell body of NEURONS. In order to record a memory, the recording agent must be able to respond within a fraction of a second to a stimulus and then keep the information indefinitely.

Some scientists believe that some older people lose their memory abilities because their bodies have stopped producing the enzymes that keep their receptors healthy.

recognition Another name for perceptual memory. One of the ways to measure how much a person remembers is by picking out the items he remembers from a group.

People may not be able to remember something but may show some evidence of remembering if recognition is used as the memory measure. A person recognizes something by acknowledging that it is familiar and that it has been seen before. (The word "recognition" means "to know again.")

An example of the test of recognition would be a multiple-choice test question: Which of the following was the first president of the United States? (a) Abraham Lincoln (b) George Washington (c) Colonel Sanders (d) John F. Kennedy.

Recognition is usually easier to do than recall, since subjects do not have to come up with the information on their own; all that is required is that it be recognized as something that has been learned.

In one study, subjects were shown 600 pairs of sentences, words and pictures. Later they were shown some of these items paired with new items and had to indicate which pair member had been seen before. Most subjects were able to identify correctly sentence pairs 88 percent of the time, words 90 percent and pictures 98 percent. Most elderly subjects performed as well as young adults in these tasks.

The reason that most people can remember a face but may have trouble with the name is that remembering a face is a task of recognition, whereas attaching the name to that face involves the more complex memory task of RECALL. (See also MEMORY FOR FACES.)

recognition memory test   See ASSESSMENT OF MEMORY DISORDERS.

reduplicative paramnesia   See AGNOSIA; CAPGRAS SYNDROME.

rehabilitation of memory   One of the greatest problems in treating organic memory loss is the fact that the brain cannot regenerate very well. When particular areas of the brain are damaged, other regions do not always take over the function of the disabled section. The ability of a brain-damaged patient to recover memory will depend on the cause and site of the damage, the individual's personality and how motivated he or she is to recover. Indeed, researchers agree there is little evidence that practice by itself will significantly improve a brain-damaged person's memory.

Internal Aids
Internal aids include MNEMONICS, rehearsal strategies or anything a patient does mentally to organize the information to be remembered.

External Aids
External aids include diaries, notebooks and calendars, alarm clocks, gadgets and computers. Environmental aids, such as painting lines on the ground to help patients find their way around, also may be used to help mold behavior in patients with severe memory problems. One of the most effective external aids is the combination of a digital alarm watch and a notebook listing the day's activities; whenever the alarm goes off, the patient consults the notebook.

The effectiveness of external aids depends on how the patient feels about using them. Some patients may benefit from counseling in order to accept use of external aids.

Brain Transplants
Initial research with rats has suggested the possibility of restoring some types of memory using brain tissue transplants. However, the moral and philosophical issues surrounding the use of brain tissue in humans presents many problems, and the fact that successful transplants depend on the availability of fetal brain tissue adds to the ethical and legal dilemma.

Rat studies have suggested that fetal brain grafts became effective parts of the grafted animal's memory system. Other studies have shown that the neural tissue taken from the same brain region in rat fetuses could improve the age-related learning impairments in rats.

Medication
While many medications and substances have been implicated in memory enhancement, the following medications actually have been studied as a treatment for memory problems.

Tetrahydroaminoacridine (THA), also known as tacrine or Cognex, is currently being tested for use in the treatment of ALZHEIMER'S DISEASE and is expected to be approved for public use in the near future. In several studies, memory loss improved in those with the disease. It is believed that THA works by increasing the production of ACETYL-CHOLINE.

The anti-inflammatory drug INDOMETHACIN used to treat arthritis shows promise for slowing the advance of Alzheimer's disease. In a recent study of 44 patients mildly to moderately affected with Alzheimer's disease, 24 patients given indomethacin showed an average memory improvement of 1.8 percent; 20 control patients continued to deteriorate an average of 8.4 percent. No patient taking indomethacin showed any memory loss during the six-month test period.

The drug NIMODIPINE, which blocks excess calcium in the part of the brain associated with memory and learning, has been used successfully to improve memory loss in stroke victims.

CENTROPHENOXINE (trade name: Lucidril) is believed to improve various aspects of memory function and may help patients whose brains are not getting enough oxygen (such as after stroke). Researchers believe the drug removes lipofuscin deposits, which increase with age and interfere with learning ability. However, the drug has not been effective in the treatment of Alzheimer's disease.

DILANTIN (phenytoin) is a well-known treatment for epilepsy that is also reputed to improve long-term memory and verbal performance in young and old alike.

HYDERGINE, an extract of the fungus ergot, is a widely used treatment for all forms of senility in the United States. It is said to increase memory, learning, recall and intelligence, inhibit free radicals, enhance brain cell metabolism, and increase blood supply and oxygen to the brain. Hydergine was the first drug that showed promise in use against Alzheimer's disease.

PHYSOSTIGMINE, a drug used to treat glaucoma (high pressure in the eyeballs) may produce mild memory improvement among Alzheimer's patients. In addition, physostigmine reverses memory loss following the administration of SCOPOLAMINE in normal subjects. It works by inhibiting acetylcholinesterase, which breaks down acetylcholine, important in a range of memory processes.

Memory Strategies

There must be about as many memory strategies as there are things to forget. They include external aids—lists, appointment diaries and calendars, "safety drills," alarms and notebook combinations. Memory strategies also can include mnemonics—rhymes ("Thirty days hath September . . ."), patterns (in birth dates, license plates, and so on), acronyms (NATO) and sayings ("Spring forward, fall back" for setting clocks to daylight savings/standard time).

Visualization and association are other types of mnemonic techniques. In the method of loci, a person links something to be remembered with a specific place and then remembers the place to recall the item. The PEG WORD SYSTEM provides pegs on which to hang unrelated words or ideas that need to be remembered. (See also LOCI, METHOD OF.)

rehearsal   The repetition of information, which is necessary for it to move from short-term to long-term memory. The importance of rehearsal in memory has been known since 400 B.C., when the Greeks advised memory students to repeat what they hear, since hearing and saying the same things transfers learning into memory.

According to researchers, rehearsal lengthens the time that information remains in short-term memory, and it appears to be the major way of transferring data into long-term memory. Often rehearsal codes information for memory by translating it into auditory images instead of visual ones. In other words, a person trying to remember a telephone number often will repeat it aloud several times before dialing. Researchers also believe that most people remember the sound of a word and not its printed shape. Studies have shown that, given a series of letters to memorize that includes the letter Q, subjects often recall the letter U instead, which sounds like Q, instead of the letter O, which looks like Q.

The best way to rehearse information to be learned is to concentrate fully, without any interfering background noise; attention is crucial to memory formation. Researchers also have found that it's better to "warm up" gradually to a task requiring concentration; therefore, before sitting down to memorize information, the subject should first read a magazine article or short story for about 10 minutes. Such a warm-up session improves concentration on the more difficult task.

relaxation and memory   Trying to recall information is easier when the person is relaxed than when he or she is nervous, according to research at Stanford University School of Medicine in Palo Alto, California. In one study, people over age 55 showed improved concentration and better success at recalling faces and names after learning relaxation techniques, such as deep breathing and progressive relaxation.

relearning as a memory test   A person who cannot recall information or even recognize that she has seen it before may still show evidence of remembering some portion of it through a measure of memory called relearning. If a person learns something and then learns it faster the second time, researchers suggest that the person must have some memory of the material. For example, a person who had once studied a foreign language and then forgot most of it will find much of the material "coming back" during the relearning phase.

In one study, a psychologist read his son Greek passages from the age of 15 months to three years, and tested the boy for retention at ages eight, 14 and 18 by having him memorize the original passages and some new material. At age eight, the boy could memorize the passages he had been exposed to already more quickly than those passages he had never heard. However, this ability decreased at 14 and again at 18, from 27 percent quicker to 8 percent to 1 percent at age 18.

remembering   The process of bringing forward memories. Remembering occurs in three stages —acquisition/encoding/recording, storage and retrieval/recall.

Encoding is the act of learning the material; storage is keeping that information "on file" in the brain until it is needed; retrieval is finding the information and getting it back when it is needed.

If a person cannot remember something, it may be because the information was never recorded in the first place (a failure of encoding); it could be that the information was never stored; or it might be that the information was not stored in a way that makes it easy to find.

Most problems in remembering occur in the retrieval stage, not the storage or encoding level. While there is not much to be done to improve retrieval directly, it can be improved indirectly by polishing the methods of recording and retaining. Such methods usually involve some type of mnemonic method that stores information in a way designed to improve its retrieval. (See MNEMONICS.)

In addition, there appear to be at least two different processes involved in memory: SHORT-TERM MEMORY (or "working" memory) and LONG-TERM MEMORY. The difference between these two types of memory is more than in the amount of time information is available. Most researchers believe these two types of memory involve two separate methods of storage or different levels of processing.

Short-term memory refers to how many things a person can pay attention to—similar to the idea of attention span. The hallmark of this type of memory is its rapid rate of forgetting; information stored in short-term memory is forgotten within 30 seconds if it is not rehearsed. In other words, a person may remember an unfamiliar telephone number from the time it is read in the phone book until it's dialed, if the number is repeated during that time. A few seconds after dialing, most people would have to look the number up once more in order to dial it again. Short-term memory also has a limited capacity, usually about seven items.

The art of remembering lies in organizing the storage of trace memories so they will be easy to find with the right cues. First, it's important to perceive in a sensory mode, integrating all five senses so that the thought processes follow categories. When there is something to be remembered, it is important to observe, select, focus, analyze and comment.

repressed memories   Memories that are unconsciously "forgotten." (Usually they are traumatic ones.) The topic of repressed memories has become controversial, because it is difficult to establish their validity. (See also FREUD, SIGMUND; FUGUE; MULTIPLE PERSONALITY DISORDER; PSYCHOGENIC AMNESIA; REPRESSION.)

repression The intentional forgetting of unpleasant memories. Repression was the underlying theme of the theories of Sigmund Freud, the father of psychoanalysis; he considered repression to be the keystone to his entire theory of neurosis. According to Freud, a person purposely pushes unacceptable, traumatic or unpleasant memories into the unconscious, where they can be forgotten. Repression of these memories is necessary to enable the person to survive mentally.

Repression is a form of coping and often occurs, Freud believed, during childhood. He also believed that childhood amnesia is caused by the repression of infantile sexuality. Many modern memory researchers say that infantile amnesia is due, instead, to the lack of early development of various mental abilities (such as language) used to cue memory.

Freud assumed that everyone stores all memories somewhere in the brain, and those who couldn't remember important things simply were not able to retrieve those hidden memories. He assumed there must be an active but known agent repressing the memory. He also assumed that if a patient could overcome a block to memory, the person would automatically remember and the memory would be accurate.

Today, researchers aren't so sure this is true. They believe that while patients may possess the courage and strength to remember, they will not necessarily be successful—especially for memories they have refused to think about for years. Also, when at last some long-buried fact is recalled, patients and therapists can't assume that the memory is historically correct. Many scientists believe that the memory will be a mixture of fact and fiction that cannot be untangled. If a person deliberately refuses to remember an episode, he or she probably will experience a lifelong amnesia for the event. If an emotional association is particularly frightening, a person can halt at memory's emotional level and remember no more, these researchers believe.

While Freud usually obtained his examples of repression from psychoanalytical interviews with mentally ill patients, he believed that the concept also applied to normal forgetting. He noted in his book *The Psychopathology of Everyday Life* (1960) that the tendency to forget what is disagreeable is universal, and the capacity to forget is probably developed to different degrees in different people.

In the early 20th century researchers tried to confirm Freud's hypothesis (the HEDONIC SELECTIVITY or the POLLYANNA HYPOTHESIS) that unpleasant memories were harder to remember than pleasant ones. The problem with the studies was that the greater recall of pleasant experiences might reflect response bias instead of a difference in the ability to recall the memory. Scientists reasoned that the fact that people remember pleasant experiences instead of unpleasant ones may be due to their reluctance to report unpleasant things, and not a failure of memory at all.

Although some parts of Freud's theories are not widely accepted today, most memory experts do believe that such motivated "forgetting" can occur.

Repression also is believed to be the unconscious defense mechanism responsible for DISSOCIATIVE DISORDERS, which segregate a group of mental or behavioral processes from the rest of a person's psychic activity. The amnesia found in these disorders is a repression of disturbing memories; once these memories are repressed (or "forgotten"), access to them is cut off temporarily. (See also AMNESIA, CHILDHOOD; FREUD, SIGMUND; FUGUE; MULTIPLE PERSONALITY DISORDER; PSYCHOGENIC AMNESIA.)

response bias A person's reluctance to report unpleasant experiences to an experimenter due to his or her reluctance to discuss them.

retention See STORAGE.

retrieval The searching and finding process that leads to recognition and or recall.

Mnemonists teach a variety of "retrieval strategies" to bring up deeply buried memories. These strategies work by bringing a memory trace (or ENGRAM) from long-term memory into consciousness by stimulating the surrounding traces of that memory. Quite often, a person who is able to retrieve part of a memory eventually can bring the full information into consciousness. If a person's face is remembered, the name should follow eventually.

There are a number of strategies that help in retrieval:

Alphabet Search Go through the alphabet to recall which letter the name or thing starts with.

Free Association Think up everything possible associated with the information.

Questions To remember details about a complicated event, a series of questions should jog memory: Who? What? Where? When? Why? How? How often? How many? How long?

Guessing Think of the length of the word, with any unusual features (double letters, funny spelling) to concentrate on.

Mood Imagine the feeling when memory was experienced.

If the memory trace is almost nonexistent, it may be possible to recall it by associating it with other information.

Retrace Go over everything that happened just before or right after the event you want to remember. If it's a thing you're trying to find, retrace all the steps you took right before you lost the object.

Causation Think of the circumstances that might have prompted the memory.

Surroundings Imagine the place where the memory was registered. What was being done, thought or said.

Return to the Scene Go to the place where the information was first learned; try to come up with features of the site that connect with the memory itself.

retroactive inhibition A type of mental interference that impedes successful memorization; it is called retroactive because the inhibition is in a backward direction. In other words, if a person studied for an anatomy test last week and studied for a physiology test last night, when he or she tries to remember the facts from the anatomy lesson, the physiology terms might get in the way. This is retroactive inhibition.

If a psychologist asked a group of subjects to memorize a string of words on list A and then asked part of the group to rest while the others memorize list B, when the time comes for the entire group to write down the remembered words from list A, the group that rested will do better. This is because the words on list B retroactively inhibited the memorization of list A. Results from studies like this have shown scientists that a key factor in successful memorization is time. A person memorizing material should rest in between task A and task B in order to give the mind time to consolidate the material, moving at least some of it from short-term to long-term memory. (See also EBBINGHAUS, HERMANN E.; INTERFERENCE THEORY; PROACTIVE INHIBITION.)

retrograde amnesia A type of AMNESIA in which the patient has a gap in memory extending back for some time from the moment of damage to the brain. This type of amnesia is principally a deficit of recall and recognition of information, and the memory gap usually shrinks over time. Retrograde amnesia also usually causes an inability to remember personal and public events instead of loss of language, conceptual knowledge or skills.

Retrograde amnesia appears to be most pronounced for the period immediately before the onset of amnesia, with less disruption of more remote memories. This means that patients with retrograde amnesia probably can describe their high school graduation but would have trouble talking about their career just before the onset of amnesia.

This phenomenon of losing most recent memories first, called RIBOT'S LAW, was first reported by Theodule-Armand Ribot in 1882 when he described his law of regression. He noted that the destruction of memory follows a logical order from the unstable to the stable.

Retrograde amnesia may occur following stroke, head injury, administration of electroconvulsive therapy or in cases of psychogenic amnesia.

Psychologists have developed tests for retrograde amnesia that can measure a patient's memory for events. By compiling a life history of the patient from relatives and friends, the tester can compile a series of questions about each period of a patient's life. The examiner also can use an autobiographical cueing procedure involving the recall of personal events in response to specific words. If the patient can recall events only from certain periods of his or her life, a diagnosis of retrograde amnesia can be made. However, this procedure may be unreliable because it is hard to determine whether the patient's memories are accurate. Retrograde amnesia also may be tested by measuring a patient's ability to remember public events, since it is assumed that memory for public and personal events has a common basis.

The most extensive test for retrograde amnesia is the BOSTON REMOTE MEMORY BATTERY, which has three parts with easy and hard questions. The easy questions may be answered on the basis of general (publicly rehearsed) knowledge, and the hard questions reflect information requiring remembering a particular time period. Unfortunately, this test is culture specific and cannot be used effectively outside the United States.

Generally, retrograde amnesia is less of a problem for patients with memory deficits than is ANTEROGRADE AMNESIA (problems acquiring new information after trauma or an illness). (See also RIBOT, THEODULE-ARMAND; SHRINKING RETROGRADE AMNESIA; TEMPORAL LOBECTOMY.)

rhetoric   The ancient practice of communication that included extensive tutoring in the art of memory. Students studied rhetoric in their training as lawyers or politicians. In modern times, however, rhetoric has shifted its emphasis from the speaker or writer to the listener or reader.

Traditionally, rhetoric is limited to the insights and methods of public speaking developed by rhetoricians in the classical period of ancient Greece (about the fifth century B.C.). Rhetoric was the center of a learning process in Europe for about two millennia, well into the 19th century. The most influential book on education ever written, *Institutio oratoria (The Training of an Orator),* by the Roman rhetorician QUINTILIAN of the first century A.D. was actually a text on rhetoric.

In early Athens, rhetoric teachers (called Sophists) offered rhetoric as a profoundly important educational discipline. By CICERO's time (106 B.C.–43 B.C.), rhetoric was divided into five sections (called "offices"): invention, disposition, elocution, pronunciation and memory. By the Middle Ages, rhetoric had moved into religion, where church

fathers were interested in marrying rhetoric with Christian oration.

rhymes   Using a rhyme to help remember information can be a very effective method in retaining data. For example, many people remember grammatical rules by recalling *"I* before *E* except after *C."* Most people also remember which months have 31 days by the rhyme: "Thirty days hath September . . ."

Basically, learning a rhyme to remember something is a way of imposing meaning as a way to enhance memory. Many people find that recalling a word that rhymes with a sought-after word is an effective cue to recalling the original word. (See also MEANINGFULNESS EFFECT; PEG WORD SYSTEM.)

rhyming-peg system   See PEG WORD SYSTEM.

Ribot, Theodule-Armand (1839–1916)   A French psychologist who described memory loss as a symptom of a brain disease by discussing principles of the evolution of memory function in the individual.

His book *Les Maladies de la mémoire (Diseases of Memory),* published in 1881, was an influential attempt to analyze abnormalities of memory in terms of physiology. In it, he outlines what came to be called RIBOT'S LAW of regression of memory (or progressive destruction), which was popular at the time and still influences contemporary thought on memory today. His law states that the destruction of memory follows a logical order, beginning with the most recent memories and ending with instinctive memory.

Ribot taught at the Sorbonne from 1885 to 1888, moving on to the College of France, where he chaired the department of experimental and comparative psychology. In later years, he became interested in affective and emotional factors in psychology.

Ribot's law   An explanation of the progressive destruction of memory described by French psychologist Theodule-Armand Ribot in his book *Les Maladies de la memoire (Diseases of Memory)* (1881). Ribot's law held that the destruction of memory follows a logical order that advances progressively from the unstable to the stable. The memory destruction begins with the most recent recollections because, since they were only lightly impressed on the "nervous elements," they were rarely repeated. Therefore, these memories had no permanent associations and represented organization in its feeblest form. The last type of memory to be lost is sensorial, instinctive memory, which, having become a permanent and integral part of a person, represents organization in its most highly developed stage.

This theory was quite popular for its time and has been applied to explain phenomena from the breakdown of memory for language (aphasia) to the gradual return of memory after a concussion. The theory also helped to strengthen the idea that as time goes on, the neural basis of memory is strengthened or consolidated.

Still, researchers investigating RETROGRADE AMNESIA (memory loss for old events) agree that Ribot's law has many exceptions. For example, patients recovering from a concussion do not always recover their most recent memories first, as Ribot's law stipulates they should. It is also difficult to separate the effects of the passage of time from those of repetition or rehearsal. (See also RIBOT, THEODULE-ARMAND.)

Ricci, Matteo (1552–1610) A 16th-century Italian Jesuit priest and master of mnemotechnics. Born to a noble family in central Italy, Ricci left for law school in Rome at age 16, but joined the Jesuits as a priest in 1571. Inspired by his superiors in the order who dedicated themselves to priestly initiative, he volunteered for work overseas and was sent to China. On a trip to convert the Chinese, he shared the European art of building MEMORY PALACES as a way of gaining his hosts' attention and respect. After building his own memory palace filled with the difficult-to-learn Chinese characters, he asked his hosts to write down a large number of different characters in no order and with no relation to each other. After reading it once, he recited the characters in perfect order—and then recited them all by memory, backward.

Ricci lived in China for 30 years, adopting the language and culture of the country and traveling to the interior, which was normally closed to foreigners.

While trying to win converts, Ricci also taught the Chinese Euclidean geometry, Western chemistry, astronomy, optics and clockmaking, wrote books and composed lyrics, and created an annotated map of the world. But he left no record of the kinds of memory palaces he created in his own mind.

Rivermead Behavioral Memory Test One of the more realistic memory tests that measures everyday aspects of forgetting and monitors change following treatment for memory deficits. It was designed to bridge the gap between laboratory-based and more natural measures of memory.

Although it is administered and scored in a standardized way, the Rivermead subtests try to provide an analog of a range of everyday memory situations that appear to cause trouble for certain patients with acquired brain damage. Its subtests include measures of remembering a name, a hidden belonging, and an appointment. The Rivermead Behavioral Memory Test also tests picture and face recognition, immediate prose recall, orientation and remembering a route and delivering a message.

These subtests were chosen on the basis of the memory problems reported by head injury patients. The items require that patients either remember to carry out some everyday task or retain the type of information needed for everyday functioning, and are combined with some conventional memory measures.

Immediately after the test items are administered, the patient is given a paired-association learning test in which six paired associates are presented verbally; patients are retested in three trials, which provides a test of long-term verbal learning. This is followed by the standard Wechsler Adult Intelligence Scale (WAIS) Digit Span (a subtest of the WAIS) in which subjects are required to repeat back sequences of digits until a point is reached at which they consistently make errors.

The Rivermead test was developed as a way of predicting which brain-damaged people are most likely to encounter everyday memory problems. Although patients with severe amnesia probably will fail all parts of the test, less-impaired patients should exhibit patterns that may correlate with various neuropsychological dysfunctions. The test is particularly useful in measuring improvement (as in head injury) or deterioration (as in Alzheimer's disease) since it can be administered in four parallel versions, which lower the practice effects through repeated testing.

rivastigmine (Exelon)   A new drug approved in spring 2000 for the treatment of ALZHEIMER'S DIS-EASE that works by helping to increase levels of the neurotransmitter ACETYLCHOLINE by blocking two enzymes that break it down. In studies, participants who took rivastigmine showed greater improvement in thinking and remembering, activities of daily living and overall functioning than did those who took placebo (inactive treatment). The drug helped slightly more than half of the people who took it.

The most common side effects were nausea, vomiting, loss of appetite, fatigue and weight loss. In most cases, these side effects were temporary and declined with continuing treatment.

It has long been known that those with Alzheimer's disease have low brain levels of the neurotransmitter acetylcholine. By slowing down the metabolic breakdown of acetylcholine, more of the brain chemical is available for communication between cells. This helps slow the progression of Alzheimer's, but it doesn't cure the disease.

In rivastigmine trials more than 90 percent of participants had (in addition to Alzheimer's disease) a variety of other illnesses common in older adults, including high blood pressure, adult-onset diabetes and arthritis. Almost all patients took other medications at the same time that they took rivastigmine.

The two other drugs already approved by the FDA to treat Alzheimer's, TACRINE (Cognex) and DONEPEZIL (Aricept), also work by boosting the availability of acetylcholine in the brain. However, none of these drugs will cure the disease.

All three are most effective if taken early in the disease when there are more functioning brain cells to produce acetylcholine. After too many cells die, the drug no longer works.

Exelon, a medication created by Novartis Pharmaceuticals, became available in pharmacies at the end of May 2000.

Roman room system   One of the most popular of the Roman mnemonic techniques. In this system, mnemonic experts imagined the entrance to their house and their room, and then filled the room with as many objects and items of furniture as they chose. Each object or piece of furniture served as a link image onto which they attached things they wanted to remember. They were particularly careful to bring order and precision to their rooms, which is essential to the proper functioning of this system. The benefit of this system is that it requires very precise structure and ordering, imagination and sensuality. (See also LOCI, METHOD OF; MEMORY PALACE.)

rosemary (Rosmariinus officinalis)   This small, perennial evergreen shrub of the mint family is known as the herb of memory. In ancient Greece, students believed that entwining a spring of rosemary in their hair would improve their memory, so they wore rosemary garlands while studying for exams. At funerals, mourners tossed fresh sprigs into the grave as a sign that the life of the departed would not be forgotten.

"I lett it runne all over my garden wall," wrote Sir Thomas More, "not onlie because my bees love it, but because 'tis the herb sacred to remembrance."

Native to the Mediterranean region, rosemary has been naturalized throughout Europe and temperate America. It is widely grown in gardens in the warmer parts of the United States and Great Britain, where an old legend states that where rosemary thrives, the mistress is master.

rote learning   Remembering information by repeating it over and over without making any of the details meaningful or using any mnemonic device to boost memory storage. The opposite of meaningful learning, since information needs to be meaningful in order to be remembered best. (See also MEANINGFULNESS EFFECT; MEMORY FOR STORIES.)

scopolamine An antispasmodic drug that blocks neurotransmission of certain chemicals in the brain, including ACETYLCHOLINE, important in the normal function of memory. If given to normal subjects, the drug causes a severe memory loss that is reversed by the administration of PHYSOSTIGMINE. Under the influence of scopolamine, retention remains intact, but effortful retrieval is impaired. Scopolamine appears to disrupt efficient encoding processes leading to a deficiency in effective retrieval of information. It has a more potent effect than sedatives or tranquilizers on human cognitive abilities, but the strength of the amnesia following scopolamine administration depends on the memory task used to define it.

screen memories Early memories that, according to psychoanalyst Sigmund Freud, are usually fabricated to block out the emotionally painful, repressed memories of infant sexuality.

For example, one subject recalled the sharp memory of a cobblestone sidewalk in front of his house when he was two years old. While he had no idea why he should remember the cobblestones, he also noted that he had contracted polio at that age, but insisted he had no memory of the onset of the illness—just the cobblestones. It could be that the image of the cobblestones was a FLASHBULB MEMORY of the moment when the reality of the illness struck him; the image persisted while the association did not. But Freud would have called this memory a screen memory, suggesting that the apparently trivial memory obscured a more painful truth as part of a deliberate repression. (See AMNESIA, CHILD-HOOD; FREUD, SIGMUND; MEMORY IN INFANCY.)

secondary memory See LONG-TERM MEMORY.

selective amnesia A type of PSYCHOGENIC AMNESIA in which a patient fails to recall some, but not all, of the events occurring during a certain period of time. (See also HYSTERICAL AMNESIA.)

selective attention Defining what one wants to remember, why and for how long.

self-testing A powerful storage aid to mentally test retention of information, especially if used soon after first seeing or hearing the information and then at gradually lengthening intervals.

semantic memory Memory for facts, such as the information that would be contained in a dictionary or encyclopedia with no connection to time or place. People don't remember when or where they learn this type of information.

Semantic memory is one of the five major human memory systems (the others are episodic, procedural, perceptual representation and short-term memory) for which evidence now exists.

Semantic memory registers and stores knowledge about the world in the broadest sense; it allows people to represent and mentally operate on situations, objects and relations in the world that aren't present to the senses. A person with an intact semantic memory system can think about things that are not here now. Because semantic memory develops first in childhood, before episodic memory, children are able to learn facts before they can remember their own experiences.

The seat of semantic memory is believed to be located in the medial temporal lobe and diencephalic structures. (See also EPISODIC MEMORY; SHORT-TERM MEMORY.)

semantic network Chunks of information connected into networks by associated meanings. Activation of any one chunk automatically "readies" others that are closely associated with it, with lessening degrees of activation spreading from one network to another. Some scientists believe the semantic network may be the main structural component of long-term memory.

senile dementia In the past, DEMENTIA was divided into two forms; presenile (affecting people under age 65) and senile (over age 65). These designations are no longer used today.

Senile dementia (or "senility") is a catchword that has been used for many years to label almost any eccentric behavior in the elderly. It has sometimes been equated with such terms as *chronic brain failure*, *chronic brain syndrome*, *organic brain syndrome* or *ALZHEIMER'S DISEASE*.

Between 50 to 60 percent of older people with impaired memories have Alzheimer's disease; approximately 20 to 25 percent of brain impairment is caused by STROKE, and the remainder is the result of other causes.

There are a number of reasons for confusion, forgetfulness and disorientation besides Alzheimer's disease. These problems could be caused by overmedication or medication interaction, chemical imbalances (lack of potassium, abnormal sugar levels, and so on), depression, sudden illness, malnutrition and dehydration or social isolation.

senility A term that once referred to changes in mental ability caused by old age. However, the term *senile* simply means "old." Therefore, senility does not really describe a disease; many people considered it to be a derogatory or prejudicial term.

Most people over age 70 suffer from some amount of impaired memory and reduced ability to concentrate. As a person ages, the risk of DEMENTIA rises to affect about one in five over age 80. Depressive illness and confusion due to physical disease are also common.

The phrases "chronic ORGANIC BRAIN SYNDROME" and "acute or reversible organic brain syndrome" have been used respectively to refer to those dementias that cannot be treated (chronic) and to

those that respond to treatment (acute). (See also AGING AND MEMORY; ALZHEIMER'S DISEASE; MILD COGNITIVE IMPAIRMENT.)

senses and memory All of the senses of a human being can evoke memory—sight, sound, touch, taste or smell—but none of them accomplish this with equal ability. Taste and smell are particularly powerful aids to remembering, partly because the olfactory fibers interact directly with the HIPPOCAMPUS and AMYGDALA. Vision requires several intermediate cell connections, whereas smell makes an immediate connection with memory structures in the brain.

sensory memory The holding of a sensory impression for a short time after it has been perceived. This type of MEMORY takes in a vast number of impressions, lasting about one second each (although the time varies for each sense); it can hold information for a maximum of about four seconds, to enable a person to select what to pay attention to for further processing in SHORT-TERM MEMORY.

sensory store The initial stage of memory that works chiefly when the sense organs (eyes, ears, tongue and nose) are stimulated. Before something can be remembered, information must be input. If it is a series of numbers, the sensory input will be visual; if it's the odor of cinnamon buns, the sensory input will be smell. Once sensory input enters the brain, it then enters short-term memory, where it is retained just long enough to be remembered briefly. From there, selected bits of information may enter long-term memory if an event called REHEARSAL takes place (that is, if the information is repeated) or if there is a strong sensory or emotional component.

sequential mental processing Mental activities involving the ability to solve a series of steps, such as solving mathematical expressions or recalling a series of items in order. It is the opposite of SIMULTANEOUS MENTAL PROCESSING.

Sequential memory processes would involve tasks such as remembering a phone or Social Security number, or the sequence of steps needed to assemble a piece of machinery.

serial position effect   The ability of people to remember serial information is affected by where in the series the information appears. Items in the middle of a list take longer to learn and are more difficult to recall than items at the beginning or end of the list. For example, the names of the first few presidents and the last few presidents are easy for most people to recall, but those who served in the middle of the list are far more difficult to remember.

In addition, the length of time after learning can affect which part of the list is the most difficult to remember. If a person tries to remember the names of the presidents immediately after learning them, she will be able to remember the last few names better than the first few. When there is a delay between learning and recall, she will be able to remember the first few presidents better. But no matter how long the interval between learning and recall, those presidents in the middle of the list still will be the most difficult to remember.

This phenomenon can be manipulated to help people remember. If items don't need to be memorized in order, arranging them with the more complex ones at the two ends of the list and the simpler ones in the middle will make the task easier. If the order can't be changed (such as in the list of presidents), people should take more time to memorize the information in the middle of the list.

serial sevens task   A component of a MENTAL STATUS EXAMINATION to determine awareness that can provide a test of attention and short-term memory. In the test, the patient begins at the number 100 and subtracts 7 at a time, backward, such as: 100, 93, 86, etc. Variations of the serial sevens task include the serial threes and serial nines tasks.

sexual abuse and traumatic memory   See CHILD ABUSE, MEMORY OF.

shass pollak   The technical term used by Jews for a memory expert who has memorized the entire contents of the Talmud (the writings constituting the body of early Jewish civil and religious law). The Talmud was memorized not just literally (that is, word for word) but also typographically (as a set of printed pages). *Shass* is the abbreviation for the Hebrew terms for the Talmud, and *Pollak* is Hebrew for "Pole."

All modern editions of the Talmud are paged alike and printed alike, with each page having the same number of words and each page beginning and ending with the same word in all editions.

Sheldrake's hypothesis   The idea that the world is kept running by nature's memory that exists as "morphic forms," not by immutable law. These forms, according to cell geneticist and Royal Society fellow Rupert Sheldrake, are patterns without energy that link to the world through resonance. Every person has his or her own morphic form, and each person resonates to other larger memory patterns in the world memory.

Morphic forms shape us, Sheldrake believes. He was fascinated by what it is that makes an oak tree an oak tree and a horse a horse. A memory pattern or morphic form rises with the first horse, and each succeeding horse resonates to the form and is shaped by it. Yet at the same time, the horse gives back its own bit of idiosyncrasy, allowing change and growth.

short-term memory   Another word for consciousness, short-term memory has a range of other names: Primary memory, immediate memory, working memory. But while some researchers describe a distinct short-term memory system of limited capacity and a long-term system of relatively unlimited capacity, others don't distinguish between the two. Instead, they suggest there is only one system with what appears to be "short-term" memory as only memory with very low levels of learning.

This type of memory storage is necessary in order to perform many tasks; for example, when reading a book, the beginning of the sentence must be kept in mind while reading the last part of the sentence in order for the whole phrase to make sense.

Short-term memory receives information from sensory memory. If not processed further, the information quickly decays; among typical subjects without any memory training, short-term memory seems as if it can deal only with about six or seven items at once for about 15 to 30 seconds at a time. Research suggests that the information in short-term storage is highly vulnerable to distraction or negative interference. (For example, when you lose your train of thought during a conversation after being interrupted.)

Once placed in short-term storage, information can then either be transferred into long-term storage (or "secondary memory") or it can be forgotten.

If a person looks up a number in a phone book, sensory memory registers the number and passes it into short-term memory. As the number is repeated over and over while dialing, it is retained in short-term memory. The limited capacity of short-term memory determines how much information a person can pay attention to at any one time. Going over information keeps it in short-term memory; after a person has looked up an unfamiliar phone number and repeated it over and over, the person could probably make a phone call without having to look up the number again in the book. However, if the person was interrupted while dialing, it is likely that the number would be forgotten when the person tried to redial.

Short-term memory also is limited in capacity to about five or ten bits of information, which can be enlarged by using MNEMONICS—strategies to help remember information. For example, grouping a phone number into segments of three, three and four makes it much easier to remember than if the number was remembered as one long continuous line of ten digits.

If data is to be transferred into long-term store, a permanent memory trace is formed that provides the basis for restoring the information to consciousness. To remember a phone number for a long period of time, it must be "encoded" and moved into LONG-TERM MEMORY—preferably using sight or sound to help remember it. A person could sing the number or think about a picture of the number to help retrieve it from long-term memory.

Short-term memory is an important part of a person's memory in that it serves as a sort of temporary notepad, briefly retaining intermediate results while we think and solve problems. It helps maintain a concept of the world by indicating what objects are in the environment and where they are located, keeping visual perceptions stable.

A person's visual perception darts around a scene taking about five retinal images per second and integrating information from all the snapshots into one sustained model of the immediate scene. New changes are included in an updated model, while old ones are discarded, thanks to short-term memory.

Short-term memory maintains the file of our intentions in "active" mode, guiding behavior toward those goals. It keeps track of topics that have been mentioned in conversations. If two friends are discussing a third acquaintance, they can refer to the person as "she" without using her name, and each will know whom the "she" refers to, because of short-term memory.

However, these early processes are extremely complex, including the necessity of word identification and object recognition. By the time information has reached short-term store, a great deal of processing has already occurred of which people are not consciously aware. What passes into consciousness and short-term store is simply the *result* of those unconscious processes. Researchers suggest that only information that has been consciously perceived is transferred from short- to long-term store.

Many researchers liken a person's short-term memory to a computer's central processing unit (CPU). Almost all computers are designed with a sort of "short-term memory" within the CPU, which receives data, stores it in memory, retrieves it and can display it on a screen or print it out. These functions are strikingly similar to short-term memory.

short-term store (STS)   See SHORT-TERM MEMORY.

shrinking retrograde amnesia   The gradual recovery from RETROGRADE AMNESIA with older memories returning first. The existence of the phenomenon of shrinking retrograde amnesia is not surprising, considering that earlier memories can be derived from a different source from that needed to recall more recent experiences.

As recovery occurs, more and more of the episodic record becomes available and more recent memories can be recalled. Researchers believe that older experiences are more broadly distributed than newer events, and a gradual recovery process will restore some component of older memories before it restores more narrowly distributed newer memories.

Simonides of Ceos (c. 500 B.C.–c. 468 B.C.)   The father of the art of trained memory, this Greek poet invented the use of loci (or place) in association with words and images to improve the memory. (See LOCI, METHOD OF.)

According to the great Roman orator Cicero, Simonides was sitting at a banquet table of the mogul Scopas, who had asked the poet to compose a lyric in his honor. Simonides informed Scopas that he would recite if he was paid (the first time a poet ever requested payment to perform); but after the recitation, in which Simonides had praised the gods Castor and Pollux, Scopas paid Simonides only half his fee. "Let the twin gods pay the rest," he retorted. Suddenly a servant appeared and told Simonides that two young men wanted to speak with him in the street; as soon as Simonides left the room, the ceiling collapsed, crushing everyone at the banquet table. (Legend holds that the two young men who saved Simonides were Castor and Pollux, come to pay their debt.)

Although the bodies were damaged beyond recognition, Simonides was able to identify all of them through his memorization of the places where they had been sitting around the table. With this experience, he realized the value of organizing a pattern in the mind. He recognized the value of this system to orators who gave speeches from memory. He invented the art of MNEMONICS and became one of the leading consultants to orators of the day.

simultaneous mental processing   Mental activities involving "all at once" processing that doesn't rely on a sequence of steps. For example, the ability to remember how many suspects a witness saw in a robbery or to remember the smell of a bakery down the street from a person's childhood home are examples of simultaneous memory tasks.

sleep and memory   In order to function with peak memory skills, it is essential to get enough sleep and rest the brain, which can be taxed by too much work during the day and poor sleeping at night.

While we sleep, our brain revises, manipulates and stores information. Anyone who has ever gone to sleep with a problem and awoken with the solution has experienced the way the brain can work out difficulties during sleep.

Of course, sleep is not the same, continuous process throughout the night. Instead, according to researchers at France's National Center for Scientific Research, consolidation of memories takes place during paradoxical sleep, which lasts for just about 20 minutes and occurs every 90 minutes in human beings. During this portion of sleep, all the senses are put on hold, disconnecting the brain from the outside world. It is then, these scientists believe, that the maturation of the memory takes place and the brain processes, reviews, consolidates and stores information.

Research has shown that depriving subjects of sleep after learning a task causes their performance to deteriorate.

But although people can't learn effectively without sleep, this doesn't mean that they can learn while sleeping. Because both the conscious and subconscious play a role in the memory process, one cannot work without the other.

Insomnia—the inability to sleep—deprives a person not just of the valuable memory consolidation periods during rest but also interferes with learning during waking hours as well. This problem affects the elderly in particular; often they have more sleep problems and get very little fourth-stage or "deep" sleep, during which the brain recharges itself. After a while the person lives in a chronic state of fatigue and finds it difficult to pay attention or register information.

sleep learning   While popular theory holds that a person can learn better while sleeping, in fact research has proven that people do not learn while they are soundly asleep: When a person is truly asleep, learning does not take place. If a person plays an educational tape while sleeping and learns some of the material, he or she actually has remembered what was heard during a waking period.

There is, however, some evidence suggesting that people can learn while they are very drowsy or even in a very light sleep. The material must be presented at just the right time: not sleepy enough and the material will wake up the subject, and too deeply asleep and the material won't make an impression at all. In addition, complex material involving reasoning or understanding can't be learned. What can be learned during this very drowsy state are nonsense syllables. Morse code, facts, dates, foreign languages and the like. Finally, sleep learning during this one period is still not enough on its own; it is effective only if used together with daytime learning.

However, some research indicates that falling asleep immediately after learning something helps someone retain the information better than if he or she stays up and engages in some activity. Further, a good night's sleep will help make people alert for memory tasks the next day.

Yet sleeping pills will not ensure that people wake up refreshed and ready to learn. The carry-over effect of these drugs makes a person less able to register new memories the next day and less susceptible to stimulation that can assist in remembering already learned information. (See also SUBLIMINAL LEARNING.)

smart drugs   Medications that are thought to enhance learning, thinking or memory. There are two basic kinds of smart drugs: NOOTROPICS and cognitive enhancers. Nootropic means "mind turning" and is used to describe nontoxic substances that may improve learning and memory without affecting the brain. "Cognitive enhancer" is a general term for any substance that might boost mental functioning.

The pyrrolidone derivatives (PIRACETAM, OXIRACETAM, aniracetam, pramiracetam, and PYROGLUTA-MATE) are the most important family of nootropics. Proponents of these drugs claim they cause remarkable improvement in memory. Although scientists don't fully understand how they work, it is generally believed that they influence nerve pathways in the brain that use ACETYLCHOLINE as a neurotransmitter. Enthusiasts say that piracetam stimulates the central nervous system. These drugs are not sold in the United States, but they can be ordered by mail or purchased over-the-counter at Mexican pharmacies.

Smith, Edwin, Surgical Papyrus of   An Egyptian medical treatise written between 2,500 and 3,000 years ago that describes how head injury can have effects throughout the body. The papyrus contains information about 48 cases; eight describe head injuries that affect other parts of the body.

Apparently intended as a textbook on surgery, the papyrus begins with the clinical cases of head injuries and works its way down the body, describing in detail the examination, diagnosis, treatment and prognosis in each case.

The papyrus was acquired in Luxor in 1862 by the American Egyptologist Edwin Smith, a pioneer in the study of Egyptian science. After his death in 1906, the papyrus was given to the New-York Historical Society, which turned it over for study to the Egyptologist James Henry Breasted in 1920. Breasted published a translation, transliteration and discussion in two volumes in 1930.

smoking and memory   While some studies have shown that nicotine can improve factual recall, smoking cigarettes containing nicotine also cuts down on the amount of oxygen that reaches the brain and in this way can interfere with memory. Studies have shown that smoking may enhance performance of simple tasks, but interferes with more complex cognitive processes.

social memory   The ability to recognize those people we have met before. Without this ability, even a person's own mother would remain a stranger. Recent research has found that the hormone oxytocin has been identified as key in forming social memories. In the past, oxytocin has been associated with maternal functions such as labor contractions, and also with male sexual behavior.

Socrates (c. 470 b.c.–399 b.c.)   An ancient Athenian philosopher who directed philosophical thought toward analyses of the character and conduct of human life, and who is remembered for his direction to "know thyself." He is best known for his method of teaching that involved a way of jogging innate memory by questioning his students in such a way that he drew information from them that they didn't know they possessed. The hidden agenda of this "Socratic method" is to draw forth the innate divine memory.

Socrates, who lived during the chaos of the Peloponnesian War, served as an infantryman during the war. Later, married with three sons, he was a conspicuous figure in Athens, where he seemed to spend all his time in the streets, the marketplace and the gymnasia. He enjoyed speaking with young men of promise and with politicians, poets and artisans about their work and their notions of right and wrong.

According to Socrates, people carried a block of wax within their soul of varying quality in different individuals—the "gift of Memory, the mother of the Muses." He believed that whenever someone hears or thinks something, this wax is held under the perceptions and thoughts, where they are imprinted upon it.

In Plato's *Phaedrus*, Socrates tells the story of the inventor of the alphabet, who believed his invention would make the Egyptians wiser and improve their memory. But according to Socrates, the god Thamus was horrified at this invention, predicting that the alphabet would only enhance forgetfulness. Thamus reasoned that when people relied on written words, they would no longer rely on improving their memory. "You have invented an elixir not of memory but of reminding," Socrates quotes Thamus in *Phaedrus*, "and you offer your pupils the appearance of wisdom, not true wisdom." Thamus warned that these students would read information without instruction, seeming to know many things but in fact being ignorant.

It has been suggested that this passage may represent a survival of the tradition of oral memory, of the time before writing was commonly used; others believe it is a description of the ancient Egyptian practice of memory as a profound discipline.

In 399 Socrates was arrested on two counts of "impiety," "corruption of the young" and "neglect of the gods whom the city worships and the practice of religious novelties." He was sentenced to death, declined an opportunity to escape and drank a fatal concoction of hemlock.

Socrates wrote nothing himself. Information about his personality and doctrines is found primarily in the words of PLATO and Zenophon's *Memorabilia*.

sodium amytal (amylbarbitone)   Also called truth serum, this drug facilitates the recall of emotionally disturbing memories. Scientists believe sodium amytal reduces anxiety so that the patient can tolerate the recollection of experiences that are too painful to recall in the normal conscious state. It is occasionally used with trauma survivors to access repressed or unconscious feelings or memories, or to help diagnose dissociative identity disorder.

sodium pentothal   A drug used to uncover buried traumatic memories of known origin (such as amnesia following combat trauma) by first sedating the patient via slow intravenous injection. This relieves any anxiety the patient may have and is followed by the onset of drowsiness. At this point, the injection is halted and the interview begins. (See also SODIUM AMYTAL [AMYLBARBITONE].)

somnambulism   A phenomenon that sometimes occurs during HYPNOSIS, in which the subject can have the outward appearance of ordinary awareness, but in fact is deeply hypnotized.

source amnesia   Loss of memory for when and where particular information was acquired.

spacing effect   Recall of items repeated immediately is far worse than spaced repetitions. This is related to the *lag effect*, in which the recall of items given spaced repetition increases as the interval between repetition increases.

SPECT (single-photon emission computerized tomography)   A type of brain scan that tracks blood flow and measures brain activity. Less expensive than PET (positron emission tomography) scans, SPECTs may be used to identify subtle injury following mild head trauma.

SPECT is a type of radionuclide scanning, a diagnostic technique based on the defection of radiation emitted by radioactive substances introduced into the body. Different types of tissue take up different radioactive substances (radionuclides) in greater concentrations; SPECT gives a clearer picture of organ function than other systems.

The radioactive substance is swallowed or injected into the bloodstream, where it accumulates in the brain. Gamma radiation (similar but shorter than X rays) is emitted from the brain. It is detected by a gamma camera, which emits light, and is used to produce an image that can be displayed on a screen; using a principle similar to CT (computerized tomography) scanning, cross-sectional images can be constructed by a computer from radiation detected by the gamma camera that rotates around the patient. Moving images can be created by using a computer to record a series of images right after the administration of the radionuclide.

Radionuclide scanning is a safe procedure requiring only tiny doses of radiation. Because the radioactive substance is ingested or injected, it avoids the risks of some X-ray procedures in which a radiopaque dye is inserted through a catheter into the organ (as in angiography). And unlike radiopaque dyes, radionuclides carry almost no risk of toxicity or allergy.

SQUID (superconducting quantum interference device)   A type of brain scanning device that senses tiny changes in magnetic fields. When brain cells fire, they create electric current; electric fields induce magnetic fields, so magnetic changes indicate neural activity.

state-dependent learning   The theory that a person performs better if learning and recalling information takes place in the same state (such as under the influence of alcohol) and poorer when trying to recall a memory when in a state different from the one in which it was registered. Therefore, a person who learns something after a few drinks can recall that information better while drunk than while sober. Or a person who learns while sober may then have difficulty recalling it when drunk. (See also ALCOHOL AND MEMORY.)

steroids   See PREGNENOLONE.

stimulus-response memory   The kind of memory involved when a dinner bell makes a trained dog salivate. This type of memory uses brain areas below the outer cortex and survives damage to regions of the brain essential for other kinds of memory.

storage   The ability to hold information in memory for a brief period of time. Traditionally, researchers have believed that in memory, the most critical problems are concerned with the physiological mechanism by which events and experiences can be retained so they can be reproduced. Most researchers believe that anything that influences the behavior of an organism leaves a trace in the central nervous system. Theoretically, as long as these traces last, they can be restimulated and the experience that established them will be remembered.

In studying retention, researchers test how well subjects learn words or sets of letters, obtaining a retention score. Future forgetting will be measured against this score. Subsequent tests of retention are then given to measure the rate at which the person forgets.

storage-deficit theories   Two types of theories explain storage deficits in memory: One states that AMNESIA is due to more rapid forgetting; the other, that amnesia is caused by a failure of consolidation. Neither of these theories, scientists say, adequately explains human amnesic syndrome.

The rapid-forgetting theorists assume that a memory is formed but that it simply decays more rapidly among amnesic patients, although research in general appears not to support this view. The second storage-deficit theory states that failure to consolidate memory is the underlying cause of amnesic syndrome.

storage vs. retrieval failure Forgetting can occur either because information was not properly stored or because of a problem in retrieval. "Storage" refers to keeping information "on file" in the brain until it is needed; "retrieval" is finding the information and getting it back when it is needed.

If a person cannot remember something, it may be because the information was never stored or because the information was not stored in a way that makes it easy to find. Most problems in remembering occur in the retrieval stage, not in storage. While there is not much to be done to improve retrieval directly, it is possible to improve retrieval indirectly by polishing the methods of recording and retaining. Such methods usually involve some type of "mnemonic method" that stores information in a way designed to improve its retrieval.

stress and memory There appears to be a relationship between stress and problems in remembering information.

St. Louis researchers found the first direct evidence that stress hormones associated with major physical or psychological problems can impair memory within a matter of days. It takes several days of stress like major surgery or severe psychological trauma in order for cortisol to produce memory impairment. After about a week after the trauma, however, memory appears to return to normal.

Researchers had already shown that synthetic stress hormones impair memory, but scientists also found that prolonged exposure to high levels of cortisol—the hormone actually produced in the body in response to high stress—has that same negative effect. Major psychological stresses, which can be different for different individuals, also could produce similar effects on memory.

For example, if a student studying for a test has just experienced a major trauma such as a death in the family, he or she might not be as good at learning new material. A few people may experience high cortisol levels in response to less profound events, such as the pressure of upcoming final exams. Moreover, there may be some effects from long-term exposure to slightly lower levels of stress hormones.

Studies with synthetic steroids show that stress hormones' effects on memory appear to be reversible.

The evidence suggests that these kinds of cortisol levels are not neurotoxic themselves. Perhaps sustained, high levels make neurons vulnerable to other types of injury, but scientists don't believe the memory impairments related to stress are in any way associated with an irreversible process.

stroke Damage to the brain caused by an interruption to its blood supply or leakage of blood outside of vessel walls. A stroke may be caused by cerebral thrombosis (clot), cerebral embolism or hemorrhage. Any area in the brain damaged by the stroke will affect further brain function, including sensation, movement and memory.

Following a stroke, serious memory problems can be caused when a large group of cells in a concentrated area die and break a memory circuit. The effects of stroke are random and depend on where the stroke occurs. Sometimes a stroke damages an area but the brain quickly recovers because the corresponding circuit in the other hemisphere continues to function. In other cases, the circuits in the two hemispheres don't appear to have developed equally, and the damage is lasting. Many causes of AGNOSIA and APHASIA are caused by stroke.

Causes

Cerebral thrombosis is a blockage by a clot that has built up on the wall of a brain artery, depriving the brain of blood; it is responsible for almost half of all strokes. Cerebral embolism is a blockage by an embolus (usually a clot) that is swept into an artery in the brain and deprives the brain of oxygen; it accounts for 30 to 35 percent of strokes. Hemorrhage is the rupture of a blood vessel and bleeding within or over the surface of the brain; it accounts for about a quarter of all strokes.

Strokes are fatal in about one-third of cases and are a leading cause of death in developed countries. In the United States, stroke will occur in about 200 out of every 100,000 people each year; incidence rises quickly with age and is higher in men than women.

Certain things can increase the risk of stroke, including high blood pressure, which weakens the walls of arteries, and atherosclerosis (thickening of the lining of arterial walls). Stroke also can be caused by conditions that cause blood clots in the heart that may migrate to the brain: irregular heartbeat (atrial fibrillation), damaged heart valves or heart attack. Conditions that increase the risk of high blood pressure and or atherosclerosis also can cause stroke; these include hyperlipidemia (fatty substances in the blood), polycythemia (high level of red blood cells in the blood), diabetes mellitus and smoking. Oral contraceptives also increase the risk of stroke in women under 50.

Symptoms

A stroke that affects the dominant of the two cerebral hemispheres in the brain (usually the left) may cause disturbance of language and speech. Symptoms that last for less than 24 hours followed by full recovery are known as TRANSIENT ISCHEMIC ATTACKS (TIAs); such attacks are warnings that part of the brain is not receiving a sufficient supply of blood.

Treatment

Unconscious or semiconscious hospital patients require a clear airway, tube feeding and regular changing of position. Any fluid accumulation in the brain may be treated with corticosteroid drugs or diuretics. A stroke caused by an embolism is treated with anticoagulant drugs to help prevent recurrences. Sometimes aspirin is prescribed or vascular surgery performed to reduce the risk of subsequent stroke.

While about half of patients recover more or less completely from their first stroke, any intellectual impairment and memory loss is usually permanent. (See also CEREBRAL VASCULAR ACCIDENT [CVA].)

Stroop, J. Ridley One of the most unusual figures in the history of experimental psychology, Stroop devised the "gold standard" of attention measures in 1936—a color word test that bears his name.

When his doctoral dissertation appeared in the *Journal of Experimental Psychology,* Stroop earned immediate prominence for his test of attention. But he published only four studies between 1932 and 1938, finally retiring from the psychology labora-

tory in favor of teaching, preaching and writing about the Bible at a small Christian college in Nashville, where he served as head of the psychology department. (See also STROOP COLOR WORD TEST; STROOP EFFECT.)

Stroop Color Word Test The best known of all methods of testing focused attention, in which subjects must sort cards on the basis of ink color. The Stroop Color Word Test is used to investigate personality, cognition, stress response, psychiatric disorders and other psychological issues.

Requiring about five minutes to administer, this screening test can effectively differentiate between normal patients, non-brain-damaged psychiatric patients and brain-damaged patients.

The Stroop consists of a Word Page with color words printed in black ink, a Color Page with Xs printed in color, and a Word-Color Page with words from the first page printed in colors from the second.

It is appropriate for anyone beyond grade 2, and is not biased toward sex or culture. (See also STROOP, J. RIDLEY; STROOP EFFECT.)

Stroop effect The inability of subjects to quickly perform a task in which they are asked to read a list of color words printed in a color different from the word. (For example, to say "green" in response to the word *purple* written in green ink.) But when asked to simply read the list of words (to say "purple" in response to the word *purple* printed in green ink), subjects can complete the task easily. This phenomenon has never been adequately explained.

More than 700 studies have investigated some aspect of the Stroop effect. Since 1969, about 20 papers a year have examined the phenomenon without reaching any concrete conclusions.

The studies have found that the Stroop effect occurs with exposure to lists of words (or other stimuli) presented singly that require variations in response. Not just colors, but also things such as the word *horse* inside a drawing of a bear interferes with the person's ability to name the pictures.

Researchers also found that words closely associated with the colors in the Stroop test interfere more with color identification than unassociated words. For example, *purple* printed in red slows down the respondents' ability to say "red" more than the word *house* printed in red.

People can name colors faster when the color words (*red*) are printed in the same color ink than when color words are printed in black ink. But this effect is weaker than the disturbance in color naming caused by mismatches of words and ink colors.

If the test presents colors and color words in different locations (such as a blue bar above the word *red* in black ink), subjects still have trouble naming the colors, but not as much as they do for the standard Stroop test.

Subjects' ability to name colors quickly slows down when a color word on one trial matches the ink color on the next trial, as when *red* in green ink precedes *purple* in red ink. Researchers believe that subjects consciously suppress the reading response *red* on the first trial, making it harder to say "red" in response to the ink color in the next trial.

However, if subjects are allowed to practice naming incompatible ink colors of various color words, they slowly can improve their ability to name colors—but they also have a harder time in reading color words printed in nonmatching colors.

Even young children experience the Stroop effect, and the effect peaks during the second and third grades as reading skills are strengthened. The amount of time it takes to name the colors then continues to decline until about age 60, when it starts to increase again. There are no differences between men and women's experience of the Stroop effect.

Some scientists believe that people read words faster than they identify colors, so when different words and colors collide in the same test, the reading response interferes with the slower color-naming response, especially when the faster response has to be ignored. But others have found that presenting various colors just before incompatible color words doesn't interfere with naming. (See also STROOP, J. RIDLEY; STROOP COLOR WORD TEST.)

subarachnoid hemorrhage   A fairly unusual type of cerebral vascular accident (or STROKE) that can cause either a temporary or a permanent memory impairment. This type of hemorrhage usually affects younger patients who are less likely to suffer from widespread cerebral vascular disease. About 8 percent of all stroke patients have this type of hemorrhage, which usually is caused by the rupture of an intercranial aneurysm that bleeds into the subarachnoid space around the brain. Common sites for these ruptures include the ANTERIOR COMMUNICATING ARTERY lying between the frontal lobes, the middle cerebral artery and the posterior communicating artery.

Shortly after the hemorrhage, the patient often will experience symptoms similar to KORSAKOFF'S SYNDROME—disorientation, confabulation and memory problems. Some patients do not develop amnesia until several days or weeks afterward.

subconscious   A term describing mental events such as thoughts, ideas or feelings that normally remain below the threshold of awareness and that a person may be unaware of temporarily, but that can be recalled under the right circumstances. In psychoanalytic theory, the subconscious refers to that part of the mind through which information passes on its way from the unconscious to the conscious mind. (See also FREUD, SIGMUND.)

subliminal learning   A type of learning that takes place below the level of consciousness and involves messages or information that is too fast or too weak for normal awareness. The idea of subliminal learning is related to sleep learning, in which material is presented when the subject is asleep.

The existence of subliminal advertising became publicized during the 1950s, when some outdoor movie theaters reported huge spurts of concession business when messages saying "Eat popcorn" and "Drink Coca-Cola" were flashed very briefly on the screen over a six-week period. Popcorn business reportedly increased 50 percent, and soda sales rose 18 percent.

Some research supports the notion that in a laboratory, subjects can process limited sensory information without conscious awareness if they are paying close attention to the task. But no scientist has succeeded in duplicating the subliminal advertising effect reported during the 1950s; other studies have found no evidence to support the ability of subliminal messages in ads or music to have any significant effect on behavior or learning.

Scientists have concluded that it is unlikely that anyone could learn or remember information if he or she is not aware that it is being presented.

substitution hypothesis A theory about eyewitness memory that explains why people report incorrect facts after an event they have witnessed. The hypothesis holds that false information presented to a witness after an event replaces or transforms the person's original memory, which is then irretrievably lost. This theory, which is supported by eyewitness expert Elizabeth Loftus's research, assumes a destructive updating mechanism in the brain and assumes that the subject would have remembered the correct information if the knowledge hadn't been replaced by false postevent information. (See also AGE AND EYEWITNESS ABILITY, EYEWITNESS TESTIMONY; MEMORY FOR EVENTS.)

substitution mnemonics A type of memory aid that substitutes words rich in images for information to be remembered. For example, to remember that Mt. Fuji is 12,365 feet tall, one might simply think of the mountain as "calendar mountain" and a calendar as 12 months and 365 days. This method also can be used to remember a person's name, by taking the name apart and linking it with a strongly visual image.

suggestibility A state of greatly enhanced receptiveness and responsiveness to suggestions and stimuli. It is characterized by the facility with which the subject can respond to either external stimuli or those from inner experience. But suggestions must be acceptable to the subject, who can just as easily reject them. By accepting and responding to suggestions, the subject can become psychologically deaf, blind, anesthetized or dissociated, and suffer from hallucinations or amnesia, or he can develop various special types of behavior (provided that he doesn't object). (See also HYPNOSIS; POSTHYPNOTIC SUGGESTIONS.)

surgical anesthesia and memory See ANESTHESIA AND MEMORY.

surroundings and memory A person remembers better when placed in the same conditions (a place or a mood) as those in which the learning occurred. In one study, researchers found that a group of subjects who learned a list of words underwater remembered more of the list when they were underwater than when they were on dry land.

In the same way, when a person feels depressed, all the memories that rise to consciousness are colored by this emotion. This is one reason why it is so difficult to "shake off" depression; all a person's associations are negative. (See also STATE-DEPENDENT LEARNING.)

synapse The point at which a nerve impulse passes from the axon of one neuron (nerve cell) to a dendrite of another. To send a signal, one neuron squirts out a chemical messenger (called a neurotransmitter) that crosses the synapsic gap between adjacent dendrites. (See NEUROTRANSMITTERS AND MEMORY.) The receiving dendrite has receptors that recognize the chemical transmitter and speeds the signal through the neuron. Many neurons have as many as 60,000 synapses.

Scientists have long believed that changes in the brain's synapses are the critical events in information storage. But researchers do not agree about how synaptic change actually represents information. One of the most widely held ideas is that the specificity of stored information is determined by the location of synaptic changes in the nervous system and by the pattern of altered neuronal interaction that these changes produce.

synaptic change and memory The theory that memory occurs as a result of functional changes in the brain's SYNAPSES caused by the effects of external stimuli prompted by training or education. Nerve cells (NEURONS) connect with other cells at junctions called synapses; they transmit electrical signals to each other by firing across this junction, which triggers the release of neurotransmitters (special signaling substances) that diffuse across the spaces between cells, attaching themselves to receptors on the neighboring nerve cell. The human brain contains about 10 billion of these nerve cells, joined together by about 60 trillion synapses.

Researchers generally have agreed that anything that influences behavior leaves a trace (ENGRAM) somewhere in the nervous system. As long as these memory traces last, theoretically they can be restimulated, and the event or experience that established them will be remembered. (See NEURO-TRANSMITTERS AND MEMORY.)

synesthesia   A sensation in one sensory modality that occurs when another is stimulated. For example, a person experiencing synesthesia would see a visual image such as colors whenever someone else speaks. While many people feel a relationship between certain sounds and light, one subject (called "S" by Russian neuroscientist Aleksandr Luria) had an incredible case of lifelong synesthesia that began at age two or three. For example, when hearing one tone, S reported that he saw a brown strip against a dark background that had red, tonguelike edges and a sense of taste similar to sweet-and-sour borscht gripped his entire tongue. Although S's descriptions were often poetic (he told one pyschologist he had a crumbly yellow voice), he was not speaking metaphorically—he actually saw yellow and felt a crumbly sensation when he heard the psychologist speak.

S's synesthesia provided not an enriched existence but a tortured one, alienating him from experience and providing a hallucinatory substitute for reality. S would get so interested in the sound, sight and taste of a person's words, for example, that he would completely lose the thread of what the person was saying. His experiences separated him from the world, and without interpretive memory, his dissociations grew bizarre. (See LURIA, ALEKSANDR R.)

syphilis   A sexually transmitted (or congenital) disease that can have devastating effects on the brain, including dementia. Syphilis of the brain, called neurosyphilis, also can cause paralysis (once called "general paralysis of the insane") in addition to dementia.

Cause
Neurosyphilis is caused by the spirochete (a type of bacterium) called *Treponema pallidum*. Usually transmitted by sexual contact, the organism enters the body via minor cuts or abrasions in the skin or mucous membranes. It also can be transmitted by infected blood or from a mother to her unborn child during pregnancy.

Neurosyphilis usually occurs 10 to 20 years after the initial infection; it is considered the tertiary (end) stage of the disease. Rarely seen today, it is encountered in elderly demented patients who were never treated properly for syphilis in their youth.

Symptoms
Symptoms include subtle changes in personality, lack of attention, poor judgment, aggression, bizarre behavior, mood swings and problems in concentration. Some patients experience delusions of grandeur, but about 50 percent have a simple dementia.

Diagnosis
Tertiary syphilis can be diagnosed with tests such as the Venereal Disease Research Laboratory test or the fluorescent treponemal antibody absorption test; it may be necessary to perform these tests on a sample of cerebrospinal fluid.

Treatment
The disease is not nearly as deadly as it once was, due to the introduction of penicillin; however, treatment of tertiary-stage syphilis takes longer. More than half of those treated suffer a severe reaction within six to 12 hours because the body reacts to the sudden annihilation of large numbers of spirochetes. Brain damage already caused by the disease cannot be reversed.

Prevention
Infection can be avoided by maintaining monogamous relationships; condoms offer some measure of protection, but do not offer absolute protection. People infected with syphilis are infectious during the primary and secondary stages, but not during the tertiary stage.

tacrine (Cognex)   The first drug approved by the U.S. Food and Drug Administration to treat some of the symptoms of ALZHEIMER'S DISEASE. The drug, which is administered four times a day, works by helping to slow the breakdown of ACETYLCHOLINE, a chemical necessary for brain-cell communication that is severely depleted in Alzheimer's disease.

However, the effects of the drug are far from dramatic, and there are unfortunate side effects. Cognex builds up an enzyme that can lead to liver damage. Generally, about half of patients who begin taking it withdraw, mostly because of side effects. In those who continue, slight improvement occurs in fewer than half of patients with mild to moderate stages of the disease. Patients taking very high dosages of the drug (160 mg per day) show the most improvement, but they also have the highest risk for liver damage. Discontinuing the drug reverses liver problems.

Liver function should be monitored regularly in individuals on tacrine. If any abnormality in liver function occurs, doctors must adjust the dosage accordingly or discontinue administration of this drug. Other frequent side effects include nausea, vomiting, diarrhea, abdominal pain, indigestion and skin rash.

tau protein   The major protein that makes up neurofibrillary tangles found in degenerating brain cells, especially in ALZHEIMER'S DISEASE. Tau is normally involved in maintaining the internal structure of the nerve cell, but in Alzheimer's disease the tau proteins begin to twist and tangle.

In the late 1980s scientists discovered that in healthy brain cells, the internal structure (called a microtubule) is formed like a parallel set of train tracks with crosspieces holding them together, which carry nutrients from the body of the cell to the ends of the axons. The crosspieces between the parallel microtubules are made of tau protein.

In cells of patients with Alzheimer's, this parallel structure collapses as the tau protein crosspieces twist into paired helical filaments. If tau doesn't function properly, the microtubules collapse and tangle together, and can no longer shuttle substances throughout the cell.

Scientists know that the development of Alzheimer's involves two normally harmless proteins in the brain, tau and BETA-AMYLOID. Alzheimer's disease develops when something triggers beta-amyloid to fold and twist into a different shape. As it changes, beta-amyloid begins forming abnormal strands that accumulate on brain cells. It also appears to induce tau protein to become a killer as well. Together, the two destroy the brain cells, forming the plaques and tangles that have been the hallmarks of the disease since it was first described in 1907 by Alois Alzheimer.

Scientists disagree about whether it's the sticky plaques of beta-amyloid in the brain or the tangles of tau protein inside brain nerve fibers that play a more central role in the destruction of brain cells. While tangles of tau have been found in the brain of people with Alzheimer's, many scientists believed that tangles were probably a secondary part of the disease. Instead, most Alzheimer's researchers have focused attention on amyloid as the substance that kills brain cells. Others think the plaques and tangles are really a marker left by nerve cells killed by some other cause.

What is known is that increases of beta-amyloid in brain tissue are associated with increasing severity of mental decline, with the highest levels of beta-amyloid found in the brains of patients with the greatest degree of dementia. (See also ALZHEIMER, ALOIS; DEMENTIA; PRESENILINS.)

temporal lobe   The part of the brain that forms much of the lower side of each half of the cerebrum (main mass of the brain). The temporal lobes are concerned with smell, taste, hearing, visual associations and some aspects of memory. Abnormal electrical activity in a lobe (such as in temporal lobe epilepsy) may cause peculiarities in any of these functions, and some scientists suspect that the phenomenon of DÉJÀ VU represents a disturbance of the temporal lobes.

While stimulating various areas of the cortex produces a range of responses from patients, only stimulation of the temporal lobes elicits meaningful, integrated experiences (including sound, movement and color) that are far more detailed, accurate and specific than normal recall. Canadian surgeon Wilder Penfield stimulated the temporal lobe area of patients during the 1950s, eliciting a range of integrated memories. Interestingly, some of the memories that popped up during stimulation were not remembered in the normal state, and stimulation of the same spot in the temporal lobe elicited the exact same memory again and again.

Research also has suggested that removing the left temporal lobe causes verbal memory deficits and removing the right lobe impairs nonverbal memory (such as remembering mazes, patterns or faces).

Direct and diffuse effects from a HEAD INJURY may cause memory deficits, and there is some evidence that the tips and undersurface of the temporal lobes are particularly vulnerable to trauma; if so, then memory problems after diffuse brain damage may indicate hippocampal damage.

temporal lobectomy   The surgical removal of both TEMPORAL LOBES. This operation is associated with severe AMNESIA when the HIPPOCAMPUS also is removed. Amnesia does not develop following surgery or damage involving the uncus or AMYGDALA as long as the hippocampus is not removed.

Removing one of the temporal lobes results in a material-specific memory deficit. (That is, patients whose left temporal lobe is removed suffer a verbal memory deficit, while those with whose right temporal lobe is removed have more problems in remembering nonverbal material, such as faces, patterns and mazes.) Left temporal lobectomies result in more problems in learning and retaining verbal material (such as paired associates, prose passages or Hebb's recurring digit sequences). In addition, stimulation of the left temporal lobe leads to a number of naming errors and impaired recall.

Patients who have undergone removal of the right temporal lobe can usually perform verbal tasks, but have problems with learning visual or tactile mazes or in figuring out whether they have seen a particular geometric shape before. They also have problems recognizing tonal patterns or faces. But those with right temporal lobectomies are impaired in maze learning and recognition for photographs only if extensive hippocampal lesions existed.

In fact, researchers have found that the more extensive the section of hippocampus removed, the greater the memory deficit. Among those whose left temporal lobe was removed, those with extensive hippocampus involvement had more problems with short-term verbal memory than those with no or little involvement.

temporal lobe epilepsy   A form of epilepsy in which abnormal electrical discharges in the brain are confined to the temporal lobe, which forms much of the lower side of each half of the cerebrum. This type of epilepsy differs from the generalized disturbance found in those with grand mal or petit mal seizures.

Temporal lobe epilepsy is usually caused by damage in one of the temporal lobes due to birth or head injury, brain tumor or abscess, or stroke. Because the temporal lobes are concerned with smell, taste, hearing, visual associations and some aspects of memory, seizures in the temporal lobes can disrupt any of these functions.

Symptoms

People with temporal lobe epilepsy suffer dreamlike states ranging from partial to total loss of awareness; they may have unpleasant hallucinations of smell or taste, or experience DÉJÀ VU.

Patients may perform tasks with no memory of them after the attack, which can last from minutes to hours. In some cases, a temporal lobe seizure progresses to a generalized grand mal seizure.

Treatment

Treatment is the same as in other types of epilepsy. Surgery has been used in some cases to remove the part of the lobe containing the irritating focus for the attacks. Operations are performed only in severe cases that have not responded to medication, because of the danger of affecting other important brain functions.

test of memory and learning (TOMAL)   A comprehensive assessment of memory and learning processes for children ages five years through 19 years 11 months. In the examination, 14 subtests yield information on verbal and nonverbal memory, composite memory and delayed recall. It also can provide information on learning, attention and concentration; sequential memory; free recall and associative recall.

thyroid function and memory   See HYPOTHYROIDISM.

thalamus   The crucial brain structure in the factual memory circuit, the thalamus (named for the Greek word meaning "chamber,") serves as the entrance chamber to the perceptual cortex. All sensory organs (except for smell) enter the cortex via the thalamus.

One of the main parts of the diencephalon, the thalamus is active during memory and is involved in many cases of memory disorder—particularly in WERNICKE-KORSAKOFF SYNDROME patients. One of the best-known cases of thalamic damage and memory problems is NA, a man who was stabbed in the thalamic region at age 22 and suffered significant memory problems.

Other cases of memory problems involving the thalamus have been reported, primarily due to tumors, which can lead to a rapidly developing dementia.

TIA   See TRANSIENT ISCHEMIC ATTACK.

tip-of-the-tongue phenomenon   An acute form of "feeling of knowing," which is a situation where we are unable to recall a piece of information, but we know that we have memorized it. Sometimes a person can recall related facts but not the specific information required. In this phenomenon, searching activates networks in a way we can feel.

The brain contains a tremendous store of information, some of which cannot be retrieved at any given moment. Problems in recovering this information is called a tip-of-the-tongue experience; a person can picture the person in the mind, or remember some part of the name or a name like it, or other related information.

For example, in trying to remember the name *Macduff*, a person might think of Scotland or Shakespeare, because of the Scottish association of the prefix "Mac" and of Macduff, a character in Shakespeare's *Macbeth*.

The brain's internal monitor will continue working on an unconscious level long after the attempt to remember has been abandoned, and the correct name or word will be remembered suddenly about 97 percent of the time, according to research.

The first research into this widespread sensation was published in the 1960s and then duplicated in the 1970s. Scientists studied the phenomenon by reading aloud definitions of unfamiliar words (such as *sampan* or *sextant*). Subjects were asked to tell what the word was or everything they could about the word. Some subjects reported words with a similar meaning or sound, or they remembered the first or last letter of the word. When given the definition of the word *sampan* (a small Chinese boat), they came up with *Siam, sarong* and *Saipan*. They also thought of words that mean nearly the same, such as *junk* or *barge*.

People in their 30s and 40s generally experience this phenomenon somewhat more often than 20-year-olds, and those over 70 have slightly more tip-of-the-tongue experiences than the middle-aged. Proper names are the biggest problem, according to research.

This phenomenon indicates that memory is a matter of degree, that it exists on a continuum—a person may remember a piece of something. Information in long-term memory may not be stored as it is expected to be. The fact that a person tries to remember something by picking up different clues about the word suggests that people remember information in pieces. Although it's possible to remember something only in part, through a series of clues, it's often possible to reach more of what has been stored. Scientists suspect older people often have the tip-of-the-tongue problem because their slower mental processing rate delays retrieval.

In addition, memory is not some sort of automatic photo-snapping process; most memories are not complete representations of information that has been learned, but are a result of the process of reconstruction.

The tip-of-the-tongue phenomenon suggests that memories are not stored in only one way; they may be filed away as an auditory memory (how many syllables a word has or how it is pronounced), in visual terms (first and last letters) or by meaning (and cross-referenced with other words similar in meaning).

To avoid the problem, one might try running through the alphabet to find a "sound trigger" for the word; if that doesn't work, one might stop thinking about it for a while. The memory may well pop into one's mind.

topectomy   A more conservative type of psychosurgery that destroys parts of the frontal cortex itself instead of the white fibers below it, as in LEUCOTOMY. The operation was designed to avoid the problems of hemorrhage, memory loss and vegetative states that often occurred after other more radical types of LOBOTOMY.

The procedure was developed by research scientist J. Lawrence Pool at Columbia University in 1947 and performed on patients at the New Jersey State Hospital in Greystone Park. (See also FREEMAN, WATER; MONIZ, ANTONIO EGAS.)

trace decay   The basis of forgetting, this theory states that anything that influences the behavior of an organism leaves a "trace" (or ENGRAM) in the central nervous system that gradually erodes as time passes, in much the way a meadow bordered by forest eventually will return to forest if it is not used. The basis of this FORGETTING is disuse; a person who has moved to a foreign country and uses

that language exclusively eventually will forget most or all of the native language.

The theory of trace decay is one of the oldest, most popular explanations of forgetting. Theoretically, as long as memory traces last, they can be restimulated and the experience that established them will be remembered.

training and eyewitness ability   While a witness's prior knowledge and expectations can influence perception and memory, researchers found there were no significant differences between the number of true detections of people and actions between police officers and civilians.

Specific face-recognition training is not effective either, according to studies of one such course. In the course, students attended three days of intensive training (lectures, slides and film demonstrations, discussions, and so on). They were taught to break the faces down into components to better discriminate among faces and better remember a face later; the best way to remember a face is to ignore any movement in the facial pattern.

But when these students were tested on their ability to remember photographed faces, results showed that the training course had no effect. When the photographed face was changed in either pose or expression, recognition dropped to 60 to 70 percent, and when the faces were disguised, performance was poor—about 30 percent. (Students who simply guessed should have been right 50 percent of the time.) Recognition training did not produce any improvement whatsoever in ability to match different versions of the same face. But surprisingly, the course did not improve either matching ability or memory ability either.

Researchers believed this particular course wrongly emphasized the importance of selecting individual facial features rather than considering the face as a whole as a way to remember it. Some evidence suggests that, in remembering a face, the basic facial framework and arrangement is even more important than individual physical features.

Many investigators have found that people are better at paying attention to the face as a whole rather than paying attention to a specific feature of a face. (See also AGE AND EYEWITNESS ABILITY; CROSS-RACIAL WITNESS IDENTIFICATION; EYEWITNESS TESTI-

MONY; GENDER AND WITNESS ABILITY; MEMORY FOR EVENTS; MEMORY FOR FACES.)

transient global amnesia   An abrupt loss of memory lasting from a few seconds to a few hours without loss of consciousness or other impairment that was first described in 1964.

During the period of amnesia, the subject cannot store new experiences and suffers a permanent memory gap. At the same time, the subject may also lose memory of many years prior to the amnesia attack; this retrograde memory loss gradually disappears, although a permanent gap in memory that usually extends backward no more than an hour before onset of the amnesia attack results.

Attacks of transient global amnesia may occur more than once and are believed to be caused by a temporary reduction in blood supply in areas of the brain concerned with memory, sometimes heralding a stoke, although several toxic substances have been associated with transient global amnesia.

Victims are usually healthy and over age 50; an attack may be precipitated by many things, including sudden changes in temperature, physical stress, eating a large meal and even sexual intercourse. This type of amnesia is not common, and it disappears within a day or two. It was first described in 1964. (See also RETROGRADE AMNESIA.)

transient ischemic attack (TIA)   A "little stroke" caused by a temporary insufficient supply of blood to the brain, which can cause brief memory problems. Even a brief interruption of the blood flow to the brain can cause a decrease in brain function. Each episode of a TIA, which is a warning that a person is at risk for a stroke, is brief and recovery afterward is complete. It may recur, however, later that same day or at a later time. Some people have only a single episode, some have recurrent episodes, and some will go on to have a full-blown stroke.

About one-third of the people who have a TIA later do have a stroke, and almost 90 percent of people who have a stroke had TIA episodes first. Approximately one-third of the people with TIA will have recurrent TIAs, and one-third will have only a single episode of TIA. The age of onset varies, but incidence rises dramatically after age 50. TIA is more common among men and African Americans.

Symptoms
Symptoms vary depending on the part of the brain affected, but often include problems with memory, vision, speech, body movements or sensation, and consciousness. If the blood flow is interrupted for longer than a few seconds, brain cells in the area are destroyed, causing permanent damage to that area of the brain or death.

Symptoms that may be confused with TIA but are not usually part of the disorder may include simple changes in consciousness caused by medications or other disorders, fainting, light-headedness or dizziness, vertigo, seizures or transient amnesia.

Cause
The loss of blood flow that triggers a TIA is most often caused by tiny blood clots in the brain. Otherwise, it may be triggered by various blood disorders, spasm of the small arteries in the brain, abnormal blood vessels, inflammation of the arteries, systemic lupus erythematosus or SYPHILIS.

Risk factors for having a TIA include high blood pressure, heart disease, migraine headaches, smoking, diabetes mellitus or increasing age.

Diagnosis
A detailed and complete history and neurologic exam is vital to the diagnosis. Blood tests, brain scans and cerebral arteriograms may rule out other causes for TIA symptoms.

Treatment
The goal of treating a TIA is to improve the blood supply to the brain so as to prevent a stroke. A person who has had a TIA within the previous 48 hours is usually admitted to a hospital to evaluate the specific cause of the TIA and to treat any underlying disease.

Blood thinners may be used to reduce clotting; aspirin is the most common medication; others include dipyridamole, heparin or Coumadin. A low-salt diet may help control high blood pressure; other diet changes also may be recommended. Cleaning out clogged carotid arteries in the neck may be appropriate for some people, particularly those whose carotid arteries are more than 70 percent closed.

transient memory disorders   A group of temporary memory disorders in which a person's memory stops functioning normally for a certain period of time. Causes include vascular disorders, closed HEAD INJURY, medications, or aftereffects of electroconvulsive therapy (ECT). Psychogenic disorders also may be of a transient nature. (See also ELECTROCONVULSIVE THERAPY AND MEMORY.)

Transient Global Amnesia   A form of sudden-onset ANTEROGRADE AMNESIA, coupled with RETROGRADE AMNESIA for recent events, disorientation in time and no loss of personal identity. Attacks may last from minutes to days and can be set off by many things, including temperature change, toxins, physical stress or even sexual intercourse. The underlying dysfunction is believed to be a temporary drop in blood supply to the memory centers of the brain.

Posttraumatic Amnesia   Most victims of closed head injury suffer only a temporary memory loss from between a few seconds to several months. It is believed that the injury interferes somehow with the transfer of information from short- to long-term memory.

ECT and Memory Loss   Many patients who undergo ECT report a temporary anterograde or retrograde amnesia that gradually fades away.

translogic   a phenomenon experienced during HYPNOSIS in which the subject shows a decrease in critical judgment. For example, during age regression to childhood, a person exhibits translogic when she takes down a complicated dictation in childish scrawl but spells all the words perfectly,

beyond the capability of any child. An adult who is consciously trying to mimic a child would not copy a complicated paragraph without remembering to insert some spelling errors. (See also AGE REGRESSION, HYPNOTIC.)

transorbital lobotomy   See LOBOTOMY.

traumatic amnesia   The inability to store new memories between an hour and a few weeks following a blow to the head. This posttraumatic confusional state also can induce a RETROGRADE AMNESIA that may extend backward for a few hours to many years; the duration of this amnesia depends on the severity of injury and the subject's age.

As the person recovers, memories often return in chronological order (as in RIBOT'S LAW), but sometimes memories return in no particular fashion and gradually become interrelated again in the brain. At times, there may be a permanent memory loss for a period of time during the injury and immediately preceding it; some researchers believe this permanent memory loss is an indication that the head injury was severe.

About 10 percent of patients admitted to a hospital following severe closed head injury suffer severe memory problems.

traumatic automatism   A dazed response following a mild head injury without loss of consciousness and no apparent change in ordinary behavior; however, the person is going through the motions of everyday life automatically and may have no memory whatever of his or her actions after the injury. (See also TRANSIENT GLOBAL AMNESIA.)

U

unclassified dementias Diseases producing dementia that are indistinguishable from ALZHEIMER'S DISEASE or PICK'S DISEASE in life; upon autopsy, no specific disease can be identified from the inspection of brain tissue. In some of these cases, depression may be the cause of the dementia; others are probably extremely rare diseases or unusual variants of more common diseases.

unconscious transference A phenomenon in which a person seen in one situation is confused with or recalled as a person seen in a second situation. For example, in one case a railroad ticket agent misidentified a sailor in a lineup as a robber. When it was later determined that the sailor had a solid alibi and could not have been the robber, the agent explained that the sailor had looked familiar. In fact, the sailor lived near the station and had purchased tickets from this agent three times before the robbery. The agent experienced unconscious transference; he mistakenly linked the familiarity of the sailor to the robbery instead of the times he sold the man tickets.

Unconscious transference is a result of the malleable nature of the human memory; a brief exposure to another person can make that person seem familiar when seen later. Unfortunately, in any given criminal case, it is almost impossible to tell whether unconscious transference has taken place. (See also AGE AND EYEWITNESS ABILITY; CROSS-RACIAL WITNESS IDENTIFICATION; EYEWITNESS TESTIMONY; GENDER AND EYEWITNESS ABILITY; MEMORY FOR EVENTS.)

unitary theory The idea that short-term, long-term and any other type of memory are all part of one system.

use-it-or-lose-it hypothesis The idea that patients can minimize losses to body and mind through vigorous mental and physical exercise. At the University of California at Berkeley, scientists discovered that rats housed in stimulating cages with plenty of interesting toys have larger nerve cells in the cerebral cortex (the thinking part of the brain) and more dendrites, or projections, from these cells. Further, researchers discovered that neuron size can be enlarged by living in a stimulating environment at any age.

Similar findings came from research at the University of California at Los Angeles, where autopsies of 20 men and women aged 18 to 79 found that those with more education and a busier social and intellectual life had longer dendrites in part of the brain than people with less stimulation. And people with more education who remain mentally active seem to have fewer cognitive declines as they get older.

vacant slot hypothesis   A theory about eyewitness memory that explains why people report incorrect facts after witnessing an event. The hypothesis holds that the original information was never stored, so that false information presented after the event was simply popped into a "vacant slot" in the memory representation.

However, many leading experts in the field, including witness expert Elizabeth Loftus, reject this hypothesis on the grounds that 90 percent of subjects who are tested immediately after witnessing an event and aren't exposed to postevent information are correct. (See also AGE AND EYEWITNESS ABILITY; CROSS-RACIAL WITNESS IDENTIFICATION; EYEWITNESS TESTIMONY; GENDER AND EYEWITNESS ABILITY; MEMORY FOR EVENTS.)

vanishing cue technique   A variant of the DIRECT PRIMING procedure, this learning method gives a patient a definition with a cued instruction; each subsequent time, the instruction is presented with one less letter than needed for the last successful recall.

variant Creutzfeldt-Jakob disease   See MAD COW DISEASE.

vascular dementia   A decrease in intellectual functioning stemming from problems in the circulation of blood to the brain. It encompasses a wide range of diseases, the principal feature of which is loss of intellectual abilities, of which loss of memory (especially short-term memory) is prominent.

Cause
The causes of all cases of vascular dementia are known, in contrast to diseases that are more elusive, such as ALZHEIMER'S DISEASE. Vascular dementia occurs when brain tissue dies from causes such as cerebral hemorrhage (bursting of a blood vessel in the brain), arteries blocked by plaques or blood clots, or poor blood flow to the brain (ischemia).

Risks
The factors associated with all forms of stroke, most importantly high blood pressure, are the most prominent risk factors for vascular dementia.

Treatment
The underlying condition can be treated; for example, medication and lifestyle changes can lower blood pressure, and medication may help dissolve blood clots.

(See also DEMENTIA.)

vasopressin   Another name for ADH (antidiuretic hormone), this chemical functions as a neurotransmitter in the brain and acts as the body's diuretic—and it also may be part of the ink with which memories are written. (See NEUROTRANSMITTERS AND MEMORY.)

Vasopressin is released from the pituitary gland and acts on the kidneys to increase their reabsorption of water into the blood. It reduces the amount of water lost in the urine and helps control the body's overall water balance. Water is continually being taken into the body in food and beverages and also is produced by the chemical reactions in cells. At the same time, water always is being lost in urine, sweat, feces and breath; vasopressin helps maintain the optimum amount of water in the body.

Its production is controlled by the HYPOTHALAMUS (located in the center of the brain), which detects changes in the concentration and volume of the blood. If the blood concentration loses water, the hypothalamus stimulates the pituitary gland to release more vasopressin, and vice versa.

External vasopressin is approved for treatment of diabetes as a way of preventing the frequent urination common in this disease. It is given via the nose or by injection; high intravenous doses cause a narrowing of blood vessels. Vasopressin also has been used to treat memory deficits of aging, senile DEMENTIA, ALZHEIMER'S DISEASE, KORSAKOFF'S SYNDROME and AMNESIA.

Research has shown that when subjects are given vasopressin, they remember long lists of words better and seem to chunk and encode better. (Chunking, or grouping, words together is a trick that memory experts teach to improve memory.) Vasopressin also is being studied as a possible memory enhancement drug.

Because cocaine, LSD, amphetamines, Ritalin (methylphenidate) and Cylert (pemoline) cause the pituitary to step up the release of natural vasopressin, abuse of these drugs can result in a depleted pool of vasopressin and a resulting mental slowness. On the other hand, alcohol and marijuana cause mental slowness by suppressing the *release* of vasopressin.

Vasopressin is available on doctor's prescription in the United States. It is available in a nasal spray bottle, and produces noticeable effect within seconds because it is absorbed by the nasal mucosa. However, it can produce a range of side effects, from congestion to headache and increased bowel movements, abdominal cramps, nausea, drowsiness and confusion. It has not been proved safe during pregnancy. Because it temporarily constricts small blood vessels, it should not be used by anyone with hypertension, angina or atherosclerosis, and should be used cautiously by epileptics. (See also ENCODING; MEMORY ENHANCEMENT.)

verbal elaboration   Comments, analysis, judgments and so on that act to enhance the recording of a memory trace, or ENGRAM. Verbal elaboration gets a person involved emotionally and intellectually, ensuring a vibrant memory trace. (See also TRACE DECAY.)

verbal memory   Also known as semantic memory, this type of memory refers to the permanent store of general world knowledge. Verbal memory can be divided into two systems, active or short-term memory and long-term memory. Active memory is a transient form of remembering that includes all of the impulses that pass through the mind during the day. Long-term memory is responsible for retaining material for years—or a lifetime. This type of memory makes learning possible. Some of the best-known strategies for boosting verbal memory include ALPHABETICAL SEARCHING and FIRST-LETTER CUEING. These strategies often are helpful in coming up with something in the wake of the TIP-OF-THE-TONGUE PHENOMENON, when something to be recalled is partially remembered. The provision of the first letter for a word not remembered may prompt memory of the entire word; thus first-letter cueing is a valuable retrieval strategy. First-letter cueing is easy to apply, since the alphabet is usually well known, and it can be written down if necessary.

Examples of first-letter cueing include remembering the notes on the stave lines by recalling "Every Good Boy Does Fine."

verbal process   One of two ways that information can be recorded, using words, numbers or names; it is opposed to the imagery process, which records information in a visual form of pictures, scenes or faces.

It's possible to see in the mind's eye a mental picture (or visual image) of a bed, or one can think of the word *bed*. Thinking of the word is an example of the verbal process.

The verbal process is best suited to represent abstract verbal information such as the word *nourishment*, whereas the visual process works better in representing a concrete form of nourishment, such as *banana*. (See also IMAGERY PROCESS AND MEMORY; VERBAL MEMORY.)

vincamine   An extract of periwinkle, this drug is a vasodilator (widens blood vessels) and increases blood flow and oxygen use in the brain. It has been used with some benefit for the treatment of memory defects.

In some studies, vincamine has been shown to cause some memory improvement in ALZHEIMER'S DISEASE patients, and it normalizes the brain wave patterns in elderly people with memory problems or with alcohol-induced ORGANIC BRAIN SYNDROME.

Vincamine also has been used to treat a variety of problems related to poor blood flow to the brain, including Ménière's syndrome, vertigo, sleep problems, mood changes, depression, hearing problems, high blood pressure and others.

However, there has been very little research on the drug and cognitive enhancement in normal subjects. (See also VINPOCETINE.)

vinpocetine   This derivative of VINCAMINE, a periwinkle extract, improves brain metabolism by improving blood flow and enhancing the use of GLUCOSE and oxygen. It is used to treat memory problems and other cerebral circulation disorders, such as STROKE, APHASIA, APRAXIA, headache and others.

Vinpocetine is used in more than 35 countries around the world to help improve the clinical outcome of stroke patients. Research suggests it may be helpful in part because of its ability to dilate brain arteries, enhancing brain blood flow in patients with cerebrovascular disease and boosting oxygen to the brain.

In a 1987 study published in the *Journal of the American Geriatric Society,* Italian researchers reported that vinpocetine was effective in treating vascular dementia in about half the patients in the study, scoring consistently better than placebo patients in all evaluations of the effectiveness of treatment.

violence and memory   According to experts, experiencing or watching violence can be so stressful that it negatively influences the ability of an eyewitness to recall the events accurately. Research has indicated that EYEWITNESS TESTIMONY about an emotionally volatile event may be more likely to be incorrect than such testimony about a less emotional incident.

In one study, subjects were shown a video of two police officers finding a criminal with the help of a third person. In the nonviolent version, there is a verbal exchange between the three people and a weak restraining movement by one police officer. In the violent version, one of the police officers physically assaults the third person. Both men and women who saw the violent version were significantly less able to recall events accurately. (See also AGE AND EYEWITNESS ABILITY; CROSS-RACIAL WITNESS IDENTIFICATION; EVENT FACTORS; GENDER AND EYEWITNESS ABILITY; MEMORY FOR EVENTS.)

visual alphabet   A way of representing letters of the alphabet by images formed in various ways, such as a picture of an object whose shape resembles letters of the alphabet. Visual alphabets are very common in memory treatises, and have come down to us from a very ancient tradition.

visual association   A memory strategy used to help make image associations in order to improve recall for many different types of information. By associating images with many contexts, it is possible to improve recall.

Visual imagery by itself is not that effective. Visual associations are most effective if they interact and if they are vivid.

To be really memorable, the two associated images must be imagined as interacting in some way with each other rather than simply sitting near each other. For example, to associate the words *horse* and *mop*, it would be better to imagine the horse mopping a floor instead of simply standing beside the mop. Researchers suggest that this interaction boosts memory because the separate interacting images are combined into one single unit; therefore, each part of the image is a cue for remembering the entire unit. However, studies show that this interactive imagery isn't much better than separate images for word pairs that are already meaningfully related, probably because they are already remembered as a unit.

In order to best remember, the images should be as clear and vivid as possible, as much like a real picture as possible. To visualize the horse with the mop, a person should try not just to think about the image, but to truly *see* the horse mopping in as detailed a picture as possible. (See also ASSOCIATION.)

visual imagery method   A type of memory technique that is basically "remembering by pictures"—either mental images or actual drawings. Visual imagery techniques include the method of loci, the VISUAL-PEG SYSTEM and the FACE-NAME ASSOCIATION METHOD.

There are a range of methods; sometimes words or sentences are read and patients are asked to make a mental image. For paired associates, a picture linking the two words is drawn for the subjects or they imagine the objects depicted by two words interacting in some way. Other procedures link the first word with the second word, the second and third with the fourth, and so on.

The visual-peg system is one popular type of visual imagery procedure that has been used since ancient times. In this system, the numbers one through ten are associated with words. (One of the best-known lists is one-bun, two-shoe). The items to be remembered are then placed on the pegs.

The face-name association method was designed specifically for learning names. In this procedure, when a subject wants to remember a name, he or she first chooses a distinctive feature of the person's face. Then the name is transformed into one or two common nouns—"Tunney" would be "ton" "knee." Finally, the distinctive features are linked with the transformed name. If the distinctive feature of Mr. Tunney is his mouth, the subject would picture Mr. Tunney with his knee shoving a ton weight into his mouth.

Research has indicated that amnesic patients can learn some paired associations more easily than others; the pairs should be based on a logical association (that is, if they rhyme or are phonetically similar). Face-name learning is one such paired associate task. In research with Korsakoff patients, subjects who were taught the face-name method were able to learn names.

A simpler type of visual imagery is simply to turn the name to be remembered into a picture, which is then drawn on a card. For example, Bill Smith could be drawn as a blacksmith with a long, rounded nose like a duck's bill. This type of system does not require mental imagery, and a person doesn't need to have any distinctive features.

Research suggests that a patient with memory problems with bilateral brain damage may be successful in using the visual imagery technique; severe damage, however, appears to interfere with successful use of visual imagery.

Research also suggests that imagery is probably of limited value in a patient's day-to-day life; it works best when patients are taught just the names of those who are regularly contacted.

The method of loci visual imagery method uses different locations to remember items. Used by the ancient Greeks and made famous by SIMONIDES OF CEOS and by ALEXSANDR R. LURIA's famous mnemonist, "S," the method is used by normal and brain-damaged patients alike.

The mental retracing of events involves retracing of a sequence of past events or actions in order to jog the memory of something that happened or to remember when someone last had something that is now lost. (See also LOCI, METHOD OF; VISUALIZATION.)

visualization   By picturing an image in one's mind, remembering it becomes easier. The more vivid, striking, silly or funny the image, the better. If a man always leaves his car keys on the counter, he might imagine the keys hopping off the counter and running after him as he heads toward the car. (See also FACE-NAME ASSOCIATION METHOD; IMAGERY PROCESS AND MEMORY; LOCI, METHOD OF; SIMONIDES OF CEOS; VISUAL IMAGERY METHOD; VISUAL-PEG SYSTEM.)

visual memory   A phenomenally vivid type of memory for images that capture a person's attention. Most people almost never forget a face (although they may well forget the name attached to that face), even if they saw the person only once, 10 years before.

Most people (about 60 percent) are predominantly visual when it comes to memorizing: They can easily visualize places, objects, faces, the pages of a book. The other 40 percent have stronger verbal memories. (They remember sounds or words, and the associations that come to their mind are often puns or rhymes.)

visual method   A type of memory learning technique used by those with memory deficits. Visual methods include ALPHABETICAL SEARCHING; ELABO-RATION; FIRST-LETTER CUEING; LOCI, METHOD OF; PQRST METHOD; VERBAL MEMORY. (See also VISUAL IMAGERY METHOD.)

visual-peg system   One popular type of VISUAL IMAGERY METHOD that has been used since ancient times. In this system, the numbers one through ten are associated with words. (One of the best-known lists is one-bun, two-shoe.) The items to be remembered are then placed on the pegs; for example, if the first thing a subject has to remember to do is mail a letter, the image could be a mailman sitting on top of a bun. If the second thing is to file some papers, the subject could imagine filing a shoe under "S" in a big filing cabinet. The visual-peg method may not work for patients with memory problems caused by brain damage on one side, as it requires remembering in two distinct stages, one involving the left hemisphere and the other, the right. (See also FACE-NAME ASSOCIATION; LOCI, METHOD OF; SIMONIDES OF CEOS.)

visual process   See IMAGERY PROCESS AND MEMORY.

vitamins and memory   Taking vitamin C and E supplements may help protect memory as you age by mopping up brain-damaging free radical particles, according to research by Hawaiian scientists. And the B vitamins are also crucial in maintaining healthy brain function.

Antioxidants
Scientists suspect that antioxidant vitamins (C and E) can ease stress in the brain cells that occurs when highly volatile forms of oxygen (free radicals) damage cell structure during normal chemical reactions that occur throughout the body.

In one recent study, vitamins C and E, which are antioxidants, were found to protect men from dementia and actually help them perform better on tests of memory, creativity and mental sharpness. While the vitamins did seem to protect the men from developing two types of dementia, the supplements didn't seem to prevent dementia related to ALZHEIMER'S DISEASE. Moreover, men who took

both vitamins for many years showed a much better improvement, which suggested that long-term use is needed to boost cognitive function later in life.

Previous research has shown that vitamin E can help prevent cardiovascular disease, increase immune response and possibly help protect against some cancers, though not all studies showed these positive effects. Because vitamin E is an antioxidant, it may aid in the breakdown of free radicals that may be damaging brain cells in individuals with Alzheimer's disease.

Columbia University researchers found that patients in the moderate stages of Alzheimer's who took either vitamin E or selegiline for two years were able to fight off more advanced stages of the disease for a longer period than those who took a placebo. The research, which appeared in the April 24, 1997, *New England Journal of Medicine,* involved 341 individuals who took selegiline (10 mg per day), vitamin E (2,000 IU per day), both, or a placebo and were followed until death, institutionalization, inability to do certain basic activities of daily living or severe dementia. Participants who took vitamin E or selegiline took significantly longer to reach one of these points than did the placebo group, although they didn't demonstrate an improvement in symptoms. Using both drugs together didn't add any benefits. It is not clear if the drugs affected the disease process or the overall health of the participants.

However, experts don't recommend vitamin E specifically for the treatment of Alzheimer's disease because there is no direct evidence that it can treat the condition. However, because previous research has demonstrated that vitamin E has other health benefits, there appears to be no reason not to take it in moderation.

B Vitamins
For some time, nutritionists have known that severe deficiencies in the B vitamins can harm cognitive ability, including memory. While many cases of memory problems are not solved by simply taking a vitamin pill, it is true that nutrition can influence the health of the brain. In particular, if the level of B vitamins dips, performance on memory tests may falter. B vitamins are found in kidney

beans, chickpeas, lentils, green leafy vegetables, grain-based food and orange juice. B$_6$ also may be found in beef, poultry and seafood.

B$_{12}$

While B$_{12}$ is widely found in foods, up to 20 percent of people over age 60—and up to 40 percent of those over age 80—can't absorb it. For this reason, older people should eat cereals fortified with B$_{12}$ or take a multivitamin supplement because this way the vitamin can be absorbed by the body.

Vitamin B$_{12}$ problems also tend to appear among vegetarians who don't eat meat, eggs, fish or dairy products, and therefore don't consume any vitamin B$_{12}$. Some diseases (such as Crohn's disease) or surgical removal of part of the intestine also can reduce the amount of B$_{12}$ absorbed into the blood.

In other research on rats, scientists at the University of North Carolina at Chapel Hill discovered that the lack of the B vitamin CHOLINE in mothers may have a permanent effect on the development of learning and memory centers in the fetal brain.

vitamin B$_3$ See NIACIN.

vocalizers People who remember things better in words than in images. Words (especially a statement or proposition) may be more efficient for abstract material, but a combination of words and images is considered to be the most effective memory system of all.

Wechsler Adult Intelligence Scale (WAIS) The best-known and commonest test used to assess general intellectual ability in adults (and also the cognitive ability of brain-damaged patients). The WAIS consists of 11 subtests, including two verbal and performance scale subtests that assess several distinct cognitive functions. The verbal scale contains tests of common knowledge, vocabulary, comprehension of common situations, arithmetic, short-term memory and abstract-thinking ability. The performance scale contains more timed tests, and high scores here depend less on previously established knowledge and problem-solving strategies.

Wechsler Memory Scale (WMS) A widely used pencil-and-paper test of memory functions designed to be used together with the Wechsler Adult Intelligence Scale (WAIS). It includes a group of six subtests used to test memory in brain-damaged patients and evaluates general knowledge, personal orientation, mental control, short-term memory, copying drawings from memory, story recall and paired associate learning. In the test, the ability to remember names is tested by showing a photo of a person and asking patients to remember the name; retention is tested 20 to 25 minutes later. Patients also are asked to remember a hidden belonging by hiding the possession and then asking for its location.

To test ability to remember an appointment, an alarm clock is set to ring 20 minutes later, and patients have to ask a specific question when the bell rings. To test picture recognition, patients are shown 10 line drawings of common objects; five minutes later patients must pick out target pictures from the sequence of 20 pictures. To test face recognition, patients view five faces; five minutes later they pick out targets from a sequence of 10 faces. To test ability to remember a route and deliver a message, the tester traces a route around a room and leaves a message at a particular point; patient's try to repeat the route.

Devised by David Wechsler in 1945, the WMS rapidly gained acceptance and is still the most widely used clinical memory test. Its value as an assessment procedure has been questioned for several reasons, however. Critics question its value as a test for organic amnesia, since it contains subtests of abilities that are not likely to be disrupted in amnesia and because it examines recall but not recognition.

The value of the WMS for measuring memory function is lessened to some extent by the fact that the test measures cognitive functions rather broadly; a low score on the test can indicate dementia rather than specific memory problems. Amnesia is diagnosed when the intelligence score exceeds the memory score. Despite its disadvantages, the WMS still is used because it has value as a quick screening procedure. (See also ASSESSMENT OF MEMORY DISORDERS.)

Wernicke, Carl (1848–1905) A 19th-century German neurologist who related nerve diseases to specific areas of the brain and also investigated the localization of memory. Wernicke is best known for his descriptions of the aphasias (disorders interfering with the ability to communicate in speech or writing).

Wernicke studied at the University of Breslau before entering practice in Berlin. He joined the faculty at Breslau, where he remained until the year before his death. He tried to relate the various aphasias to impaired psychic processes in different parts of the brain and included the first accurate description of a sensory aphasia in the temporal lobe. Wernicke showed that auditory word images appear to be located in a memory bank separate from that containing the images of the articulated words. He also noted a second language center farther back in the brain known today as Wernicke's area, which contains the records of individual words.

Wernicke went on to elaborate on different clinical syndromes in terms of damage to either Wernicke's area or the area of the brain discovered by Paul Broca.

In his *Textbook of Brain Disorders (Lehrbuch der Gehirnkrankheiten;* 1891), Wernicke tried to illustrate cerebral localization for all brain disease. Among the disorders he described was Wernicke's encephalopathy, which is caused by a thiamine deficiency. (See also WERNICKE-KORSAKOFF SYNDROME; WERNICKE'S [RECEPTIVE] APHASIA.)

Wernicke-Korsakoff syndrome   This acute neurological condition is an uncommon brain disorder almost always due to the malnutrition that occurs in chronic alcohol dependence, although it also can occur in other conditions, such as cancer with malnutrition. Typically, Wernicke-Korsakoff syndrome gradually affects people between 40 and 80 years old. The syndrome is actually two disorders that may occur independently or together. Wernicke's disease (or Wernicke's encephalopathy) damages multiple nerves throughout the body. It may also include symptoms caused by alcohol withdrawal. The cause is generally attributed to malnutrition, especially lack of vitamin B$_1$ (thiamine), which is a common problem of alcoholics. The second disorder, KORSAKOFF'S SYNDROME (also called Korsakoff psychosis), impairs memory and interferes with problem solving or learning, along with multiple symptoms of nerve damage. The most distinguishing symptom is "confabulation," where the person makes up detailed, believable stories about experiences or situations to cover the gaps in the memory. Korsakoff psychosis involves damage to areas of the brain.

Symptoms

In Wernicke encephalopathy, the patient usually develops symptoms suddenly, including abnormal eye movements, problems in coordinating body movements, slowness and confusion. There are also signs of neuropathy, such as loss of sensation, pins and needles or impaired reflexes. The level of consciousness progressively falls, and without treatment, this syndrome may lead to coma and death.

Korsakoff's syndrome may follow if treatment is not instituted soon enough. In this stage, sufferers experience severe amnesia, apathy and disorientation. Recent memories are affected more than distant memory; often patients cannot remember what they did even a few moments before and they may make up stories to cover for their loss of memory.

Causes

The disease is caused by a deficiency of thiamine (vitamin B$_1$), which affects the brain and nervous system. This deficiency is probably caused by poor eating habits or an inherited defect in thiamine metabolism.

Diagnosis

A doctor may examine the nervous/muscular system for evidence of damage to multiple nerve systems, and abnormal reflexes. Personal history may reveal a history of alcohol abuse. Tests of gait and coordination may indicate weak muscles and damage to portions of the brain that control muscle coordination. Eye exams may show eye movement problems. A nutritional assessment may confirm a malnourished state, and a blood test will be done to check B$_1$ levels, pyruvate and alcohol levels. A brain scan rarely shows changes in the tissue of the brain indicating Wernicke-Korsakoff syndrome, however.

Treatment

Wernicke's encephalopathy is a medical emergency requiring large doses of intravenous thiamine if the diagnosis is even suspected. Often such treatment can reverse the symptoms within a few hours. In the absence of treatment, however, the disease will progress to Korsakoff's psychosis and at this stage is usually irreversible. Patients will experience permanent impairment of memory and are in need of constant supervision. Total alcohol abstinence is important to prevent the progressive loss of brain function and nerve damage.

Wernicke's (receptive) aphasia   A type of comprehension problem caused by damage to Wernicke's area in the brain, a particular area in the dominant cerebral hemisphere. Speech is fluent, but "internal speech" is impaired because of the impaired comprehension, and speech content includes many errors in word selection and grammar. Writing also is impaired, and spoken or written commands are not understood. Wernicke's aphasia is associated with difficulty in accessing the meaning of words such as nouns.

Wernicke's encephalopathy   See WERNICKE-KORSAKOFF SYNDROME.

wide-range assessment of memory and learning (WRAML)   A comprehensive assessment of memory and learning for ages five through 17. The three verbal, three visual and three learning subtests can provide information on verbal memory, visual memory and learning. Results from all three subtests combined give an assessment of "general memory."

Williams Scale for Measurement of Memory   See ASSESSMENT OF MEMORY DISORDERS.

Wisconsin card sorting test   One of the most common ways to assess frontal lobe damage. The subject is given a deck of cards marked by a pattern with various symbol shapes, numbers and colors. A card might have three blue stars or one red star or two green triangles.

The tester's comments provide hints as to how the cards should be sorted (such as by placing all the cards with green triangles in one pile). A normal person quickly learns what the proper sorting method is; once the subject has learned to sort by the rule, the rule is changed and the subject must figure out what the new sorting rule is. Patients with frontal lobe damage or KORSAKOFF'S SYNDROME tend to make a perseveration error at this point, continuing to sort the cards by the first rule. They have not lost the ability to understand that the rules have changed, but their understanding does not improve their behavior. They continue to sort by color although each error brings the news that the action was wrong. Their mistake is not one of imagination, reasoning or any other type of intelligence, but is an inflexibility in voluntary motor behavior. It is as if once they have decided to touch their finger, it becomes impossible to touch their nose.

They can recognize the problem because they have suffered no damage to their perceptual cortex, but purposeful action is controlled in the brain's frontal areas. When that region is damaged, they may not be able to adapt their actions no matter how normal their perceptions are. A normal interpretive memory depends on a loop that brings the separate regions of the brain into harmony. (See also ASSESSMENT OF MEMORY DISORDERS.)

witness perception   See EYEWITNESS TESTIMONY.

working memory   A borderline area between short-term and long-term memory where, some theorists believe, material needed only for a brief period is stored. It is sometimes confused as a synonym for SHORT-TERM MEMORY.

xanthinol nicotinate   A form of NIACIN that passes into cells much more easily where it increases the rate of glucose metabolism and improves blood flow to the brain.

In recent studies, it was found to improve the performance of healthy elderly subjects on a variety of short- and long-term memory tasks. Like niacin, however, excess doses can cause flushing and a variety of other mild symptoms.

Z

zatosetron A drug that increases the release of ACETYLCHOLINE, a neurotransmitter linked to improved learning and memory and deficient in many types of memory impairment. By selectivity blocking serotonin (a brain substance that inhibits the release of acetylcholine), zatosetron increases acetylcholine release and enhances memory and performance, according to some research. Initial research suggests that zatosetron, like its cousin ONDANSETRON, may improve memory in some healthy older adults with AGE ASSOCIATED MEMORY IMPAIRMENT.

Scientists at the Memory Assessment Clinics in Bethesda, Maryland, and Scottsdale, Arizona, are testing zatosetron in preliminary double-blind studies of 200 subjects over age 50 with age associated memory impairment.

APPENDIXES

APPENDIX I
ASSOCIATIONS DEALING WITH MEMORY PROBLEMS

ALCOHOLISM

Al-Anon and Ala-Teen
Al-Anon Family Group Headquarters, Inc.
1600 Corporate Landing Parkway
Virginia Beach, VA 23454-5617
http://www.al-anon.alateen.org/
(888) 4AL-ANON

Support groups for the family and friends of alcoholics.

Alcoholics Anonymous
A.A. World Services, Inc.
P.O. Box 459
New York, NY 10163
http://www.alcoholics-anonymous.org
(212) 870-3400.

Information and links to support groups.

AMYOTROPHIC LATERAL SCLEROSIS

The ALS Association National Office
27001 Agoura Road, Suite 150
Calabasas Hills, CA 91301-5104
http://www.alsa.org
Information and Referral Service: (800) 782-4747
All others: (818) 880-9007

ALZHEIMER'S DISEASE

ADEAR/Alzheimer's Disease Education & Referral Center
NIH
P.O. Box 8250
Silver Spring, MD 20907-8250
http://www.alzheimers.org/
e-mail: adear@alzheimers.org
(800) 438-4380; (301) 495-3311
(301) 495-3334

Information about Alzheimer's disease and related disorders.

The ADEAR Center is a service of the National Institute on Aging.

The NIA is one of the National Institutes of Health under the U.S. Department of Health and Human Services.

Alzheimer's Association
919 N. Michigan Avenue
Suite 1100
Chicago, IL 60611-1676
http://www.alz.org
e-mail: info@alz.org
(312) 335-8700; (800) 272-3900
Fax: (312) 335-1110

Offers information on publications available from the association, refers callers to local chapters and support groups.

APHASIA

National Aphasia Association
156 Fifth Avenue, Suite 707
New York, NY 10010
http://www.aphasia.org/
(800) 922-4622

Education, research, rehabilitation and support services to assist people with aphasia and their families.

CAREGIVERS

Family Caregiver Alliance
690 Market Street
Suite 600
San Francisco, CA 94104
http://www.caregiver.org
e-mail: info@caregiver.org
(415) 434-3388; (800) 445-8106 (CA)
Fax: (415) 434-3508

Family Caregiver Alliance supports and assists caregivers of brain-impaired adults through education, research, services and advocacy.

CHRONIC FATIGUE AND IMMUNE DYSFUNCTION

The CFIDS Association of America
P.O. Box 220398
Charlotte, NC 28222-0398
http://www.cfids.org/
Info Line: (800) 442-3437
Resource Line: (704) 365-2343
Fax: (704) 365-9755
e-mail: info@cfids.org

Advocacy, information, research and encouragement for the Chronic Fatigue and Immune Dysfunction Syndrome community.

CREUTZFELDT-JAKOB DISEASE

Creutzfeldt-Jakob Disease Foundation
P.O. Box 611625
Miami, FL 33261-1626
http://www.cjdfoundation.org
e-mail: crjakob@aol.com.
Fax: (954) 436-7591

HUNTINGTON'S DISEASE

Huntington's Disease Society of America
158 W. 29th St.
7th Floor
New York, NY 10001-5300
http://www.hdsa.org
(212) 242-1968 extension 10 for the receptionist
(800) 345-HDSA
Fax: (212) 239-3430
e-mail: hdsainfo@hdsa.org

Provides information on disease; referrals to physicians and support groups; answers questions on presymptomatic testing.

INFECTIOUS DISEASES

CDC National Prevention Information Network
(800) 458-5231

Information about AIDS and other infectious diseases.

MULTIPLE SCLEROSIS

National Multiple Sclerosis Society
733 3rd Avenue
6th Flr.
New York, NY 10017-3288
www.nmss.org
(212) 986-3240; (800) 344-4867 (FIGHTMS)
e-mail: nat@nmss.org

PARKINSON'S DISEASE

National Parkinson Foundation
Bob Hope Parkinson Research Center
1501 N.W. 9th Avenue
Bob Hope Road
Miami, Florida 33136-1494
(305) 547-6666; (800) 327-4545
http://www.parkinson.org
e-mail: mailbox@npf.med.miami.edu
(800) 327-7872; (800) 433-7022 (FL)

Information, referrals, written material.

PICK'S DISEASE

National Niemann-Pick Disease Foundation, Inc.
N1590 Fairview Lane
Ft. Atkinson, WI 53538
http://www.nnpdf.org
(877)-CURE-NPC

APPENDIX II
HELPFUL WEBSITES

GENERAL INFORMATION

http://www.nih.gov/nia/health/agepages/forget.htm

Forgetfulness: It's Not Always What You Think.

A National Institute on Health informational page with link to the Alzheimer's Disease Education and Referral Center (ADEAR).

http://www.mayohealth.org/mayo/common/htm/alzheimers.htm

Memory Loss: Not Always Permanent

Informative site that is part of the Mayo Clinic Health Oasis. The Alzheimer's Center link leads to information for caregivers and quizzes to test your knowledge of the disease.

http://www.brain.nwu.edu/core/define.htm

Definitions for the medical terms you might hear while seeking treatment for memory loss.

http://www.brain.nwu.edu/core/caregive.htm

Information for caregivers of those with Alzheimer's and memory disorders.

http://www.alz.uci.edu/CausesofDementia.html

A list of the possible causes of dementia.

http://alzheimers.about.com/health/alzheimers/msubmemory.htm

A useful site with links to the many aspects of the impact of memory loss.

AIDS DEMENTIA COMPLEX

http://alzheimers.about.com/health/alzheimers/library/blaidsrelateddementia.htm

A definition of AIDS Dementia Complex.

http://www.natip.org/memory.html

Memory, thinking and behavior problems associated with AIDS.

http://www.cdc.gov/hiv/pubs/faq/faq5.htm

How can I tell if I'm infected with HIV? What are the symptoms?

ALZHEIMER'S DISEASE

http://www.ahcpr.gov:80/clinic/alzcons.htm

A patient and family guide to early Alzheimer's, published by the Agency for Healthcare Research and Quality.

http://www.alzheimers.com/

Practical information that supports prevention and treatment of Alzheimer's disease and the efforts of caregivers who deal with those who are affected by it.

http://www.ohioalzcenter.org/warn.html

Ten warning signs of Alzheimer's disease.

http://www.brain.nwu.edu/core/dementia.htm

A clear definition of dementia, covering Alzheimer's and its 10 warning signs.

http://www.drkoop.com/dyncon/article.asp?at=&id=1223

A definition of Alzheimer's from a site under the name of the former Surgeon General of the United States, C. Everett Koop.

http://www.drkoop.com/dyncon/article.asp?at=&id=6149

Wellness and prevention of Alzheimer's disease.

http://www.drkoop.com/dyncon/article.asp?at=&id=4037

How a diagnosis of Alzheimer's disease is reached.

http://www.drkoop.com/dyncon/article.asp?at=&id=5906

Treatment and management of Alzheimer's disease.

http://home.mira.net/~dhs/ad3.html

The Alzheimer's Web. A site devoted to Alzheimer's research. This site is for patients and physicians but takes a more academic approach.

http://www.alzheimer.ca/

The site for the Alzheimer Society of Canada.

http://www.ahaf.org/alzdis/about/adsymp.htm

The symptoms of Alzheimer's disease from the American Health Assistance Foundation.

http://www.ahaf.org/aFlzdis/about/adcare.htm

Practical information on creating a safe environment and solving day-to-day problems for caregivers of those with Alzheimer's.

http://www.alzheimers.org/pubs/adcdir.html

A list of national Alzheimer's disease centers.

http://alzheimers.about.com/health/alzheimers/library/weekly/aa051300a.htm?terms=MEMORY+LOSS

Coping with memory loss and links to other information.

BEHCET'S DISEASE

http://www.ninds.nih.gov/health and medical/disorders/behcet doc.htm

A fact sheet from the National Institute of Neurological Disorders and Stroke.

CHRONIC FATIGUE SYNDROME AND FIBROMYALGIA

http://familydoctor.org/handouts/031.html

How Do I Know If I Have Chronic Fatigue Syndrome. A series of questions with links to informational sites about the syndrome.

http://www.cdc.gov/ncidod/diseases/cfs/cfshome.htm

Chronic Fatigue Syndrome information and links to support groups from the Center for Disease Control.

http://chronicfatigue.about.com/health/chronicfatigue/library/weekly/aa051999.htm

Information, support and links.

http://chronicfatigue.about.com/health/chronicfatigue/msubfmdef.htm?terms=fibromyalgia

Links to definitions of fibromyalgia, information and how to tell if you might have the condition.

CREUTZFELDT-JAKOB DISEASE

http://www.ninds.nih.gov/health_and_medical/pubs/creutzfeldt-jakob_disease_fact_sheet.htm

A fact sheet containing information about Creutzfeldt-Jakob disease from the National Institute of Neurologic Disorders and Stroke.

http//members.aol.com/larmstr853/cjdvoice/facts.htm

A fact sheet on Creutzfeldt-Jakob disease from the CJD-Voice, an e-mail based support and discussion group.

DEMENTIA WITH LEWY BODIES

http://www.ninds.nih.gov/health_and_medical/disorders/dementiawithlewybodiesdoc.htm

A page defining Dementia with Lewy Bodies, a dementia with elements of both Alzheimer's and Parkinson's.

DEPRESSION

http://onhealth.com/conditions/resource/conditions/item,291.asp

A definition of the condition and description of symptoms.

http://onhealth.com/conditions/in-depth/item/item,14931_1_1.asp

Depression checklist.

http://www.nimh.nih.gov/publicat/depressionmenu.cfm

Information on depression from the National Institute of Mental Health.

ELECTROCONVULSIVE THERAPY

http://www.ect.org/effects.shtml

The effects of electroconvulsive therapy.

HUNTINGTON'S DISEASE

http://alzheimers.about.com/health/alzheimers/msubhuntingtons.htm

Links to information and support.

http://www.noah.cuny.edu/neuro/
hunting.html

Ask NOAH (New York Online Access to Health) about Huntington's. Useful information and links.

LEWY BODY DEMENTIA

Lewy-Net

http://www.ccc.nottingham.ac.uk/~mpzjlowe/
lewy/lewyhome.html

LYME DISEASE

http://library.LymeNet.org/domino/file.nsf

Links to information about the effects and treatment of Lyme Disease.

http://www/geocities.com/HotSprings/Oasis/
6455/lyme-links.html

Lots of links to exhaustive information about Lyme disease.

MEMORY QUIZZES AND MEMORY IMPROVEMENT INFORMATION

http://www.nymemory.org/devig/
memoryquiz.html

Memory Quiz from the New York Memory and Healthy Aging Services.

http://www.alzheimers.com/health
library/risk/risk_04_sharp.html

How to Stay Mentally Sharp for Life, Part I.

http://www.alzheimers.com/health
library/risk/risk_05_sharp2.html

How to Stay Mentally Sharp for Life, Part II.

http://www.alzheimers.com/health
library/risk/risk_06_quiz.html

Memory Quiz: How Sharp Are You?

http://www.brain.nwu.edu/core/memory.htm

A memory test offered by the Cognitive Neurology and Alzheimer's Disease Center of Northwestern University.

MENOPAUSE

http://www.nymemory.org/devig/index.html

A site for women addressing memory loss in menopause, the effect of estrogen therapy and Alzheimer's.

http://www.alzheimers.com/health
library/treatment/treatment_02_estro.html

Estrogen therapy in women and its apparent effect on Alzheimer's.

http://pharmacology.about.com/health/
pharmacology/library/weekly/aa980815.htm

Definition of and treatment for menopause.

MILD COGNITIVE IMPAIRMENT

http://www.mayohealth.org/mayo/9903/htm/
memorylo.htm

Definition of Mild Cognitive Impairment. A state of memory loss somewhere between that associated with normal aging and that of Alzheimer's disease.

MULTIPLE SCLEROSIS

http://www.htinet.com/msen.html

The online Multiple Sclerosis Education Network.

http://www.ninds.nih.gov/health_and_
medical/disorders/multiple_sclerosis.htm

Information on multiple sclerosis from the National Institute of Neurological Disorders and Stroke.

NIEMANN-PICK-DISEASE

http://easyweb.easynet.co.uk/vob/alzheimers/
information/picks_disease.htm

What is Pick's Disease?

http://www.ninds.nih.gov/health_and_
medical/disorders/niemann.doc.htm

Information on Niemann-Pick's disease from the National Institute of Neurological Disorders and Stroke.

NUTRITIONAL DEFICIENCY DEMENTIA

http://www.alzheimers.com/health
library/diagnosis/diagnosis_12_nutri.html

A short overview of the condition.

PARKINSON'S DISEASE

http://www.ninds.nih.gov/health_and_
medical/pubs/parkinson_disease_htr.htm

A thorough look at Parkinson's Disease from the National Institute of Neurologic Disorders and Stroke.

http://www.ninds.nih.gov/health_and_ medical/pubs/parkinson_disease_htr.htm#early symptoms

The early symptoms of Parkinson's Disease.

http://alzheimers.about.com/health/alzheimers/ msubparkinsons.htm

Links to information and support.

PRIMARY PROGRESSIVE APHASIA

http://www.brain.nwu.edu/core/PPA.HTM

A site defining Primary Progressive Aphasia.

http://www.cdc.gov/hiv/pubs/faq/faq5.htm

What is Primary Progressive Aphasia?

PSEUDODEMENTIA OF DEPRESSION

http://midwestneuro.com/deg/ dd pseudodemen.htm

The difference between dementia and pseudodementia.

http://midwestneuro.com/deg/dd_ pseudodemen.htm

A test for pseudodementia.

STROKE/MULTI-INFARCT DEMENTIA

http://www.ninds.nih.gov/health and medical/ pubs/stroke_hope_through_research.htm

An exhaustive brochure on stroke—types, causes and therapies.

http://www.alzheimers.com/healthlibrary/ diagnosis/diagnosis 08 mid.html

Information on multi-infarct dementia.

http://www.ninds.nih.gov/health_and_medical/ disorders/multi-infarctdementia_doc.htm

A mini fact sheet on multi-infarct dementia from the National Institute of Neurological Disorders and Stroke.

WERNICKE-KORSAKOFF SYNDROME (ALCOHOL-RELATED DEMENTIA)

http://www.caregiver.org/factsheets/wks.html

A definition of alcohol-related dementia plus information on treatment and recommendations for caregivers.

http://my.webmd.com/content/asset/Miller_ keane_35782

Definition and information about symptoms.

http://netwellness.org/mhc/top/000771.htm

Causes, incidence and risk factors.

WILSON'S DISEASE

http://www.ninds.nih.gov/health_and_ medical/disorders/wilsons_doc.htm

An information sheet on Wilson's Disease from the National Institute of Neurological Disorders and Stroke.

APPENDIX III
READ MORE ABOUT IT

AIDS/HIV

Ford, Michael Thomas. *100 Questions & Answers About AIDS: What You Need to Know Now.* New York: William Morrow & Co, 1993.

Stine, Gerald J. *AIDS Update 2000.* Upper Saddle River, NJ: Prentice Hall 1999.

Ward, Darrell E. *The Amfar AIDS Handbook: The Complete Guide to Understanding HIV and AIDS.* New York: W.W. Norton & Company, 1998.

ALZHEIMER'S DISEASE

Bellenir, Karen (ed). *Alzheimer's Disease Sourcebook: Basic Consumer Health Information About Alzheimer's Disease, Related Disorders, and Other Dementias.* Detroit, MI: Omnigraphics, Inc., 1999.

Cohen, Elwood. *Alzheimer's Disease: Prevention, Intervention, and Treatment.* New Canaan, CT: Keats Publishing, 1999.

Davies, Helen D., Jensen, Michael P. *Alzheimer's: The Answers You Need.* Forest Knolls, CA: Elder Books, 1998.

Gray-Davidson, Frena. *Alzheimer's Disease Frequently Asked Questions: Making Sense of the Journey.* Lowell, MA: Lowell House, 1999.

Hay, Jennifer. *Alzheimer's & Dementia: Questions You Have . . . Answers You Need.* Allentown, PA: Peoples Medical Society, 1996.

Kuhn, Daniel, Bennett, David A. *Alzheimer's Early Stages: First Steps in Caring and Treatment.* Alameda, CA: Hunter House, 1999.

Lindemann Nelson, James Lindemann, Nelson, Hilde. *Alzheimer's: Answers to Hard Questions for Families.* New York: Main Street Books, 1997.

Molloy, William, Caldwell, Paul. *Alzheimer's Disease.* Willowdale, ONT, Canada: Firefly Books, 1998.

Rogers, Joseph. *Candle and Darkness: Current Research in Alzheimer's Disease.* Chicago: Bonus Books, 1998.

Snyder, Lisa LCSW. *Speaking Our Minds: Personal Reflections from Individuals With Alzheimer's.* New York: W. H. Freeman & Co., 1999.

CAREGIVERS' BOOKS

Dowling, James R., Mace, Nancy L. *Keeping Busy: A Handbook of Activities for Persons With Dementia.* Baltimore: Johns Hopkins University Press, 1995.

Driskoll, Eileen. *Alzheimer: A Handbook for the Caretaker.* Boston: Branden Publishing Co., 1994.

Edwards, Allen Jack. *When Memory Fails: Helping the Alzheimer's and Dementia Patient.* Cambridge, MA: Perseus Press, 1994.

Gray-Davidson, Frena. *The Alzheimer's Sourcebook for Caregivers: A Practical Guide for Getting Through the Day.* Los Angeles: Lowell House, 1996.

Gruetzner, Howard. *Alzheimer's: A Caregiver's Guide and Sourcebook.* New York: John Wiley & Sons, 1992.

Haisman, Pam. *Alzheimer's Disease: Caregivers Speak Out.* Fort Myers, FL: Chippendale House Publishers, 1998.

Hamdy, R. C., Turnbull, James M., Edwards, Joellyn, and Turnball, James M. (eds). *Alzheimer's Disease: A Handbook for Caregivers.* St. Louis: Mosby, 1997.

Hodgson, Harriet. *Alzheimer's: Finding the Words: A Communication Guide for Those Who Care.* New York: John Wiley & Sons, 1995.

MacE, Nancy L., Rabins, Peter V. MD, McHugh, Paul R. *The 36-Hour Day: A Family Guide to Caring for Persons with Alzheimer Disease, Related Dementing Illnesses, and Memory Loss in Later Life.* Baltimore: Johns Hopkins University Press, 1999.

Sheridan, Carmel B. *Failure-Free Activities for the Alzheimer Patient: A Guidebook for Caregivers.* Forest Knolls, CA: Elder Books 1987.

CHRONIC FATIGUE

Bell, David S. *The Doctor's Guide to Chronic Fatigue Syndrome.* Cambridge, MA: Perseus Press, 1995.

DEMENTIA

Rabens, Peter, et.al. *Practical Dementia Care.* Oxford: Oxford University Press, 1999.

DEPRESSION

Mondimore, Francis Mark. *Depression: The Mood Disease (Johns Hopkins Health Book)* Baltimore: Johns Hopkins University Press, 1995.

Perry, Angela R. (ed). *Essential Guide to Depression: American Medical Association.* New York: Pocket Books, 1998.

LYME DISEASE

Lang, Denise. *Coping With Lyme Disease: A Practical Guide to Dealing With Diagnosis and Treatment.* New York: Henry Holt, 1997.

MEMORY IMPROVEMENT

Crook, Thomas H. and Adderly, Brenda D. *The Memory Cure.* New York: Pocket Books, 1999.

Green, Cynthia R. *Total Memory Workout: 8 Steps to Maximum Memory Fitness.* New York: Bantam Doubleday Dell, 1999.

Lorayne, Harry and Lucas, Jerry. *The Memory Book.* New York: Ballantine Books, 1996.

Mark, Vernon H., MD, Mark, Jeffrey P. *Reversing Memory Loss: Proven Methods for Regaining, Strengthening, and Preserving Your Memory.* Boston: Houghton Mifflin Co., 2000.

Turkington, Carol A. *12 Steps to a Better Memory.* New York: Plume, 1996.

Yutsis, Pavel and Toth, Lynda. *Why Can't I Remember?: Reversing Normal Memory Loss.* East Rutherford, NJ: Avery Publishing Group, 1999.

MENOPAUSE

Warga, Claire L. *Menopause and the Mind: The Complete Guide to Coping with Memory Loss, Foggy Thinking, Verbal Confusion, and Other Cognitive Effects of Perimenopause and Menopause.* New York: Simon & Schuster, 1999.

MULTIPLE SCLEROSIS

Barnes, David, McDonald, Ian. *Multiple Sclerosis: Questions and Answers.* Coral Springs, FL: Merit Publishing International 2000.

PARKINSON'S DISEASE

Cram, David L. *Understanding Parkinson's Disease: A Self-Help Guide.* Omaha, NE: Addicus Books, 1999.

Hutton, J. Thomas (ed). Dippel, Raye Lynne (ed). Slewett, Nathan. *Caring for the Parkinson Patient: A Practical Guide.* Amherst, NY: Prometheus Books, 1999.

STROKE

Caplan, Louis R., Dyken, Mark L., Easton, J. Donald. *American Heart Association Family Guide to Stroke Treatment, Recovery, and Prevention.* New York: Times Books, 1996.

Tanner, Dennis C. *Family Guide to Surviving Stroke and Communication Disorders, The.* Needham Heights, MA: Allyn & Bacon, 1998.

APPENDIX IV
PERIODICALS THAT PUBLISH
RESEARCH IN MEMORY

American Journal of Clinical Hypnosis
American Society of Clinical Hypnosis
130 East Elm Ct.
Suite 201
Roselle, IL 60172-2000
630-980-4740
Fax: 630-351-8490
e-mail: info@asch.net
www.asch.net/journal.htm

American Journal of Psychiatry
American Psychiatric Association
1400 K St., NW
Washington, DC 20005
(202) 682-6020
Fax: 202-682-6850
e-mail: apa@psych.org
www.ajp.psychiatryonline.org

Presents clinical research and discussion on current psychiatric issues.

American Journal of Psychology
University of Illinois Press
1325 South Oak St.
Champaign, IL 61820-6903
217-333-0950
Fax: 217-244-8082
e-mail: uipress@illinois.edu
www.press.uillinois.edu/journals/ajp.html

American Journal of Physiology
American Physiological Society
9650 Rockville Pike
Bethesda, MD 20814
301-530-7071
http://ajpcon.physiology.org

APA Monitor
American Psychological Association
750 First St., NE
Washington, DC 20002-4242
202-336-5500

800-374-2721
www.apa.org/monitor

American Psychologist
American Psychological Association
750 First St., NE
Washington, DC 20002
202-336-5500
800-374-2721
http://www.apa.org/journals/amp.html

Annals of the New York Academy of Science
New York Academy of Science
2 E. 63rd St.
New York, NY 10021
212-838-0230
e-mail: nyas@nyas.org
www.nyas.org

Annual Review of Neuroscience
Annual Reviews, Inc.
4139 El Camino Way
Box 10139
Palo Alto, CA 94303-0139
800-523-8635
650-493-4400
Fax: 650-424-0910 or 650-855-9815

Presents original reviews of critical literature and current developments in neuroscience

Annual Review of Psychology
Annual Reviews, Inc.
4139 El Camino Way
Box 10139
Palo Alto, CA 94303
650-493-4400
Fax: 650-424-0910 or 650-855-9815

Apasiology
Taylor and Francis, LTD
Rankine Rd.
Basingstoke, Hants
England RG24 8PR

+44(0) 1256 813000
Fax: +44 (0) 1256 479438
e-mail: Enquiry@taudf.co.uk
www.taylorandfrancis.com/jnls/aph.htm

Presents information on all aspects of brain damage-related language problems.

Journal of Comparative Psychology
American Psychological Association
750 First St., NE
Washington, DC 20002-4242
202-336-5500
800-374-2721

Presents laboratory and field studies of behavioral patterns of various species as they relate to development, evolution, etc.

Journal of Experimental Child Psychology
Academic Press
Journals Division
525 B Street
Suite 1900
San Diego, CA 92101-4495
619-231-0926
800-321-5068
http://www.academicpress.com/jecp

Covers all aspects of behavior in children.

Journal of Experimental Psychology
American Psychological Association
750 First St., NW
Washington, DC 20002-4242
202-336-5500
800-374-2721
http://www.apa.org/journals/xge.html

Journal of Experimental Psychology: Learning, Memory & Cognition
American Psychological Association
750 First St., NE
Washington, DC 20002-4242
202-336-5500
800-374-2721
http://www.apa.org/journals/xlm.html

Presents experimental studies of fundamentals of encoding, transfer, memory and cognition processes in human behavior.

Journal of General Psychology
Heldref Publications
1319 18th St. NW
Washington, DC 20036-1802
202-296-6267
800-365-9753
Fax: 202-296-5149
e-mail: tkelly@heldref.org
www.heldref.org

Journal of General Psychology
Heldref Publications
1319 18th St. NW
Washington, DC 20036-1802
202-296-6267
800-365-9753
Fax: 202-296-5149
e-mail: tkelly@heldref.org
www.heldref.org

Journal of Geriatric Psychiatry
International Universities Press
Journals Dept.
59 Boston Post Rd.
P.O. Box 1524
Madison, CT 06443-1524
203-245-4000

Presents research in the field of geriatric psychiatry, Alzheimer's disease.

Journal of Gerontology
Gerontological Society of America
1030 15th St. NW
Suite 250
Washington, DC 20005-1503
202-842-1275
Fax: 202-842-1150
www.geron.org/journals/gsapub.html

Journal of Mind and Behavior
Institute of Mind and Behavior
Box 522
Village Station, NY 10014
212-595-4853

Presents articles on the theory of consciousness, mind and body epistemology, etc.

Journal of Nervous and Mental Disease
Lippincott Williams and Wilkins
2107 Insurance Way
Hagerstown, MD 21740
www.jonmd.com.custserv/ww.com

Presents studies in social behavior and neurological science.

Journal of Neurology, Neurosurgery and Psychiatry
BMJ Publishing Group
BMA House
Tavistock Square
London, England WC1H 9JR
+44 (0) 171 387 4499
http://jnnp.bmjjournals.com

Presents reports on clinical neurology, neurosurgery, neuropsychology, neuropsychiatry

Journal of Neuroscience
Society for Neuroscience

11 Dupont Circle NW
Suite 500
Washington, DC 20036
202-462-6688
Fax: 202-462-1547
e-mail: Jn@sfn.org
www.jneurosci.org

Allschwilerstr. 10
P.O. Box CH4009
Basel Switzerland
061-3061111

Presents information on the neural bases of cognitive dysfunction (such as in Parkinson's disease, Alzheimer's disease, Huntington's disease).

Developmental Psychbiology
John Wiley & Sons
Journals
605 3rd Ave.
New York, NY 10158-0012
212-850-6000

Developmental Psychology
American Psychological Association
750 First St., NE
Washington, DC 20002-4242
202-336-5500
800-374-2721
http://www.apa.org/journals/dev.html

Experimental Neurology
Academic Press
525 B Street
Suite 1900
San Diego, CA 92101
619-231-0926
800-321-5068
http://www.academicpress/com/en

Presents original research in neuroscience.

International Journal of Neuroscience
Gordon & Breach, Science Publishers
P.O. Box 32160
Newark, NJ 07102
800-545-8398

Journal of Abnormal Psychology
American Psychological Association
750 First St.
Washington, DC 20002-4242
202-336-5500
800-374-2721
http://www.apa.org/journals.abn.html

Articles on basic research and theory in abnormal behavior.

Journal of Applied Developmental Psychology
Ablex Publishing Co.

355 Chestnut St.
Norwood, NJ 07648
201-767-8450

Journal of Applied Psychology
American Psychological Association
750 First St., NE
Washington, DC 20002-4242
202-336-5500
800-374-2721
http://www.apa.org/journals/apa.html

Presents research on applications of psychology in work settings.

Journal of Child Psychology and Psychiatry and Allied Disciplines
Pergamon Press
Journals Division
660 White Plains Rd.
Tarrytown, NY 10591-5153

Primarily concerned with child and adolescent psychiatry and psychology.

Journal of Clinical Psychiatry
Physician's Postgraduate Press
P.O. Box 752870
Memphis TN 38175
901-751-3800
Fax: 901-751-3444

Presents original material on psychiatric behavior and neurological science.

Journal of Clinical Psychology
Clinical Psychology Publishing Co.
4 Conant Square
Branden, VT 05733
802-247-6871

Journal of Cognitive Neuroscience
MIT Press
5 Cambridge Center
Cambridge, MA 02142-1493
617-253-5646
Fax: 617-258-6779

Presents research on the brain and behavior.

Archives of Child Neuropsychology
Pergamon Press
Journals Division
660 White Plains Rd.
Tarrytown, NY 19591-5153

Archives of General Psychiatry
American Medical Association
515 N. State St.
Chicago, IL 60610
312-464-0183
http://archneur.ama-assn.org

Behavioral Brain Research
Elsevier Science Publishing Co.
655 Avenue of the Americas
New York, NY 10010-5107
212-633-3730
Fax: 212-633-3680
e-mail: Usinfo-f@elsevier.com

Behavioral Neuroscience
American Psychological Association
750 First St., NE
Washington, DC 20002-4242
202-336-5500
800-374-2721
http://www.apa.org/journals/bne.html

Biological Psychiatry
Elsevier Science Publishing Co.
655 Avenue of the Americas
New York, NY 10010-5107
212-633-3730
Fax: 212-633-3680
e-mail: Usinfo-f@elsevier.com

Covers the whole range of psychiatric research.

Brain Research
Elsevier Science Publishing Co.
655 Avenue of the Americas
New York, NY 10010-5107
212-633-3730
Fax: 212-633-3680
e-mail: Usinfo-f@elsevier.com

Presents information on behavioral science and neurology.

Brain Research Bulletin
Pergamon Press
Journals Division
660 White Plains Rd.
Tarrytown, NY 10591-5153

Presents a broad spectrum of articles in neuroscience.

Clinical Neurology and Neurosurgery
Elsevier Science Publishing Co.
655 Avenue of the Americas
New York, NY 10010-5107
212-633-3680
Fax: 212-633-3680
e-mail: Usinfo-f@elsevier.com

Cognition
Elsevier Science Publishing Co.
655 Avenue of the Americas
New York, NY 10010-5107
212-633-3680
Fax: 212-633-3680
e-mail: Usinfo-f@elsevier.com

Cognitive Development
Ablex Publishing Co.
355 Chestnut St.
Norwood, NJ 07648

Cognitive Psychology
Academic Press
Journals Division
525 B Street
Suite 1900
San Diego, CA 92101-4495
619-231-0926
800-321-5068
http://www.academic.press.com/cogpsych

Cognitive Science
Ablex Publishing Co.
355 Chestnut St.
Norwood, NJ 07648

Journal of Neuroscience Research
John Wiley & Sons
Journals
605 3rd Ave
New York, NY 10158-0012
212-850-6000

Presents basic research in molecular cellular aspects of neuroscience.

Journal of Psychology: Interdisciplinary and Applied
Heldref Publications
1319 18th St. NW
Washington, DC 20036-1802
202-296-6267
800-365-9753
Fax: 202-296-5149
e-mail: Tkelly@heldref.org
www.heldref.org

The Lancet
655 Avenue of the Americas
New York, NY 10010
800-462-6198
212-633-3850
e-mail: custserv@lancet.com
www.thelancet.com

Neurobiology of Aging
Pergamon Press
Journals Division
660 White Plains Rd.
Tarrytown, NY 10591-5153

Neuropsychology
American Psychological Association
750 First St., NE
Washington, DC 20002-4242
202-336-550

800-374-2721
http://www.apa.org/journals/neuro.html

Presents information in clinical neuropsychology, especially neuropsychological measurement techniques and psychosocial adjustment of patients.

New England Journal of Medicine
Massachusetts Medical Society
860 Winter St.
Waltham Woods Corporate Center
Waltham, MA 02451-1411
781-893-3800
www.nejm.org

Proceedings of the National Academy of Science
National Academy of Science
2102 Constitution Ave.
Washington, DC 20418
202-334-2672
Fax: 202-334-2739

Psychiatry Research
Elsevier Science Publishing Co.
655 Avenue of the Americas
New York, NY 10010-5107
212-633-3730
e-mail: Usinfo-f@elsevier.com

Psychological Bulletin
American Psychological Association
750 First St., NW
Washington, DC 20002-4242
202-336-5500
800-374-2721
http://www.apa.org/journals/bul.html

Psychology and Aging
American Psychological Association
750 First St., NE
Washington, DC 20002-4242
http://www.apa.org/journals/pag.html

Surgical Neurology
Elsevier Science Publishing Company
655 Avenue of the Americas
New York, NY 10010-5107
212-633-3730
Fax: 212-633-3680
e-mail: Usinfo-f@elsevier.com

Trends in Neuroscience
Elsevier Science Publishing Co.
655 Avenue of the Americas
New York, NY 10010-5107
212-633-3730
Fax: 212-633-3730
e-mail: Usinfo-f@elsevier.com

GLOSSARY

acetylcholine A neurotransmitter that appears to be involved in learning and memory. Acetylcholine is severely diminished in the brains of persons with Alzheimer's disease.

activities of daily living (ADLs) Personal care activities necessary for everyday living, such as eating, bathing, grooming, dressing and toileting. People with dementia may not be able to perform necessary functions without assistance. Professionals often assess a person's ADLs to determine what type of care is needed.

allele One or two or more alternative forms of a gene; for example, one allele of the gene for eye color codes for blue eyes, while another allele codes for brown eyes.

amino acids The basic building blocks of proteins. Genes contain the code for the production of the 20 amino acids necessary for human growth and function.

amyloid A protein deposit associated with tissue degeneration; amyloid is found in the brains of individuals with Alzheimer's.

amyloid plaque Abnormal cluster of dead and dying nerve cells, other brain cells and amyloid protein fragments. These plaques are one of the characteristic abnormalities found in the brains of people with Alzheimer's disease. The presence of amyloid plaques and neurofibrillary tangles on autopsy positively diagnose Alzheimer's disease.

amyloid precursor protein (APP) A normal protein found in the brain, heart, kidneys, lungs, spleen and intestines from which beta amyloid protein is formed. In Alzheimer's disease, APP is cut and releases beta amyloid protein, which then forms clumps called amyloid plaques.

apolipoprotein E (ApoE) A protein that ferries cholesterol through the bloodstream. The ApoE gene has three variants, E2, E3, and E4. Each person inherits one variant from each parent. ApoE4 is the form of the gene that occurs more often in people with Alzheimer's disease than in the general population. E2 and E3 may protect against the disease.

axon The tubelike arm of a nerve cell that normally transmits outgoing signals from one cell body to another. Each nerve cell has one axon.

beta-amyloid protein A specific type of protein normally found in humans and animals. In Alzheimer's disease, it is found in the core of plaques in the brain.

blood-brain barrier The selective barrier membrane that controls the entry of substances from the blood into the brain.

cell The smallest unit of a living organism that is capable of functioning independently.

central nervous system (CNS) One of the two major divisions of the nervous system. Composed of the brain and spinal cord, the CNS is the control network for the entire body.

cerebral cortex The outer layer of the brain, consisting of nerve cells and the pathways that connect them. The cerebral cortex is the part of the brain in which thought processes (including learning, language and reasoning) take place.

cerebrospinal fluid (CSF) The fluid that fills the areas surrounding the brain and spinal cord.

choline A natural substance required by the body that is obtained from various foods, such as eggs; an essential component of acetylcholine.

choline acetyltransferase (CAT) An enzyme that controls the production of acetylcholine.

cholinergic system The system of nerve cells that uses acetylcholine as its neurotransmitter.

cholinesterase An enzyme that breaks down acetylcholine, so that its parts can be recycled.

chromosome An H-shaped structure inside the cell nucleus made up of tightly coiled strands of genes. Each chromosome is numbered (in humans, 1–46), and contains DNA, sequences of which make up genes.

cognitive abilities Mental abilities such as judgment, memory, learning, comprehension and reasoning.

cortisol The major natural glucocortocoid (GC) in humans. It is the primary stress hormone.

dendrites Branched extensions of the nerve cell body that receive signals from other nerve cells. Each nerve cell usually has many dendrites.

enzyme A protein produced by living organisms that promotes or otherwise influences chemical reactions.

free radicals Also called oxygen free radicals, these are oxygen molecules with an unpaired electron that is highly reactive, combining easily with other molecules and sometimes damaging other cells. Antioxidants deactivate free radicals.

gene The biological unit of heredity. Each gene is located at a specific spot on a particular chromosome, and is made up of a string of chemicals arranged in a certain sequence along the DNA molecule.

hippocampus An area buried deep in the forebrain that helps regulate emotion and is important for learning and memory.

myelin sheath A protein-based membrane surrounding the body of the nerve cell that acts as insulation. The growth of the myelin sheath is associated with increased efficiency in the neuron's ability to carry nerve impulses. Brain damage frequently takes the form of destruction of the myelin sheath, causing death of the neuron.

nerve cell (neuron) The basic working unit of the nervous system. The nerve cell is typically composed of a cell body containing the nucleus, several short branches (dendrites), and one long arm (the axon) with short branches along its length and at its end.

nerve growth factor A substance that occurs naturally in the body and enhances the growth and survival of cholinergic nerves.

neurotransmitter A specialized chemical messenger (e.g., acetylcholine, dopamine, norepinephrine, serotonin) that sends a message from one nerve cell to another. Most neurotransmitters play different roles throughout the body, many of which are not yet known.

nucleus basalis of Meynert A small group of cholinergic nerve cells in the forebrain and connected to areas of the cerebral cortex.

protein A molecule made up of amino acids arranged in a certain order. Proteins include neurotransmitters, enzymes and many other substances.

receptor A site on a nerve cell that receives a specific neurotransmitter; the message receiver.

synapse The tiny gap across which a signal is transmitted from one nerve cell to another, usually by a neurotransmitter.

REFERENCES

Adler, Tina. "Additional Information Can Distort Memories." *APA Monitor* (October 1989): 12–3.

———. "Implicit Memory Seems to Age Well." *APA Monitor* (February 1990): 8.

———. "Ability to Store Memory Linked to Glucose Levels." *APA Monitor* (September 1990): 5–6.

———. "Encoding Is Achilles' Heel for Dyslexic Kids." *APA Monitor* (November 1990): 4.

———. "Infants' Memories May Be Specific, Retrievable." *APA Monitor* (November 1990): 9.

———. "Psychologists Examine Aging, Cognitive Change." *APA Monitor* (November 1990): 4–5.

Aks, D.J. "Influence of exercise on visual search: implications of remediating cognitive mechanisms," *Perceptual and Motor Skills* 1 (December 1998): 771–83.

Alkon, Daniel L. "Memory Storage and Neural Systems: Electrical and Chemical Changes Which Accompany Conditioning Applied to Artificial Network Designs." *Scientific American* 261 (July 1989): 42–51.

Allman, W.F. *Apprentices of Wonder Inside the Neural Network Revolution.* New York: Bantam Books, 1989.

Allport, Susan. *Explorers of the Black Box: The Search for the Cellular Basis of Memory.* New York: W.W. Norton & Co., 1986.

"Alzheimer's Report in Dispute." *Philadelphia Inquirer,* January 31, 1991.

Amaducci, L. "Phosphatidylserine in the Treatment of Alzheimer's Disease: Results of a Multicenter Study." *Psychopharmacology Bulletin* 24 (1988): 130–34.

Amaducci, L., et al. "Use of Phosphatidylserine in Alzheimer's Disease." *Annals of the New York Academy of Sciences* 640 (1991): 245–49.

Anderson, J.R. *Cognitive Psychology and Its Implications.* New York: Freeman Press, 1985.

Arnold, M.B. *Memory and the Brain.* Hillsdale, NJ: Lawrence Erlbaum Associates, 1984.

Arsten, A., and Goldman-Rakic, Pl. "Catecholamines and Cognitive Decline in Aged Nonhuman Primates." *Annals of the New York Academy of Sciences* 444 (1985): 218–34.

———. N"2-Adrenergic Mechanisms in Prefrontal Cortex Associated with Cognitive Decline in Nonhuman Primates." *Science* 230 (1985): 1273–76.

Axelrod, B.N., Putnam, S.H., Woodard, J.L., and Adams, K.M. "Cross-validation of predicted Wechsler memory scale-revised scores," *Psychological Assessment* 8 (1996): 73–75.

Babikian, V. and Ropper, A. "Binswanger's disease: A review," *Stroke,* 18:1 (January–February 1987): 2–12.

Bachvalier, J., and Mishkin, M. "An Early and a Late Developing System for Learning and Retention in Infant Monkeys." *Behavioral Neuroscience* 98 (1984): 770–78.

Baddeley, Alan. *The Psychology of Memory.* New York: Basic Books, 1976.

———. "Working Memory." *Science* 255 (1992): 556–59.

Bagne, C.A., et al. *Treatment Development Strategies of Alzheimer's Disease.* New Caanan, CT: Mark Powley Associates, 1986.

Baker, Robert A., Haynes, Brikan, and Patrick, Bonnie. "The Effect of Suggestion on Past-Lives Regression." *American Journal of Clinical Hypnosis* 25 (July 1982): 71–76.

———. "Hypnosis, Memory and Incidental Memory." *American Journal of Clinical Hypnosis* 25 (April 1983): 253–62.

———. "The Aliens Among Us: Hypnotic Regression Revisited." *The Skeptical Inquirer* 12 (Winter 1987–88): 147–63.

Ballard, Clive, Grace, Janet and Holmes, Clive. "Neuroleptic sensitivity in dementia with Lewy bodies and Alzheimer's disease." *Lancet* 351 (April 4, 1998): 1032–33.

Barinaga, Marcia, "Is Apoptosis Key in Alzheimer's Disease?" *Science* (August 28, 1998).

Barnes, C.A., et al. "Acetyl-L-carnitine, 2: Effects on Learning and Memory Performance of Aged Rats in Simple and Complex Mazes." *Neurobiological Aging* 11, no. 5 (September–October 1990): 499–506.

Barr, W.B. "Receiver operating characteristic curve analysis of Wechsler memory scale—revised scores in epilepsy surgery candidates," *Psychological Assessment,* 9 (1997): 171–176.

Bartlett, F.C. *Remembering.* Cambridge: Cambridge University Press, 1932.

Bartus, R.T. "Four Stimulants of the Central Nervous System: Effects on Short-term Memory in Young Versus

Aged Monkeys." *Journal of American Geriatrics Society* 27 (1979): 289–98.

Bartus, R.T., et al. "Profound Effects of Combining Choline and Piracetam on Memory Enhancement and Cholinergic Function in Aged Rats." *Neurobiology of Aging* 2 (1981): 105–11.

Bartus, R.T., et al. "The Cholinergic Hypothesis of Geriatric Memory Dysfunction." *Science* 217 (1982): 408.

Belli, R.F. "Influences of Misleading Postevent Information: Misinformation Interference and Acceptance." *Journal of Experimental Psychology* 118 (1989): 72–85.

Bennett, Dawn. "Baby's Memory." *APA Monitor* (October 1985): 25.

Bernal, J., et al. "Visual Evoked Potentials, Attention and Mnemonic Abilities in Children." *International Journal of Neuroscience* 66, nos. 1–2 (September 1992): 45–51.

Birkmayer, W., et al. "L-deprenyl Plus L-phenylalanine in the Treatment of Depression." *Journal of Neural Transmission* 59 (1984): 81–87.

Birnbaumer, N. "Slow Potentials of the Cerebral Cortex and Behavior." *Physiological Review* (January 1990): 1–41.

Birren, J.E., and Schaie, K.W. *Handbook of the Psychology of Aging.* New York: Van Nostrand Reinhold, 1977.

Blakeslee, Sandra. "Pervasive Chemical, Crucial to the Body, Is Indicted as an Agent in Brain Damage." *New York Times,* November 29, 1988.

———. "Memories Are Made of This." *New Choices for the Best Years* 29 (November 1989): 41–45.

Bliss, E.L. "A Reexamination of Freud's Basic Concepts from Studies of Multiple Personality Disorder." *Dissociation* 1 (1988): 36–40.

Blumenthal, J.A., and Madden, D.J. "Effects of Aerobic Exercise Training, Age and Physical Fitness on Memory-search Performance." *Psychology and Aging* 3 (1988): 280–85.

Blundon, G., Smits, E. "Cognitive rehabilitation: a pilot survey of therapeutic modalities used by Canadian occupational therapists with survivors of traumatic brain injury," *Canadian Journal of Occupational Therapy* 67/3 (June 2000): 184–96.

Boller, K., and Rovee-Collier, C. "Contextual Coding and Recoding of Infant Memory." *Journal of Experimental Child Psychology* 52 (1992): 1–23.

Bolles, Edmund Blair. *So Much to Say.* New York: St. Martin's Press, 1982.

———. *Remembering and Forgetting: Inquiries into the Nature of Memory.* New York: Walker and Co., 1988.

Bologa, L., Sharma, J., and Roberts, E. "Dehydro-epiandrosterone and Its Sulfated Derivative Reduce Neuronal Death and Enhance Astrocytic Differentiation in Brain Cell Cultures." *Journal of Neuroscience Research* 17, no. 3 (1985): 225–34.

Bompani, R., and Scali, G. "Fipexide, an Effective Cognition Activator in the Elderly: A Placebo-controlled, Double-blind Clinical Trial." *Current Medical Research and Opinion* 10, no. 2 (1986): 99–196.

Bonavita, E. "Study of the Efficacy and Tolerability of L-acetylcarnitine Therapy in the Senile Brain." *Journal of Clinical Pharmacology, Therapy and Toxicology* 24 (1986): 511–16.

Bornstein, R.F. "Implicit Perception, Implicit Memory and the Recovery of Unconscious Material in Psychotherapy." *Journal of Nervous and Mental Disease* 181, no. 6 (June 1993): 337–44.

Botwinick, Jack, and Storandt, Martha. *Memory, Related Functions and Age.* Springfield, IL: Charles C. Thomas, 1974.

Bower, Bruce. "Neural Networks: The Buck Stops Here." *Science News* (August 6, 1988): 85.

———. "The Brain in the Machine: Biologically Inspired Computer Models Renew Debates Over the Nature of Thought." *Science News* 134 (November 26, 1988): 344–45.

———. "Boosting Memory in the Blink of an Eye," *Science News* 135 (February 11, 1989): 86.

———. "Investigating Eyewitnesses' Memory Mishaps." *Science News* 135 (March 4, 1989): 134.

———. "Weak Memories Make Strong Comeback." *Science News* 138 (July 21, 1990): 36.

———. "Gone But Not Forgotten: Scientists Uncover Pervasive, Unconscious Influences on Memory." *Science News* 138 (November 17, 1990): 312–15.

———. "Focused Attention Boosts Depressed Memory." *Science News* 140 (September 7, 1991): 151.

———. "Infant Memory Shows the Power of Place." *Science News* 141 (April 18, 1992): 244–45.

———. "Schizophrenic Kids' Memory Muddle." *Science News* 141 (May 23, 1992): 351.

———. "Some Lasting Memories Emerge at Age 2." *Science News* 143 (June 12, 1993): 143.

Bradley, W., et al. (eds). *Neurology in Clinical Practice: Principles of Diagnosis and Management, vol. II,* Boston: Butterworth-Heinemann, Boston, 1991.

Branconnier, R. "The Efficacy of the Cerebral Metabolic Enhancers in the Treatment of Senile Dementia." *Psychopharmacology Bulletin* 19, no. 2 (1983): 212–20.

Braude, Stephen E. "Some Recent Books on Multiple Personality and Dissociation." *Journal of the American Society for Psychical Research* 82 (October 1988): 39–52.

Brayne, C., and Calloway, D. "Normal Aging, Impaired Cognitive Function and Senile Dementia of the Alzheimer's Type: A Continuum?" *Lancet* 1 (1988): 1265–66.

Bremness, Lesley. *Herbs.* Pleasantville, NJ: The Readers Digest Association, 1990.

Breuer, J., and Freud, S. *Studies on Hysteria.* In *The Standard Edition of the Complete Psychological Works of Sigmund Freud,* ed. J. Strachey, vol. 2, London: Hogarth Press, 1955. (Originally published 1895).

Brewer, W.F., and Treyens, J.C. "Role of Schemata in Memory for Places." *Cognitive Psychology* 13 (1981): 207–30.

Brooks, D.N. *Closed Head Injury.* Oxford: Oxford University Press, 1984.

Brown, H.D., and Kosslyn, S.M. "Cerebral Lateralization." *Current Opinions in Neurobiology* 3, no. 2 (April 1993): 183–86.

Brown, N.R., Rips, L.J., and Shevell, S.K. "The Subjective Dates of Natural Events in Very Long-term Memory." *Cognitive Psychology* 17 (1985): 139–77.

Burg, Bob. "Six Steps to Remembering What's-His-Name." *ABA Banking Journal* 82 (September 1990): 92.

———. *The Memory System: Remember Everything You Need When You Need It.* Shawnee Mission, KS: National Seminars Publications, 1992.

Buccafusco, J.J., Jackson, W.J., Terry Jr. A.V., Marsh, K.C., Decker, M.W. and Arneric, S.P. (1995) "Improvement in performance of a delayed matching-to-sample task by monkeys following ABT-418: a novel cholinergic channel activator for memory enhancement," *Psychopharmacology* 120 (1995): 256–266.

Butters, M.A., Glisky, E.L., and Schacter, D.L. "Transfer of New Learning in Memory-impaired Patients." *Journal of Clinical and Experimental Neuropsychology* 15, no. 2 (March 1993): 219–30.

Butterworth, B., Campbell, R., and Howard, D. "The Uses of Short-term Memory: A Case Study." *Quarterly Journal of Experimental Psychology* 38A (1986): 705–38.

Buzan, Tony. *Use Your Perfect Memory.* New York: E.P. Dutton, 1984.

Bylinsky, G. "Medicine's Next Marvel: The Memory Pill." *Fortune,* January 20, 1986.

"Caffeine Can Increase Brain Serotonin Levels." *Nutrition Review* 46 (October 1988): 366–67.

Campi, N., Todeschini, G.P., and Scarzella, L. "Selegiline Versus L-acetylcarnitine in the Treatment of Alzheimer-type Dementia." *Clinical Therapy* 12, no. 4 (July–August 1990): 306–14.

Carey, C.J., et al. "Ondansetron and Arecoline Prevent Scopolamine-induced Cognitive Deficits in the Marmoset." *Pharmacology, Biochemistry Behavior* 42, no. 1 (1992): 75–83.

Carey, John, and Baker, Stephen. "Brain Repair Is Possible." *Business Week,* November 18, 1991.

Carillo, M.C., et al. "(-)Deprenyl Induced Activities of Both Superoxide Dismutase and Catalase in Young Male Rats." *Life Science* 48 (1991): 517.

Casale, R., Giorgi, I., and Guarnaschelli, C. "Evaluation of the Effect of Vincamine Teprosilate on Behavioral Performances of Patients Affected with Chronic Cerebrovascular Disease." *International Journal of Clinical Pharmacology Research* 4, no. 4 (1984): 313–19.

Cermak, Laird S. *Human Memory Research and Theory.* New York: The Ronald Press Co., 1972.

———. *Human Memory and Amnesia.* Hillsdale, NJ: Erlbaum, 1982.

Chase, Marilyn. "Scientists Work to Slow Human Aging." *Wall Street Journal,* March 12, 1992.

Chase, W.G., and Simon, H.A. "Perception in Chess." *Cognitive Psychology* 4 (1973): 55–81.

Chi, M.T.H., and Koeske, R.D. "Network Representation of a Child's Dinosaur Knowledge." *Developmental Psychology* 19 (1983): 29–39.

Christensen, H., and Mackinnon, A. "The Association Between Mental, Social and Physical Activity and Cognitive Performance in Young and Old Subjects." *Age and Ageing* 22, no. 3 (May 1993): 175–82.

Clark, Linda. *Help Yourself to Health.* New York: Pyramid Books, 1976.

Claustrat, B., et al. "Melatonin and Jet Lag: Confirmatory Result Using a Simplified Protocol." *Biological Psychiatry* 32, no. 8 (1992): 705–11.

Cohen, Gillian. *Memory in the Real World.* London: Lawrence Erlbaum Associates, 1989.

Colombo, C., et al. "Memory Function and Temporal-limbic Morphology in Schizophrenics." *Psychiatry Research* 50, no. 1 (April 1993): 45–56.

Colombo, Michael, et al. "Auditory Association Cortex Lesions Impair Auditory Short-term Memory in Monkeys." *Science* 247 (January 19, 1990): 336–38.

Concar, David. "Brain Boosters," *New Scientist* (February 8, 1997): 32–36.

Conrad, C.D., and Roy, D.J. "Selective Loss of Hippocampal Granule Cells Following Adrenalectomy: Implications for Spatial Memory." *Journal of Neuroscience* 13, no. 6 (June 1993): 2582–90.

Constantinidis, J. "The Zinc Deficiency Theory for the Pathogenesis of Neurofibrillary Tangles: Possibility of Preventive Treatment by a Zinc Compound." *Neurobiology of Aging* 11 (1990): 282.

Cotton, P. "Constellation of Risks and Processes Seen in Search for Alzheimer's Clues," *Journal of the American Medical Association* 271 (1994): 89–91.

Crook, T.H., et al. "Effects of Phosphatidylserine in Age-associated Memory Impairment." *Neurology* 41 (May 1991): 644–49.

Crook, T., et al. "Effects of Phosphatidylserine in Alzheimer's Disease." *Psychopharmacology Bulletin* 28 (1992): 61–66.

Cullum, C.M., Thompson, L.L., and Smernoff, E.N. "Three-word Recall as a Measure of Memory." *Journal of Clinical and Experimental Neuropsychology* 15, no. 2 (March 1993): 321–29.

Czerwinski, A.W., et al. "Safety and Efficacy of Zinc Sulfate in Geriatric Patients." *Clinical Pharmacology and Therapeutics* 15 (1974): 436–41.

Dantzer, R., and Bluthe, R.M. "Vasopressin and Behavior: From Memory to Olfaction." *Regulatory Peptides* 45, nos. 1–2 (April 29, 1993): 121–25.

Darling, W.G., and Miller, G.F. "Transformations Between Visual and Kinesthetic Coordinate Systems in Reaches to Remembered Objects, Locations and Orientations." *Experimental Brain Research* 93, no. 3 (1993): 534–47.

DeAngelis, Tori. "Dietary Recall Is Poor, Survey Study Suggests." *APA Monitor* (December 1988): 14.

———. "Children in Court: Studies Explore Custody Disputes, Technique to Aid Memory of Events." *APA Monitor* (December 1990): 31.

Deberdt, Walter. "Interaction Between Psychological and Pharmacological Treatment in Cognitive Impairment," *Life Sciences* 55: 25/26 (1994): 2057–66.

de Koning, I., Dippel, D.W., van Kooten, F., Koudstaal, P.J. "A Short Screening Instrument for Poststroke Dementia: The R-CAMCOG," *Stroke* 31/7 (July 2000): 1502–08.

DeNoble, V.J., et al. "Vinpocetine: Nootropic Effects on Scopolamine-induced and Hyposia-induced Retrieval Deficits of a Step-through Passive Avoidance Response in Rats." *Pharmacology Biochemistry and Behavior* 24 (1986): 1123–28.

Denton, Laurie. "Memory Subsystems in Precarious Balance." *APA Monitor* (August 1987): 26.

———. "Mood's Role in Memory Still Puzzling." *APA Monitor* (November 1987): 18.

———. "Memory: Not Place, but Process." *APA Monitor* (November 1988): 4.

Deyo, Richard Al, Straube, Karen T., and Disterhoft, John F. "Nimodipine Facilitates Associative Learning in Aging Rabbits." *Science* 243, no. 4892 (February 10, 1989): 809–11.

Diagram Group, The. *The Brain: A User's Manual.* New York: G.P. Putnam & Sons, 1982.

Dilman, V.M., and Dean, W. *The Neuroendocrine Theory of Aging and Degenerative Disease.* Pensacola, FL: The Center for BioGerontology, 1992.

Dimond, Stuart J. and Brouwers, E.Y.M., "Increase in the Power of Human Memory in Normal Man through the Use of Drugs," *Psychopharmacology* 49 (1976): 307–309.

Dixon, R.A., Hertzog, C., and Hultsch, D.F. "The Multiple Relationships Among Metamemory in Adulthood Scales and Cognitive Abilities in Adulthood." *Human Learning* 5 (1986): 165–78.

Dobkin, Bruce. "Present Tense." *Discover* 13 (August 1992): 74–76.

Druckman, D., and Swets, J.A. *Enhancing Human Performance.* Washington, DC: National Academy Press, 1988.

Dysken, M.W., et al. "Milacemide: A Placebo-controlled Study in Senile Dementia of the Alzheimer Type." *Journal of the American Geriatrics Society* 40 (1992): 503–6.

Ebbinghaus, Hermann. *Memory: A Contribution to Experimental Psychology.* New York: Dover Publications, 1964.

Edson, Lee. *How We Learn.* New York: Time-Life Books, 1975.

Eichenbaum, H., and Otto, T. "Long-term Potentiation and Memory: Can We Enhance the Connection?" *Trends in Neuroscience* 16, no. 5 (May 1993): 163–64.

Eisdorfer, Carol, and Friedel, Robert O., eds. *Cognitive and Emotional Disturbances in the Elderly: Clinical Issues.* Chicago: Year Book Medical Publishing, Inc., 1977.

Erdelyi, M.H. *Psychoanalysis: Freud's Cognitive Psychology.* New York: W.H. Freeman, 1985.

Erikson, G.C., et al. "The Effects of Caffeine on Memory for Word Lists." *Physiology and Behavior* 35 (1985): 47–51.

Evans, C.D., ed. *Rehabilitation After Severe Head Injury.* Edinburgh: Churchill Livingstone, 1981.

Ezzel, Carol. "Memories Might Be Made of This: Closing in on the Biochemistry of Learning." *Science News* 139 (May 25, 1991): 328–330.

———. "Monitoring Memories Moving in the Brain." *Science News* 141 (May 2, 1992): 294.

Faglioni, P., Bertolani, L., Botti, C., Merelli, E. "Verbal learning strategies in patients with multiple sclerosis," *Cortex* 36/2 (April 2000): 243–63.

Finali, G., et al. "L-deprenyl Therapy Improves Verbal Memory in Amnesic Alzheimer Patients." *Clinical Neuropharmacology* 14, no. 6 (1991): 526–36.

Finkel, M.M. "Phenytoin Revisited." *Journal of Clinical Therapeutics* 6, no. 5 (1984): 577–91.

Fisher, Kathy. "Studies Strengthen Role of Amygdala in Memory." *APA Monitor* (October 1984): 20.

———. "Learning and Memory: Brain Structure." *APA Monitor* (September 1990): 3, 6, 7.

Fisher, Ronald P., Geiselman, R. Edward, and Amador, Michael. "Field Test of the Cognitive Interview: Enhancing the Recollection of Actual Victims and Witnesses of Crime." *Journal of Applied Psychology* 74 (October 1989): 722–28.

Fitzgerald, J.M., and Lawrence, R. "Autobiographical Memory Across the Life Span." *Journal of Gerontology* 39 (1984): 692–98.

Flood, J.F., and Cherkin, A. "Effect of Acute Arecoline, Tacrine and Arecoline Tacrine Post-training Administration on Retention in Old Mice." *Neurobiology of Aging* 9 (1985): 5–8.

Flood, J.F., and Roberts, E. "Dehydroepindrosterone Sulfate Improves Memory in Aging Mice." *Brain Research* 447, no. 2 (1988): 269–78.

Florer, F.L., Allen, G. "Feelings of knowing in the Ranschburg effect," *American Journal of Psychology* 113/2 (summer 2000): 179–98.

Forrest-Pressley, D.L., MacKinnon, G.E., and Waller, T.G. *Metacognition, Cognition and Human Performance,* vols. 1 and 2. New York: Academic Press, 1985.

Frankel, F.H. "Adult Reconstruction of Childhood Events in Multiple Personality Disorder." *American Journal of Psychiatry* 150, no. 6 (June 1993): 954–98.

Freeman, W., and Watts, J. *Psychosurgery.* Springfield, IL: Charles C. Thomas, 1942; (2nd ed. 1950).

Freud, S. *The Psychopathology of Everyday Life,* ed. James Strachey. New York: W.W. Norton, 1960.

Friedman, E., et al. "Clinical Response to Choline Plus Piracetam in Senile Dementia: Relation to Red-cell Choline Levels." *New England Journal of Medicine* 304 (1981): 1490–91.

Frith, C., Bloxham, C., and Carpenter, K. "Impairments in the Learning and Performance of a New Manual Skill on Patients with Parkinson's Disease." *Journal of Neurology, Neurosurgery and Psychiatry* 46 (1986): 661–68.

Fünfgeld, E.W.; Baggen, M.; Nedwidek, P.; et al. "Double-blind study with phosphatidylserine (PS) in Parkinsonian patients with senile dementia of Alzheimer's type (SDAT)," *Progress in Clinical Biological Research* 317 (1989): 1235–46.

Furst, Bruno. *Stop Forgetting.* Garden City, NY: Doubleday and Co., 1979.

Gade, A. "Amnesia After Operations of Aneurysms of the Anterior Communicating Artery." *Surgical Neurology* 18 (1982): 46–49.

Gallant, Roy A. *Memory: How It Works and How to Improve It.* New York: Four Winds Press, 1980.

Gardner, Howard. "Mind Explorers Merge Their Maps." *New York Times,* February 8, 1991.

Garand, L., Buckwalter, K.C., Hall, G.R. "The biological basis of behavioral symptoms in dementia," *Issues in Mental Health Nursing* 21/1 (January–February 2000): 91–107.

Gatz, M., Lowe, B., Berg, S., et al. "Dementia: Not Just a Search for the Gene," *The Gerontologist* 34 (1994): 251–255.

George, M.S.; Gudotti, A.; Rubinow, D.; et al. "CSF Neuroactive Steroids in Affective Disorders: Pregnenolone, Progesterone, and DBI," *Biological Psychiatry* 35 (1994): 775–80.

Ghirardi, O., et al. "Active Avoidance Learning in Old Rats Chronically Treated with Levocarnitine Acetyl." *Physiological Behavior* 52, no. 1 (July 1992): 185–87.

Gilling, Dick, and Brightwell, Robin. *The Human Brain.* New York: Facts On File, 1982.

Glasgow, R.E., et al. "Case Studies on Remediating Memory Deficits in Brain-damaged Individuals." *Journal of Clinical Psychology* 33 (1977): 1049–54.

Gleick, James. "Brain at Work Revealed Through New Imagery," *New York Times,* August 18, 1987.

Glick, L.J. "Use of Magnesium in the Management of Dementias." *Medical Science Research* 18 (1990): 831–33.

Goad, D.L., et al. "The Use of Selegiline in Alzheimer's Patients with Behavior Problems." *Journal of Clinical Psychiatry* 52, no. 8 (August 1991): 342–54.

Gold, Philip E. "Glucose Modulation of Memory Storage Processing." *Behavioral Neural Biology* 45 (1986): 342–49.

———. "Sweet Memories." *American Scientist* 75 (1987): 151–55.

Goldberg, Joan. "The Cutting Edge: Peptide Power." *American Health* (June 1990): 35–41.

Goleman, Daniel. "In Memory, People Re-create Their Lives to Suit Their Images of the Present." *New York Times,* June 23, 1987.

———. "Open to Suggestion: Recall of Anesthetized Patients May Aid Recovery." *Reader's Digest* 136 (February 1990): 23–24.

Gomez-Pinilla, F.; Dao, L.; and So, V. "Physical exercise induces FGF-2 and its mRNA in the hippocampus," *Brain Research* 1/764 (August 1997): 1–8.

Gordon, James S., Jaffe, Dennis, and Bresler, David. *Mind, Body and Health: Toward an Integral Medicine.* New York: Human Sciences Press, 1984.

Gose, Kathleen, and Levi, Gloria. *Dealing with Memory Changes As You Grow Older.* New York: Bantam Books, 1988.

Gothard, K.M.; Skaggs, W.E. and McNaughton, B.L. "Dynamics of mismatch correction in the hippocampal ensemble code for space: interaction between path integration and environmental cues," *Journal of Neuroscience* 16/24 (1996): 8027–40.

Grafman, J., et al. "Analysis of Neuropsychological Functioning in Patients with Chronic Fatigue Syndrome." *Journal of Neurology, Neurosurgery and Psychiatry* 56, no. 6 (June 1993): 684–89.

Gray, J. *The Neuropsychology of Anxiety.* Oxford: Oxford University Press, 1982.

Greene, E., and Nartanjo, J. "Thalamic Role in Spatial Memory." *Behavioral Brain Research* 19 (1986): 123–31.

Grobe-Einsler, R., and Traber, J. "Clinical Results with Nimodipine in Alzheimer's Disease." *Clinical Neuropharmacology* 15, suppl. 1, pt. A (1992): 416A–17A.

Gruneberg, Michael, Morris, P.E., and Sykes, R.N., eds. *Practical Aspects of Memory.* Chichester: John Wiley and Sons, 1988.

Gupta, Uma. "Effects of Caffeine on Recognition Pharmacology," *Biochemistry and Behavior* 44 (1993): 393–396.

Gunning-Dixon, F.M., Raz, N. "The cognitive correlates of white matter abnormalities in normal aging: a quantitative review," *Neuropsychology* 14/2 (April 2000): 224–32.

Hamilton, E. *Plato: The Collected Dialogues.* New York: Bollingen Foundation, 1961.

Handelmann, G.E., et al. "Milacemide, a Glycine Prodrug, Enhances Performance of Learning Tasks in Normal and Amnestic Rodents." *Pharmacology, Biochemistry and Behavior* 34 (1989): 823–28.

Harris, J.E., and Morris, P.E., eds. *Everyday Memory, Actions and Absent-Mindedness.* London: Harcourt Brace Jovanovich, 1984.

Hart, R.P., and O'Shanick, G.J. "Forgetting Rates for Verbal, Pictorial and Figural Stimuli." *Journal of Clinical and Experimental Neuropsychology* 15, no. 2 (March 1993): 245–65.

Harvard Editors. "When to Worry About Forgetting." *Harvard Health Letter* (July 1992): 1–3.

Harwood, D.G., Barker, W.W., Ownby, R.L., Bravo, M., Aguero, H., Duara, R. "Predictors of positive and negative appraisal among Cuban American caregivers of Alzheimer's disease patients," *International Journal of Geriatric Psychiatry* 15/6 (June 2000): 481–7.

Harwood, D.G., Barker, W.W., Ownby, R.L., Mullan, M.J., Duara R. "Family history of dementia and current depression in nondemented community-dwelling older adults," *Journal of Geriatric Psychiatry and Neurology* 13/2 (summer 2000): 65–71.

Hayne, H. "The Effect of Multiple Reminders on Long-term Retention In Human Infants." *Developmental Psychobiology* 23 (1990): 453–77.

Heck, E.T., and Bryer, J.B. "Superior Sorting and Categorizing Ability in a Case of Bilateral Frontal Atrophy: An Exception to the Rule." *Journal of Clinical Psychology* 8 (1986): 313–16.

Heiss, W.D.; Kessler, J.; Mielke, R.; et al. "Long-term effects of phosphatidylserine, pyritinol, and cognitive training in Alzheimer's disease," A neuropsychological, EEG, and PET investigation," *Dementia* 5 (1994): 88–98.

Herrmann, Douglas J. *Super Memory: A Quick-Action Program for Memory Improvement.* Emmaus, PA: Rodale Press, 1991.

Heston, Leonard L., and White, June A. *Dementia: A Practical Guide to Alzheimer's Disease and Related Illnesses.* New York: W.H. Freeman and Co., 1983.

Higbee, Kenneth L. *Your Memory: How It Works and How to Improve It.* New York: Simon & Schuster, 1988.

Hilgard, Ernest R. *Psychology in America: A Historical Survey.* New York: Harcourt Brace Jovanovich, 1987.

Hilts, Philip. "A Brain Unit Seen as Index for Recalling Memories." *New York Times,* September 24, 1991.

———. "Photos Show Mind Recalling a Word." *New York Times,* November 11, 1991.

Hines, William. "Brain Tumors and Their Many Different Paths." *Washington Post Health Magazine,* April 7, 1987.

Hirst, W., et al. "Recognition and Recall in Amnesics." *Journal of Experimental Psychology: Learning, Memory and Cognition* 12 (1986): 445–51.

Hoffer, A. "A Case of Alzheimer's Treatment with Nutrients and Aspirin." *Journal of Orthomolecular Medicine* 8, no. 1 (1993): 43–44.

Hoffer, A. and Walker, M. *Smart Nutrients.* Garden City Park, NY: Avery, 1994.

Holmes, G.L., et al. "Effects of Kindling on Subsequent Learning, Memory, Behavior and Seizure Susceptibility." *Developmental Brain Research* 73, no. 1 (May 21, 1993): 71–77.

Horel, J. "Some comments on the special cognitive function claimed for the hippocampus," *Cortex* 30 (1994): 269–280.

Horel, J., Voytko, M., and Salsbury, K. "Visual Learning Suppressed by Cooling the Temporal Pole." *Behavioral Neuroscience* 98 (1984): 310–24.

Hostetler, A.J. "Exploring the 'Gatekeeper' of Memory: Changes in Hippocampus Seen in Aging, Amnesia, Alzheimer's." *APA Monitor* (April 1988): 3.

———. "Try to Remember . . . A Computer Battery Is Helping Test Drugs' Effects on Alzheimer's." *APA Monitor* (May 1987): 18.

Howard Rosanne. "Mild Head Injury: Challenging Emergency Room Decisions." *Headlines* 3 (March/April 1991): 6–7.

"How the Brain Works." *New York Times,* October 9, 1988.

Impastato, D.J. "The Story of the First Electroshock Treatment." *American Journal of Psychiatry* 116 (1960): 1113–14.

Isseroff, A., et al. "Spatial Memory Impairments Following Damage to the Mediodorsal Nucleus of the Thalamus in Rhesus Monkeys." *Brain Research* 232 (1982): 97–113.

Izumi, Yukitoshi, Clifford, David B., and Zorumski, Charles F. "Inhibition of Long-term Potentiation by NMDA-mediated Nitric Oxide Release." *Science* 257 (August 28, 1992): 1273–76.

James, W. *The Principles of Psychology*. New York: Henry Holt, 1890.

Jerusalinsky, Diana; Kornisiuk, Edgar and Izquierdo, Ivan. "Cholinergic Neurotransmission and Synaptic Plasticity Concerning Memory Processing," *Neurochemical Research* 22/4 (1997): 507–15.

Job, Eena. *Fending Off Forgetfulness: A Practical Guide to Improving Memory*. London: University of Queensland Press, 1985.

Johnson, George. *In the Palaces of Memory: How We Build the Worlds Inside Our Heads*. New York: Alfred A. Knopf, 1991.

Jones, David P. "Ritualism and Child Sexual Abuse." *Child Abuse and Neglect* 15 (1991): 161–69.

Kagan, J., and Hamburg, M. "The Enhancement of Memory in the First Year." *Journal of Genetic Psychology* 138 (1981): 3–14.

Karayamidis, F., et al. "Event-related Potentials and Repetition Priming in Young, Middle-aged and Elderly Normal Subjects." *Brain Research* 1, no. 2 (April 1993): 123–34.

Kavanau, J.L. "Mental malfunction and memory maintenance mechanisms," *Medical Hypotheses* 54/4 (April 2000): 678–83.

Kearsley, Greg. "Think Tanks: Bell Laboratories." *APA Monitor* (November 1981): 1, 4, 12.

Klatzky, Robert L. *Human Memory: Structures and Processes*. New York: W.H. Freeman, 1980.

Klivington, K. *The Science of Mind*. Cambridge, MA: MIT Press, 1989.

Kolb, B., and Whishaw, Ian Q. *Fundamentals of Human Neuropsychology*, 2nd ed. New York: W.H. Freeman, 1985.

Knoll, J. "The Striatal Dopamine Dependency of Lifespan in Male Rats." *Mechanisms of Aging and Development* 46 (1988): 237–62.

———. "Extension of Lifespan of Rats by Long-term (-)Deprenyl Treatment." *Mount Sinai Journal of Medicine* 55 (1988): 67–74.

———. "(-)Deprenyl-medication: A Strategy to Modulate the Age-related Decline in the Striatal Dopaminergic System." *Journal of the American Geriatric Society* 40, no. 8 (August 1992): 839–47.

Kolata, Gina. "FDA Panel Rejects Alzheimer's Drug." *New York Times*, March 17, 1991.

———. "Mental Gymnastics." *New York Times Magazine*, October 6, 1991.

Kopelman, M.D. "The Cholinergic Neurotransmitter System in Human Memory and Dementia: A Review." *Quarterly Journal of Experimental Psychology* 38A (1986): 535–74.

Kra, Siegfried. *Aging Myths: Reversible Causes of Mind and Memory Loss*. New York: McGraw-Hill, 1986.

Krassner, Michael B. "Diet and Brain Function." *Nutrition Reviews*: suppl. (May 1986): 12–15.

Krauthammer, Charles. "Disorders of Memory." *Time*, July 3, 1989.

Kruck, T.P.A., et al. "Molecular Shuttle Chelation—Studies on Desferrioxamine-based Chelation of Aluminum for Neurobiological Applications: Alzheimer's Disease." *Neurobiology of Aging* 11 (1990): 342.

Krupa, D.J., Thompson, J.K., and Thompson, R.F. "Localization of a Memory Trace in the Mammalian Brain." *Science* 260, no. 5110 (May 14, 1993): 989–91.

Lambert, J.C., Perez-Tur J., Dupire M.J., et al. "Distortion of allelic expression of apolipoprotein E in Alzheimer's disease," *Human Molecular Genetics* 6/12 (1997): 2151–2154.

Landauer, T.K. "How Much Do People Remember? Some Estimates of the Quantity of Learned Information in Long-term Memory." *Cognitive Science* 10 (1986): 477–94.

Landers, Susan. "Memories of Elderly Found to be Accurate in Surveys." *APA Monitor* (October 1987): 15.

Langley, M.S., and Sorkin, E.M. "Nimodipine: A Review of Its Pharmacodynamic and Pharmacokinetic Properties, and Therapeutic Potential in Cerebrovascular Disease." *Drugs* 37 (1989): 669–99.

Lapp, Danielle. *(Nearly) Total Recall: A Guide to a Better Memory at Any Age*. Stanford, CA: Stanford Alumni Association, 1992.

Larkin, Marilyn. "Treating Head Pain Resulting from Subtle Brain Injury." *Headlines* 3 (March/April 1991): 14–20.

Lashley, M.E. "The Painful Side of Reminiscence." *Geriatric Nursing* 14, no. 3 (May/June 1993): 138–41.

Lee, E.H.Y. and Ma, Y.L. "Amphetamine Enhances Memory Retention and Facilitates Norepinephrine Release From the Hippocampus in Rats," *Brain Research Bulletin* 4 (1995): 411–16.

Leiner, H., Leiner, A. and Dow, R. "Does the Cerebellum Contribute to Mental Skills?" *Behavioral Neuroscience* 100 (1986): 443–54.

Levin, H., High, W., and Eisenberg, H. "Learning and Forgetting During and After Post-traumatic Amnesia in Head-injured Patients." *Society for Neuroscience Abstracts* 13 (1987): 205.

Lisanby, S.H., Maddox, J.H., Prudic, J., Devanand, D.P., Sackeim, H.A. "The effects of electroconvulsive therapy on memory of autobiographical and public events," *Archives of General Psychiatry* 57/6 (June 2000): 581–90.

Loftus, Elizabeth. *Eyewitness Testimony*. Cambridge, MA: Harvard University Press, 1979.

————. *Memory: Surprising New Insights Into How We Remember and Why We Forget.* Reading, MA: Addison-Wesley Publishing Co., 1980.

Loftus, E.F., and Greene, E. "Warning: Even Memory for Faces May Be Contagious." *Law and Human Behavior* 4 (1980): 323–34.

Loftus, E.F., and Loftus, G.R. "On the Permanence of Stored Information in the Human Brain." *American Psychologist* 35 (1980): 421–34.

Loftus, E.F. and Marburger, W. "Since the Eruption of Mt. St. Helens Has Anyone Beaten You Up? Improving the Accuracy of Retrospective Reports with Landmark Events." *Memory and Cognition* 2 (1983): 114–20.

Lorayne, Harry, and Lucas, Jerry. *The Memory Book.* New York: Dorset Press, 1974.

Luria, A.R. *The Mind of a Mnemonist.* New York: Basic Books, 1968.

Lynch, G. "What Memories Are Made Of: A Chemical Called Calpain Records the Events of a Lifetime." *Sciences* (September–October 1985): 38–43.

Mace, Nancy, and Rabins, Peter. *The 36 Hour Day: A Guide to Caring for Persons with Alzheimer's Disease and Related Dementing Illnesses.* Baltimore: Johns Hopkins University Press, 1991.

Maestroni, G.J., Conti, A., and Pierpaoli, W. "Pineal Melatonin, Its Fundamental Immunoregulatory Role in Aging and Cancer." *Annals of the New York Academy of Science* 521 (1988): 140–48.

Mahler, M. and Cummings, J. "Behavioral Neurology of Multi-Infarct Dementia." *Alzheimer Disease and Associated Disorders* 5:2 (1991): 122–30.

Maina, G., et al. "Oxiracetam in the Treatment of Primary Degenerative and Multi-infarct Dementia: A Double-blind, Placebo-controlled Study." *Neuropsychobiology* 21, no. 3 (1989): 141–45.

Mantyla, T. "Knowing but Not Remembering: Adult Age Differences in Recollective Expression." *Memory and Cognition* 21, no. 3 (May 1993): 379–88.

Mark, Vernon, and Mark, Jeffrey P. "Why We Forget: Ten Common and Reversible Causes of Memory Loss." *Modern Maturity* 33 (August–September 1990): 70–74.

Markowitsch, H.J. "Hypotheses on Mnemonic Information Processing by the Brain." *International Journal of Neuroscience* 15 (1985): 189–287.

Martin, E.M., et al. "Speed of Memory Scanning Not Affected in Early HIV-1 Infection." *Journal of Clinical and Experimental Neuropsychology* 15, no. 2 (March 1993): 311–20.

Martinez, J.L., and Kesner, R.P. *Learning and Memory: A Biological View.* Orlando, FL: Academic Press, 1986.

Masaki, K.; Losondzy, M.; Izmirlian, G.; et al. "Association of vitamin E and C supplement use with cognitive function and dementia in elderly men," *Neurology* 54 (March 23, 2000): 1265–72.

Matlock, James G. "Age and Stimulus in Past Life Memory: A Study of Published Cases." *Journal of the American Society for Psychical Research* 83 (October 1989): 303–16.

Maugh, Thomas H., II. "Researchers Observe Brain's Memory-forming Process." *Philadelphia Inquirer,* November 12, 1991.

————. "Steroid Found to Aid Memory in Lab Mice; Human Tests Planned." *Philadelphia Inquirer,* March 21, 1992.

Mayes, Andrew R. *Human Organic Memory Disorders.* Cambridge: Cambridge University Press, 1988.

Mayo, W; Dedhu, E; Robel, P.; et al. "Infusion of Neurosteroids into the Nucleus Basalis Magnocellularis Affects Cognitive Processes in the Rat," *Brain Research* 607 (1993): 324–28.

McDougall, G.J. "Memory improvement in assisted living elders," *Issues in Mental Health Nursing* 21/2 (March 2000): 217–33.

McEnroe, Colin. "Sub-total Recall; Having Trouble Remembering Names, Faces, Facts? Welcome to Your 40s." *Men's Health* 6 (April 1991): 12.

McEntee, W.J., and Mair, R.G. "Memory Enhancement in Korsakoff's Psychosis by Clonidine: Further Evidence for a Noradrenergic Deficit." *Annals of Neurology* 7 (1980): 466–70.

McKenna P., and Warrington, E.K. "Testing for Nominal Dysphasia." *Journal of Neurology, Neurosurgery and Psychiatry* 43 (1980): 781–88.

McKenzie, Aline. "Gone to Pot: Marijuana Use and Short-term Memory Problems." *Reader's Digest/Canadian,* 137 (December 1990): 92.

Merzenich, M.M., and Sameshima, K. "Cortical Plasticity and Memory." *Current Opinions in Neurobiology* 3, no. 2 (April 1993): 187–96.

Meurs, E.J., and Hes, R. "Deja Vu and Holographic Images." *American Journal of Psychiatry* 150, no. 4 (April 1993): 679–80.

Milwain, E. "Mild cognitive impairment: further caution," *Lancet* 355/9208 (March 18, 2000): 1018.

Minninger, Joan. *Total Recall: How to Boost Your Memory Power.* Emmaus, PA: Rodale Press, 1984.

Mishkin, Mortimer, and Appenzeller, Tim. "The Anatomy of Memory." *Scientific American* 256 (June 1987): 80–89.

Mitiguy, Judith. "New Applications of Diagnostic Techniques." *Headlines* 3 (March/April 1992): 2–5, 8–10.

Mondadori, Cesare. "In Search of the Mechanism of Action of the Nootropics: New Insights and Potential Clinical Implications," *Life Sciences* 55: 25/26 (1994): 2171–78.

Monzani, F., et al. "Subclinical Hypothyroidism: Neurobehavioral Features and Beneficial Effect of L-thyroxine Treatment." *Clinical Investigator* 71, no. 5 (May 1993): 367–71.

Moscovitch, M., ed. *Advances in the Study of Communication and Affect: Vol. 9. Infant Memory.* New York: Plenum Press, 1984.

"Mouse Models Created for Alzheimer's Disease." *New York Times,* July 23, 1991.

Myers, N.A., Clifton, R.K., and Clarkson, M.G. "When They Were Very Young: Almost-threes Remember Two Years Ago." *Infant Behavior and Development* 10 (1987): 123–32.

Naatanen, R., et al. "Development of a Memory Trace for a Complex Sound in the Human Brain." *Neuroreport* 4, no. 5 (May 1993): 503–6.

Nakamura, H., Nakanishi, M., Hamanaka, T., Nakaaki, S., Yoshida, S. "Semantic priming in patients with Alzheimer and semantic dementia," *Cortex* 36/2 (April 2000): 151–62.

Nauta, Walle J.H., and Feirtag, Michael. *Fundamental Neuroanatomy.* New York: W.H. Freeman, 1986.

Neisser, Ulric. *Memory Observed: Remembering in Natural Contexts.* San Francisco: W.H. Freeman and Company, 1982.

———. "Interpreting Harry Bahrick's Discovery: What Confers Immunity Against Forgetting?" *Journal of Experimental Psychology* 113 (1984): 32–35.

Nicholson, C. "Pharmacology of nootropics and metabolically active compounds in relation to their use in dementia," *Psychopharmacology* 101 (1990): 147–59.

Nigro, G., and Neisser, U. "Point of View in Personal Memories." *Cognitive Psychology* 15 (1983): 465–82.

Norman, D.A. *Learning and Memory.* New York: W.H. Freeman, 1982.

Ohno, M., Yamamoto, T., and Watanabe, S. "Blockage of Hippocampal Nicotinic Receptors Impairs Working Memory But Not Reference Memory in Rats." *Pharmacology, Biochemistry and Behavior* 45, no. 1 (May 1993): 89–93.

Oler, J.A., Markus, E.J. "Age-related deficits in episodic memory may result from decreased responsiveness of hippocampal place cells to changes in context," *Annals of the New York Academy of Science* 911 (June 2000): 465–70.

Ostrander, Sheila, and Schroeder, Lynn. *Super-Memory: The Revolution.* New York: Carroll & Graf Publishers, 1991.

Pan, Y., Anthony, M., Watson, S., Clarkson, T.B. "Soy phytoestrogens improve radial arm maze performance in ovariectomized retired breeder rats and do not attenuate benefits of 17beta-estradiol treatment," *Menopause* 7/4 (July–August 2000): 230–5.

Parent, M.E., Krondl, M., and Chow, R.K. "Reconstruction of Past Calcium Intake Patterns During Adulthood." *Journal of the American Dietetic Association* 93, no. 6 (June 1993): 649–52.

Parkin, Alan J. *Memory and Amnesia.* Oxford: Basil Blackwell, Ltd., 1987.

Parkinson Study Group, The. "Effect of Deprenyl on the Progression of Disability in Early Parkinson's Disease." *New England Journal of Medicine* 321 (November 16, 1989): 1364–71.

Parnetti, L., et al. "Mental Deterioration in Old Age—Results of 2 Multicenter Clinical Trials with Nimodipine." *Clinical Therapeutics* 15, no. 2 (March/April 1993): 394–406.

Pelton, R., and Pelton, T.C. *Mind Food & Smart Pills.* New York: Doubleday, 1989.

Perri, R., Carlesimo, G.A., Loasses, A., Caltagirone, C. "Deficient intentional access to semantic knowledge in patients with severe closed-head injury," *Cortex* 36/2 (April 2000): 213–25.

Petkov, V. "Effects of Standardized Ginseng Extract on Learning, Memory and Physical Capabilities." *American Journal of Chinese Medicine* 15, no. 1 (1987): 19–29.

Pettinati, Helen M., ed. *Hypnosis and Memory.* New York: Guilford Press, 1988.

Piaget, J., and Inhelder, B. *Memory and Intelligence.* New York: Basic Books, 1973.

Piccinin, G.L., Finali, G., and Piccirilli, M. "Neuropsychological Effects of L-deprenyl in Alzheimer's Type Dementia." *Clinical Neuropharmacology* 13, no. 2 (April 1990): 147–63.

Pipitone, Paul. "Brain Reorganization Explored in Stroke Recovery." *Headlines* 3 (March/April 1991): 27.

———. "Study on Substance Abuse and Brain Injury." *Headlines* 3 (March/April 1991): 27.

Polani, P.E. "Olfactory dysfunction in Alzheimer's disease," *Lancet.* 355/9208 (March 18, 2000): 1015.

Pool, J.L. *Nature's Masterpiece: The Brain and How It Works.* New York: Walker and Company, 1987.

Poole, Robert, ed. *The Incredible Machine.* Washington, DC: National Geographic Society, 1986.

Poon, L.W. "A Systems Approach for the Assessment and Treatment of Memory Problems." In *The Comprehensive Handbook of Behavioral Medicine,* ed. J.M. Ferguson and C.B. Taylor, vol. 1. Great Neck, NY: PMA Publishing Corp., 1980.

Prevention Magazine Editors. *Future Youth: How to Reverse the Aging Process.* Emmaus, PA: Rodale Press, 1987.

Procter, A.W., et al. "Glutamate/Aspartame-Releasing Neurones in Alzheimer's Disease," *New England Journal of Medicine* 314 (1986): 1711–12.

Proctor A., Wilson B., Sanchez, C., and Wesley, E. "Executive function and verbal working memory in adolescents with closed head injury," *Brain Injury* 14/7 (July 2000): 633–47.

Proust, M. *Remembrance of Things Past,* trans. C.S. Moncrieff and T. Kilmartin. New York: Random House, 1981.

Psychology Today Editors. "Buried Memories (Experiments on Memory in Infants)." *Psychology Today* 23 (April 1989): 12.

Putnam, F.W. "Dissociation as a Response to Extreme Trauma." In *Childhood Antecedents of Multiple Personality,* ed. R. Kluft. Washington, DC: American Psychiatric Press, 1985.

Raeburn, Paul. "Memory Tea." *American Health* (January–February 1990): 126.

Rai, G., et al. "Double Blind, Placebo Controlled Study of Acetyl-L-carnitine in Patients with Alzheimer's Dementia." *Current Medical Research and Opinion* 11, no. 10 (1990): 638–47.

Reason, James T., and Mycielska, Klara. *Absent-Minded? The Psychology of Mental Lapses and Everyday Errors.* Englewood Cliffs, NJ: Prentice-Hall, 1982.

Recer, Paul. "FDA Panel Declines to Support Approval for Alzheimer's Drug." *Philadelphia Inquirer,* March 16, 1991.

Reed, B.R., Jagust, W.J., and Coulter, L. "Anosognosia in Alzheimer's Disease: Relationships to Depression, Cognitive Function and Cerebral Perfusion." *Journal of Clinical and Experimental Neuropsychology* 15, no. 2 (March 1993): 231–44.

Reed, Graham. *The Psychology of Anomalous Experience: A Cognitive Approach.* Buffalo, NY: Prometheus Books, 1988.

Restak, Richard. *The Brain.* New York: Bantam Books, 1984.

Richardson, John T.E. *Mental Imagery and Human Memory.* New York: St. Martin's Press, 1980.

Richman, Barbara. "Memorable Mnemonic." *APA Monitor* (October 1986): 16.

Rizzo, M., Anderson, S.W., Dawson, J., Nawrot, M. "Vision and cognition in Alzheimer's disease," *Neuropsychologia* 38/8 (2000): 1157–69.

Roberts, H.J. *Aspartame (NutraSweet): Is It Safe?* Philadelphia: The Charles Press, 1990.

Rolls, E.T., et al. "Response of Single Neurons in the Hippocampus of the Macaque Related to Reorganization Memory." *Experimental Brain Research* 93, no. 2 (1993): 299–306.

Roman, G. "Senile dementia of the Binswanger type," *Journal of the American Medical Association* 258:13 (October 1987): 1782–88.

Rosenfield, Israel. *The Invention of Memory: A New View of the Brain.* New York: Basic Books, 1989.

Roses, A.D. "Apolipoprotein E alleles as risk factors in Alzheimer's disease," *Annual Review of Medicine* 47 (1996): 387–400.

Rosse, R.B., et al. "An Open-label Trial of Milacemide in Schizophrenia: An NMDA Intervention Strategy." *Clinical Neuropharmacology* 13, no. 4 (1990): 348–54.

Routtenberg, A., Cantallops, I., Zaffuto, S., Serrano, P., Namgung, U. "Enhanced learning after genetic overexpression of a brain growth protein," *Proceeds of the National Academy of Science* 97/13 (June 20, 2000): 7657–62.

Rovee-Collier, Carolyn. "The Capacity for Long-term Memory in Infancy." *Current Directions in Psychological Science* 2 (August 1993): 130–35.

———. "Infants' Eyewitness Testimony: Effects of Postevent Information on a Prior Memory Representation." *Memory & Cognition* 21 (1993): 267–79.

Rovee-Collier, Carolyn, and Hayne, H. "Reactivation of Infant Memory: Implications for Cognitive Development." In *Advances in Child Development and Behavior.* New York: Academic Press, 1987.

Ryan, E.B., and See, S.K. "Age-based Beliefs About Memory Changes for Self and Others Across Adulthood." *Journal of Gerontology* 48, no. 4 (July 1993): 199–201.

Sabelli, H.C. "Rapid Treatment of Depression with Selegiline-phenylalanine Combination." *Journal of Clinical Psychiatry* 53, no. 3 (March 1991): 137.

Sakai, K., and Miyashita. "Memory and Imagery in the Temporal Lobe." *Current Opinions in Neurobiology* 3, no. 2 (April 1993): 166–70.

Saletu, B., and Grunberger, J. "Memory Dysfunction and Vigilance: Neurophysiological and Psychopharmacological Aspects." *Annals of the New York Academy of Sciences* 444 (1985): 406–27.

Saletu, B., Grunberger, J., and Linzmayer, L. "Acute and Subacute CNS Effects of Milacemide in Elderly People: Double-blind, Placebo-controlled Quantitative EEG and Psychometric Investigations." *Archives of Gerontology and Geriatrics* 5 (1986): 165–81.

Saline, Carol. "Remembrance of Things, uh . . . uh. well, hmm . . ." *Philadelphia Magazine* (May 1992): 49–53.

Salzman, C. "The Use of ECT in the Treatment of Schizophrenia." *American Journal of Psychiatry* 137 (1980): 1032–34.

Sangiorgio, Maureen, Gutfeld, Greg, and Rao, Linda. "Aerobic Memory: Exercises and Memory." *Prevention* 44 (February 1992): 14–15.

Sartori, G., et al. "Category-specific Form of Knowledge Deficit in Patients with Herpes Simplex Virus Encephalitis." *Journal of Clinical and Experimental Neuropsychology* 15, no. 2 (March 1993): 280–99.

Schatz, J., Kramer, J.H., Ablin, A., Matthay, K.K. "Processing speed, working memory, and IQ: a developmental model of cognitive deficits following cranial radiation therapy," *Neuropsychology* 14/2 (April 2000): 189–200.

Schmeck, Harold M. "Study Identifies Part of Brain as Important Site for Anxiety." *New York Times,* February 24, 1989.

Schoenthaler, S.J. "Diet and IQ." *Nature* 352 (1991): 292.

Schoenthaler, S.J., et al. "Controlled Trial Vitamin-mineral Supplementation: Effects on Intelligence and Performance." *Personality and Individual Differences* 12, no. 4 (1991): 351–62.

Schooler, J., and Loftus, E. "Memory." *McGraw-Hill Encyclopedia of Science and Technology,* vol. 10. New York: McGraw-Hill, 1987.

Schwartz, B. et al. "Glycine Pro-drug Facilitates Word Retrieval in Humans." *Neurology* 41 (1991): 1341–43.

———. "The Effects of Milacemide on Item and Source Memory." *Clinical Neuropharmacology* 15 (1992): 114–19.

Schwartz, Evan I. "This Software Can Help Restore Lost Memory—for Humans." *Business Week,* December 24, 1990.

Schwartz, G.E., Russek, L.G., Bell, I.R., Riley, D. "Plausibility of homeopathy and conventional chemical therapy: the systemic memory resonance hypothesis," *Medical Hypotheses* 54/4 (April 2000): 634–7.

Science News Editors. "Marijuana Mangles Memory." *Science News* 136 (November 18, 1989): 332.

———. "Lights Out for Some Flashbulb Memories." *Science News* 139 (February 2, 1991): 78.

Sera, G., et al. "Effect of Fipexide on Passive Avoidance Behavior in Rats." *Pharmacological Research* 21, no. 5 (1989): 603–8.

Sher, L. "Memory creation and the treatment of psychiatric disorders," *Medical Hypotheses* 54/4 (April 2000): 628–9.

Skinner, Karen J. "The Chemistry of Learning and Memory." *Chemical & Engineering News* 69 (October 7, 1991): 24–42.

Simons, Marlise. "Le Brain Jogging." *New York Times Magazine,* October 6, 1991.

Smith, Charles. "Your Memory: Don't Leave Home Without It." *American Salesman* 35 (October 1990): 3–5.

Smith, D.A., Browning, M., and Dunwiddie, T.V. "Cocaine Inhibition of Hippocampal Long-term Potentiation." *Brain Research* 608, no. 2 (April 16, 1993): 259–65.

Smith, M.E., and Guster, K. "Decomposition of Recognition Memory Event-related Potential Yield Target

Repetition and Retrieval Effects." *Electroencephalography and Clinical Neurophysiology* 86, no. 5 (May 1993): 335–43.

Souetre, E., et al. "Abnormal Melatonin Response to 5-methoxypsoralen in Dementia." *American Journal of Psychiatry* 146, no. 8 (August 1989): 1037–40.

Spence, J.D. *The Memory Palace of Matteo Ricci.* New York: Viking Press, 1984.

Squire, Larry R., and Zola-Morgan, Stuart. "Mechanisms of Memory," *Science,* 232 (June 27, 1986): 1612–19.

———. *Memory and Brain.* New York: Oxford University Press, 1987.

———. "The Medial Temporal Lobe Memory System." *Science* 253 (September 20, 1991): 1380–87.

Squire, Larry R., and Butters, N. *Neuropsychology of Memory.* New York: Guilford Press, 1984.

Staiger, E.H. "Probing More of the Mind." *ChemTech* (October 1986): 588–91.

Stevenson, I. "The phenomenon of claimed memories of previous lives: possible interpretations and importance," *Medical Hypotheses* 54/4 (April 2000): 652–59.

Sullivan, E.V., Rosenbloom, M.J., Lim, K.O., Pfefferbaum, A. "Longitudinal changes in cognition, gait, and balance in abstinent and relapsed alcoholic men: relationships to changes in brain structure," *Neuropsychology* 14/2 (April 2000): 178–88.

Sunderland, T., et al. "Reduced Plasma Dehydroepiandrosterone Concentrations in Alzheimer's Disease." *Lancet* 2 (1989): 1335–36.

Tarazi, Linda. "An Unusual Case of Hypnotic Regression with Some Unexplained Contents." *Journal of the American Society for Psychical Research* 84 (October 1990): 309–44.

Tariiot, P.N., et al. "L-deprenyl in Alzheimer's Disease: Preliminary Evidence for Behavioral Change with Monoamine Oxidase B Inhibitors." *Archives of General Psychiatry* 44 (May 1987): 427–33.

Tierney, M.C., Szalai, J.P., Dunn, E., Geslani, D., McDowell, I. "Prediction of probable Alzheimer disease in patients with symptoms suggestive of memory impairment. Value of the Mini-Mental State Examination," *Archives of Family Medicine* 9/69 (June 2000): 527–32.

Tortora, G.J., and Anagnostakos, N.P. *Principles of Anatomy and Physiology.* New York: Harper & Row, 1990.

Toufexis, Anastasia. "When Can Memories Be Trusted?" *Time,* October 28, 1992.

Treffert, D. "The Idiot Savant: A Review of the Syndrome." *American Journal of Psychiatry* 145 (1988): 563–72.

Trotter, Bob. "Better Memory Through Chemistry." *American Health: Fitness of Body and Mind* (April 1991): 12.

Tulving, E. *Elements of Episodic Memory.* Oxford: Clarendon Press, 1983.

———. "How Many Memory Systems Are There?" *American Psychologist* 40 (1984): 385–98.

Turkington, Carol. "Hypnotic Memory Is Not Always Accurate." *APA Monitor* (March 1982): 46–74.

———. "Disorders Highlight Differences in Learning, Memory Functions." *APA Monitor* (October 1983): 28.

———. "Memory Found Under Anesthesia." *APA Monitor* (May 1984): 33.

———. "Enkephalins Tied to Plasma." *APA Monitor* (October 1985): 10.

Ullman, Montague. "Dreams, Species-connectedness and the Paranormal." *Journal of the American Society for Psychical Research* 84 (April 1990): 105–25.

van Dyck C.; Newhouse, P.; Falk, W.; Mattes, J. "Extended-release physostigmine in Alzheimer disease," *Archives of General Psychiatry* 57 (February 2000): 157–64.

Verhaeghen, P., Marcoen, A., and Goossens, L. "Facts and Fiction About Memory and Aging: A Quantitative Integration of Research Findings." *Journal of Gerontology* 48, no. 4 (July 1993): 157–71.

Watson, Ronald R. "Caffeine: Is It Dangerous to Health?" *American Journal of Health Promotion* 2 (Spring 1988): 13–21.

Wearden, J.H., and Ferrara, A. "Subjective Shortening in Human's Memory for Stimulus Duration." *Quarterly Journal of Experimental Psychology* 46, no. 2 (May 1993): 163–86.

Weiner, R.D. "Retrograde amnesia with electroconvulsive therapy: characteristics and implications," *Archives of General Psychiatry* 57/6 (June 2000): 591–92.

Weintraub, Pamela. "Total Recall: Ways to Improve Your Memory." *American Health* (March 1992): 77–73.

Weiss, R. "Human Brain Neurons Grown in Culture." *Science News* 137 (May 5, 1990): 276.

Welte, P.O. "Indices of Verbal Learning and Memory Deficits After Right Hemisphere Stroke." *Archives of Physical Medicine and Rehabilitation* 74, no. 6 (June 1993): 631–36.

"What Causes Memory Loss?" *USA Today* (magazine) 119 (October 1990): 3.

"What Does Your Memory Smell Like?" *USA Today* (magazine) 120 (January 1992): 6.

"What REALLY Causes Amnesia?" *USA Today* (magazine) 117 (April 1989): 13.

White, N.M. and McDonald, R.J. "A triple dissociation of memory systems: hippocampus amygdala and dorsal striatum," *Behavioral Neuroscience* 107 (1993): 3–22.

White, N.M., Packard, M.G., and Seamans, J. "Memory Enhancement by Post-training Peripheral Administration of Low Doses of Dopamine Agonists." *Behavioral and Neural Biology* 59, no. 3 (May 1993): 230–41.

Whittington, C.J., Podd, J., Kan, M.M. "Recognition memory impairment in Parkinson's disease: power and meta-analyses," *Neuropsychology* 14/2 (April 2000): 233–46.

Williams, P. and Lord, S.R., "Effects of group exercise on cognitive functioning and mood in older women," *Australian and New Zealand Journal of Public Health* 21/1 (February 1997): 45–52.

Wilson, B. *The Rehabilitation of Memory.* New York: Guilford Press, 1987.

Wilson, B., and Moffat, N. *Clinical Management of Memory Problems.* Rockville, MD: Aspen Systems, 1984.

Wilson, F.A., Scalardhe, S.P., and Goldman-Rakic, P.S. "Dissociation of Object and Spatial Process Domains in Primate Prefontal Cortex." *Science* 260 (1993): 1876.

Winston, J. "Biology and Function of REM Sleep." *Current Opinions in Neurobiology* 3, no. 2 (April 1993): 243–48.

Wolinsky, Joan. "Responsibility Can Delay Aging." *APA Monitor* (March 1982): 14, 41.

Woods, N.F., Mitchell, E.S., and Adams, C. "Memory functioning among midlife women: observations from the Seattle Midlife Women's Health Study," *Menopause* 7/4 (July/August 2000): 257–65.

Wuethrich, B. "Higher Risk of Alzheimer's Linked to Gene." *Science News* 144, no. 7 (August 14, 1993): 108.

Yalch, Richard F. "Memory in a Jingle Jungle: Music as a Mnemonic Device in Communicating Advertising Slogans." *Journal of Applied Psychology* 76 (April 1991): 268–75.

Yates, Frances A. *The Art of Memory.* Chicago: University of Chicago Press, 1966.

Yesavage, J.A., and Rolf, J. "Effects of Relaxation and Mnemonics on Memory, Attention and Anxiety in the Elderly." *Experimental Aging Research* 10 (1984): 211–14.

Young, Walter C. "Patients Reporting Ritual Abuse in Childhood: A Clinical Syndrome." *Child Abuse and Neglect* 15 (1991): 181–89.

Zalla, T., Sirigu, A., Pillon, B., Dubois, B., Agid, Y., Grafman, J. "How patients with Parkinson's disease retrieve and manage cognitive event knowledge," *Cortex* 36/2 (April 2000): 163–79.

Zatorre, R.J., and Halpern, A.R. "Effect of Unilateral Temporal Lobe Excision on Perception and Imagery of Songs." *Neuropsychologia* 31, no. 3 (March 1993): 221–32.

Zhong, Y., Nishijo, H., Uwano, T., Tamura, R., Kawanishi, K., Ono, T. "Red ginseng ameliorated place navigation deficits in young rats with hippocampal lesions and aged rats," *Physiology and Behavior* 69/4-5 (June 1, 2000): 511–25.

INDEX

from repeated blows 56
scans of 139
from syphilis 219
transplants and 43
brain-derived neurotrophic factor (BDNF)
85–86
Brainerd, C. J. 96
brain scans **42**. *See also specific brain scanning
techniques*
for AIDS dementia complex 10
for Alzheimer's disease 15
for Parkinson's disease 176
plasticity and 183
for transient ischemic attack 225
for tumors 44
brain stem 38, 43–44, 71, 102, 129, 131,
137
brain tumor **43–44,** 145
agnosia from 8
agraphia from 9
amnesia from 22, 25, 41
apraxia from 30
Broca, Paul on 44
Capgras syndrome and 48
CT scan of 55
dementia from 66, 67–68
elderly with 6
endogenous brain damage from 82
Korsakoff's syndrome from 125
plasticity and 184
temporal lobe epilepsy from 222
brain waves 39
BRAT battery **44**
breast cancer 20, 63
Breasted, James Henry 212
breathing 25, 28, 56, 200
Breslau University 12
Breuer, Josef 27, **44,** 73
Brigham and Women's Hospital 6, 20
Broca, band of 52
Broca, Paul **44–45,** 236
bromocriptine 176
Brown-Peterson task **45**
Brown University 43
bruising 60, 102
Buddha 151
burns 3
Buschke Selective Reminding Test *165*
buspirone (Buspar) 19
Butler, Robert 7

C

caffeine **47,** 168
calcitonin 48
calcium 17, **47–48,** 50, 91, 167, 181, 189,
199
calculations 15, 35, 44, 129, 153, 163
calendar calculators. *See savants, autistic*
calendars 35, 41, 159, 198, 199
calpain 47, **48,** 166
camphor 80
Canby, Margaret 60
cancer 13, 20, 44, 63, 187, 233, 236
Capgras, Jean Marie Joseph 48
Capgras syndrome 9, **48,** 96, 156
carbidopa 176
carbohydrates 72
carbon monoxide poisoning 23, 41, **48–49,**
50, 67, 157, 172

Case Western Reserve University 22
catecholamines, catecholamine system 26,
52, 74
catharsis **49**
Catholic Church 106
CAT scan. *See computerized axial tomography (CAT) scan*
caudate nucleus 38, **49,** 107, 108, 144
causation 202
CDC (Centers for Disease Control, U.S.) 10
celiac ganglion 99
cell assembly 57
cell phones **49**
central nervous system (CNS). *See also
nervous system*
AIDS and 9–10
anticholinergics and 28
declarative memory and 63
James, William on 33
multiple sclerosis and 160–161
nootropic drugs and 167–168
piracetam for 212
storage, memory and 214
trace decay and 224
transmissible spongiform
encephalopathies and 136
centrophenoxine **49–50,** 199
cerebellar degeneration 68
cerebellopontine angle 43–44
cerebellum 43–44, 107, 149
cerebral hemispheres
agnosia and 8, 92
aphasia and 29, 99
Recognition Memory Test for 32
stroke and 216
tumor of 43
writing and 9
cerebropathia psychica toxemica **50,** 124
cerebrospinal fluid (CSF) 10, 15, 68, 169,
192, 219. *See also spinal fluid*
cerebrovascular accident (CVA) 41, **50,**
217. *See also stroke*
cerebrum **50.** *See also specific parts of cerebrum*
abscess on 40
alexia and 11
Alzheimer's disease and 15
aphasia and 167, 237
apraxia and 30
Capgras syndrome and 48
dementia and 65
head injury and 101, 102
Kluver-Bucy syndrome and 124
Korsakoff's syndrome and 125
Wernicke, Carl on 236
Cerletti, Ugo 80
chaining 38, **50,** 149
chanting 171
Charcot, Jean-Martin 111
Charmadas 185
ChAT. *See choline acetyltransferase*
chemicals **50–51.** *See also specific chemicals*
chemistry, body 15–16, 64. *See also neuro-
transmitter(s)*
chemotherapy 44, *163,* 171
chess **51**
child abuse **51**
childbirth 112
childhood

autobiographical memory and 35
Binet, Alfred on 39
brain during 184
Freud, Sigmund on 94–95, 166, 201
hypnotic age regression to 4–5, 112,
226
long-term memory and 132
multiple personality disorder and 160,
192
overlearning and 173
of Proust, Marcel 189–190
simultaneous mental processing and
211
smells from 148, 189–190
children
with ADHD 3
with AIDS dementia complex 10
with autism 35
with delirium 64
diet of 71
with dyslexia 75–76
eidetic memory of 78, 142
engrams and 83
eyewitness ability of 4, 88
forgetting by 93
with Huntington's disease 108
implicit memory of 116
Klüver, Heinrich on 123
magnetic resonance imaging on 137
memory storage by 143
with meningitis 154
with multiple personalities 73
Nakkane's mnemonics and 163
Piaget, Jean on 181–182
semantic memory of 207
Stroop effect and 217
test of memoral and learning (TOMAL)
for 223
chlordiazepoxide 64
chloride 91, 181
chlorpromazine 64
cholesterol 17, 29, 63, 187
choline 15, **52,** 72, 127–128, 168, 183, 234
choline acetyltransferase 2, 15, 50, **52**
cholinergic agonists 99, 168
cholinergic basal forebrain 27, **52**
cholinergic system 168, 187, 193
cholinomimetic agents **52**
chromosomes 17, 18, 29, 108, 187
chronic brain failure, chronic brain syndrome 208
chunking, process of **52–53,** 132, 134, 141,
148, 152, 157, 208, 230
Cicero 4, **53,** 106, 132, 155, 179, 195, 203,
211
cigarettes. *See smoke, smoking*
cingulate gyrus 3, 129, 130, 131
circadian rhythm **53**
circulation 21, 29, **53,** 172. *See also blood
flow*
City of Hope Medical Center 187
CJD. *See Creutzfeldt-Jakob disease*
clioquinol **53–54,** 75
clonidine 52
clumsiness 107, 159
cocaine 230
"cocktail party effect" 34
Coenzyme Q10 **54**
coexistence hypothesis **54,** 65, 145

from alcohol abuse 11
from Alzheimer's disease 15
from anticholinergic syndrome 28
from apraxia 30
caffeine and 47
cerebellum and 149
from dementia 10, 67
from huffing 107
from Wernicke-Korsakoff syndrome 236
copper 72
Cornex 198–199
corpus callosum 43, 58
cortex, cerebral **58, 106.** *See also specific parts of cerebral cortex*
abstract memory in 1
acetylcholine and 1–2
adrenal 2, 168, 193
aging and 5
Alzheimer's disease in 13
amnesic syndrome in 25
blood flow to 105
Broca's aphasia in 45
cell loss in 5
of children 24
EEG of 34
effortful processing in 78
event memory in 85
explicit memory in 86
ginseng and 98
head injury and 102
hologram theory and 106
huffing and 107
Huntington's disease in 107
Korsakoff's syndrome in 237
Lashley, Karl on 127
learning and 130
lesions of 25, 78
leucotomy on 128, 158
memory storage in 146
Penfield, Wilder on 178–179
Pick's disease in 183
psychosurgery on 224
quantitative EEG of 80
retrieval and 3
stimulation of 79
use-it-or-lose-it hypothesis and 227
cortisol 5, 215
cortisone 133
cough, hysterical 27
Coumadin 225
cramming 8
cramps 113, 230
Creutzfeldt-Jakob disease 18, **58–59,** 66, 67, 135, 136, 188
Crohn's disease 234
cryptococcus 67
cryptomnesia **59–60**
CT scan. *See* computerized tomography (CT) scan
cues, cueing 172
amnesia and 118, 202
anxiety and 28
children and 24, 117, 166

for dementia 68
dyslexia and 75
elderly and *8*
encoding and 6
first-letter **90,** 147, 230, 233
forgetting and **60,** 93
free recall and 94
hippocampus and 104
infants and 143, 150, 151
kinesthetic memory and 123
language for 201
in memory palace 152
in music 147
PQRST method and 186
recall and 6, 139, 200
rhymes as 203
vanishing cue technique and 229
Cushing, Harvey 60
Cushing's syndrome **60–61**
CVA. *See* cerebrovascular accident (CVA)
Cylert 230
Cyrus 185
cytosine 84

D

dates 212
daydreams 89
deafness 9, 144, 218. *See also* hearing
death. *See also* suicide
from alcohol abuse 11
from Alzheimer's disease 12, 13, 14
from Binswanger's disease 39
from carbon monoxide poisoning 49
from Creutzfeldt-Jakob disease 58, 136
from Cushing's syndrome 60
from encephalitis 103, 124
from familial insomnia 136
fear of 138
forgetting and 128, 151
from huffing 107
from Huntington's disease 108
infantile amnesia and 117
Lewy body dementia and 130
from lupus erythematosus 133
from meningitis 154
from Pick's disease 183
from pneumonia 130
of Socrates 213
from stroke 215
from Wernicke-Korsakoff syndrome 236
decay theory **63,** 93
deceptions, memory 175
decision making 50, 107, 116
declarative memory **63,** 86, 99, 107, 143, 189

defense mechanism 27, 58, **63,** 69, 73, 78, 113, 190, 191, 201
degenerative diseases 68, 135–136, 175–177, 203–204. *See also specific degenerative diseases*
dehydration 71, 154, 208
dehydroepiandrosterone **63**
déjà vu **63–64,** 121, 123, 175, 190, 222
delayed matching/nonmatching to sample **64**
delayed memory 51, 54
delayed recall task **64**
delirium 28, **64,** 68, 133, 156, 172
delirium tremens **64–65**
delusions. *See also* illusion(s)
from Alzheimer's disease 14
from anticholinergic syndrome 28
from Cushing's syndrome 60
from delirium tremens 64
from dementia 65, 129
denial and 69
from Ganser's syndrome 97
misidentification syndromes and 156–157
from organic brain syndrome 172
from syphilis 219
demand characteristics hypothesis **65,** 145–146
dementia(s) **65–69.** *See also specific kinds of dementia*
amnesia and 22, 23, 113, 124
brain damage from 41
from brain tumor 44, 142
centrophenoxine for 49
cognition and 144
from Creutzfeldt-Jakob disease 135, 136
delirium and 64
depression and 70
diet and 29
from Down syndrome 18
drugs for 168
electroconvulsive therapy for 80
exercise and 29
from folic acid deficiency 91
fugue and 96
from Huntington's disease 107
from hypothyroidism 113
language and 166
from lupus erythematosus 133
from meningitis 154
mental stimulation for 19
mild cognitive impairment and 156
mini-mental state examination and 156
nimodipine and 167
normal-pressure hydrocephalus and 169

organic mental syndromes and 172
from Pick's disease 182, 183
praecocissiima **69**
praecox 12, **69**
pugilistica 192
from syphilis 219
tau protein and 16
from thalamus tumor 223
unclassified **227**
vascular **229,** 231
vitamins for 233
Wechsler Memory Scale and 235
demoic acid 16
demyelination, subcortical 58
dendrites
nerve growth factor and 109
in neurons 82, 164, 227
NMDA on 167
receptors in 197, 218
stimulation and 6, 7, 140
vitamins for 72
denial 63, **69**
De oratore (Cicero) 195
depersonalization disorder 73, 74
deprenyl 15–16, **69–70**
depression **70**
acetylcholine and 2
aging and 5
Alzheimer's disease and 14
amnesia and 23, 24, 113
Binswanger's disease and 39
Cushing's syndrome and 60
dementia and 9, 10, 68, 159, 208, 227
DMAE and 73
electroconvulsive therapy for 79, 80
folic acid for 91
fugue and 96, 191
from hypothyroidism 113
leucotomy for 128
from Lewy body dementia 129
limbic system and 130
from malnutrition 137, 181
from multiple sclerosis 161
as neurosis 166
pseudosenility from 190
registration and 144
surroundings and 218
thiamine deficiency and 67
vincamine for 231
De Sanctis, Sante 69
Descartes, René 31, 106
desegregation 73, 122
despair, feelings of 68
details, detail salience 4, 6, 11, **70–71,** 79, 85, 88
detection failure 148
DHEA **63**
diabetes **71**
Alzheimer's disease and 17, 29, 205
hypoglycemia and 112–113